# Community Integration Program

## Second Edition

Missy Armstrong, MS, CTRS
Sara Lauzen, CTRS

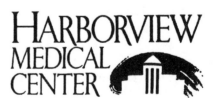

Royalties from this manual will be dedicated to meeting the continuing education and research needs of Therapeutic Recreation staff, Division of Occupational/Therapeutic Recreation, Department of Rehabilitation Medicine, Harborview Medical Center, Seattle, Washington.

**Published by**

Idyll Arbor, Inc.

PO Box 720, Ravensdale, WA  98051  (425) 432-3231

Published and distributed by

Idyll Arbor, Inc.

PO Box 720, Ravensdale, WA 98051 (425) 432-3231

ISBN 1-882883-03-9     Three Ring Notebook
ISBN 1-882883-09-8     Perfect Bound

# Table of Contents

Acknowledgments.............................................................................................................. v
Author's Notes............................................................................................................... vi

**Section 1**
**Setting Up a Community Integration Program**......................................................... 1
  1. Introduction.............................................................................................................. 3
     Purpose of the CIP............................................................................................... 3
     History of the CIP............................................................................................... 4
     What's in this Book............................................................................................. 7
     Scope of Service ................................................................................................. 8
  2. Overview.................................................................................................................. 11
  3. Why It Works........................................................................................................... 13
     Usability .............................................................................................................. 13
     In Support of Community Integration Training................................................. 15
     Smith-Armstrong Study .................................................................................... 25
  4. Program Management ............................................................................................. 31
     Modules to Use ................................................................................................... 31
     Approaches To Follow........................................................................................ 33
        Individual or Group .................................................................................. 33
        Formal, Informal, or Independent ........................................................... 34
     Documenting the CIP ......................................................................................... 35
        Documentation of Patient Functional Skill Level and Ability ................ 36
        Establishment of The Course of Treatment............................................. 36
        Establishment of a Data Base for Efficacy Studies ................................ 36
        Standardizing Documentation ................................................................. 37
     Adapting the CIP................................................................................................ 39
  5. Clinical Information ................................................................................................ 43
     Team Membership............................................................................................... 44
     Proficiency Checklist.......................................................................................... 45
     Basic Goals of Good Skin Care ......................................................................... 47
     Pressure Sores.................................................................................................... 48
     Treatment of Pressure Sores.............................................................................. 49
     Severity of Tissue Injury ................................................................................... 51
     New ASIA Standards for Classifying SCI ........................................................ 52
     Thoracic Lumbar Sacral Orthosis (TLSO) Body Jacket Protocol ..................... 55
     Quad Coughing................................................................................................... 56
     Types of Contractures ........................................................................................ 57
     Terms of Movement............................................................................................ 58
     Range of Motion................................................................................................. 59
     Muscle Strength.................................................................................................. 60
     Sensation............................................................................................................ 60
     The Bladder After Spinal Cord Injury............................................................... 61
     Autonomic Dysreflexia ...................................................................................... 63
     Traumatic Brain Injury ...................................................................................... 64
     Executive Function ............................................................................................ 66
  6. Equipment and Supply List .................................................................................... 69

## Section 2
**CIP Modules**................................................................................................................**71**

7. Related Forms....................................................................................................73
    Initial Screening and Initial Assessment.......................................................73
    Discharge Summary ......................................................................................80
8. Community Environment...................................................................................83
    Module 1A Environmental Safety...................................................................88
    Module 1B: Emergency Preparedness............................................................96
    Module 1C Basic Survival Skills ..................................................................98
9. Cultural Activities...........................................................................................101
    Module 2A Theater .....................................................................................103
    Module 2B Restaurant.................................................................................105
    Module 2C Library......................................................................................107
    Module 2D Sporting Event ..........................................................................109
10. Community Activities ....................................................................................111
    Module 3A Shopping Mall ..........................................................................113
    Module 3B Grocery Store ...........................................................................115
    Module 3C Downtown.................................................................................122
    Module 3D Bank ........................................................................................124
    Module 3E Laundromat...............................................................................126
11. Transportation ..............................................................................................129
    Module 4A Personal Travel.........................................................................131
    Module 4B Taxi/Taxi Vans.........................................................................133
    Module 4C Train.........................................................................................135
    Module 4D Air Travel.................................................................................138
    Module 4E City Bus ...................................................................................141
    Module 4F Bus Station................................................................................145
12. Physical Activity ..........................................................................................149
    Module 5A Aquatics...................................................................................150
    Module 5B Wheelchair Sports.....................................................................155
    Module 5C Leisure Activities .....................................................................156
13. Independent Plan ..........................................................................................159
    Module 6A Independent Patient Plan ...........................................................161
14. Summary .....................................................................................................163

## Section 3
**Related Information**.......................................................................................**165**

15. Glossary......................................................................................................167
16. Americans with Disabilities Act Fact Sheet....................................................199
17. Americans with Disabilities Act Accessibility Guidelines................................207
    Introduction ...............................................................................................208
    Survey Instructions.....................................................................................213
18. Transportation Safety ...................................................................................299
19. Air Travel ...................................................................................................305
References ........................................................................................................319

# *Acknowledgments*

This publication is the result of years of work and input from many people. We would like to recognize those who have made a significant contribution — although we realize that it would be impossible to recognize everyone. For those whose names are not here — it does not mean that we did not value your input — it just means that we are human.

- The original members of the treatment team who developed the first CIP: Missy Armstrong, MS, CTRS, Lindsey Coan Ford, MA, TRS, Edward O'Shaughnessy, MD, Roy Fowler, PhD, and Tracie Acsell Fike,

- All the current and past members of the Division of Therapeutic Recreation at Harborview Medical Center, especially, Gaby Bell, CTRS, Barbara Bond-Howard, CTRS, Jennifer Forbes, CTRS, Kathleen Jones, TRS, Patricia Maarhuis, CTRS, Donna Seim, CTRS, and Debbie Beckmeyer. MA, CTRS.

- All contributing authors, most of whom are associated with the Rehabilitation Medicine team at Harborview Medical Center.

- Past and present members of the Rehabilitation Medicine team at Harborview Medical Center; the Divisions of Occupational, Physical, and Speech Therapy, Nutrition, Nursing, Medicine, Vocational Rehabilitation, Psychology, and Social Work.

- Pat Mitsuda, MS, CCC, Peter Esselman, MD, Barbara deLateur, MD, Cynthia Chasan, RPT, and Gerri Furuta, OT, Kathy Michael, CRRN, Ross Baarslag-Benson, MS, CCC and Joyce Hedges, MS, CCC, who, as members of the team, provided editorial support and professional encouragement.

- The families of the primary authors.

- Students, past and present, who raised questions, requested clarification and have now spread the program throughout the nation.

- Patients and family members who participated, provided feedback, and pronounced the program a success.

- We thank all of those Therapeutic Recreation Specialists who provided feedback and written material, now incorporated into this document, including Laree Shandra, CTRS and Hal Smith, Ph.D.

# *Author's Notes*

- Every therapist has stories of their favorite or not so favorite experiences in the field. We laughed ourselves to tears thinking about patients, students, and family members who participated in those oh, so memorable "outings from hell." It is our hope that by sharing some of those experiences we can provide clarity to the theory and practice of the program.

  Despite our emphasis on prior planning to ensure successful participation, we know that situations will become uncontrollable, patients medically unstable, dysfunctional families unglued. As therapists we need to be challenged by community integration. Please note, however, that these stories cover a time period in which we have made great strides in the development of treatment protocols for therapists and in recognition of the needs of people with disabilities. We have become part of the process.

- This is not a textbook. Instead it contains the perspectives of two Certified Therapeutic Recreation Specialists and their personal experiences with community integration. If it's casual in its presentation, then we have achieved our goal. If you have questions, please feel free to write to us in care of Idyll Arbor (PO Box 720, Ravensdale, WA, 98051).

- This program was designed for an acute care facility but experience at other facilities has shown that it can be adapted for other populations. Our use of the word patient versus client or resident or some other title is only because of our particular experience.

- We do not wish to enter the battle over the name of the profession. At Harborview Medical Center we use the name Therapeutic Recreation and the initials TR. This choice is practical rather than philosophical because we are part of a trauma facility and RT is used by Respiratory Therapy during a stat intervention. When we consider the question, we consider ourselves to be therapeutic recreation specialists who provide recreation therapy services. In this book we have used the title CTRS (Certified Therapeutic Recreation Specialist) for all references to individual therapists and Therapeutic Recreation to discuss our profession.

- Some may feel that we are encroaching on other discipline's territory. We emphasize that at Harborview Medical Center this has been established as our unique treatment domain. We are recognized by the team as the community experts.

  We do not co-lead. We do co-treat but through the process of team goal setting. We do cooperate with all disciplines through regular communication with individual disciplines, rounds re-check, and family conferences. In addition, we provide inservices for the other health care professionals in our hospital to keep them up to date on the practice of therapeutic recreation and how this may impact the delivery of their services. We support our treatment team and are relieved that the trend in health care is for closer interdisciplinary team work and less defense of "professional territory."

- The depth of coverage in the modules may seem more detailed than necessary. The severity of disability of the patients seen at Harborview Medical Center sometimes requires this much depth. You may find that your facility does not require as much.

# Section 1

# Setting Up a Community Integration Program

## Long, long ago...

in a city far, far away a young man was discharged after a six month rehabilitation program in a well known facility to the home he shared with his long time girlfriend. They lived in a small apartment. After a snow skiing accident, the man found himself with a C5 quadriplegia.

During his hospitalization, he and his girlfriend had left the facility only once. The only other attention they gave to community participation and leisure lifestyle was to sit on the sidelines watching a wheelchair basketball game, and to practice car transfer training with a portable hoyer lift.

With a large group of friends providing support, these two attempted to return to a leisure lifestyle appropriate for their age and interest. They learned the hard way how it was best accomplished (and often not accomplished).

Together they struggled with little money, few accessible locations to visit and many biases in attitude. They were refused service in restaurants, kicked off reserved airline flights and other modes of public transportation and locked out of theaters because of architectural barriers. They were refused access to buildings and shows because the wheelchair was considered a fire hazard.

With much trial and error, a vehicle that required a hoyer lift, many run ins with architectural barriers, the girlfriend dropping him all over town (in driveways, out of the car, and out of bed), and the invaluable help of their friends, they succeeded — at least as well as they could with the architectural barriers still in place. A leisure lifestyle was created and managed.

Later with the relationship over, the girlfriend decided to go back to graduate school. Her new career — therapeutic recreation and community education — had a distinct bias toward community integration using leisure opportunities. She started work at Harborview Medical Center and the Community Integration Program, in concept, was born.

# 1. Introduction

This book is about the Community Integration Program (CIP) at Harborview Medical Center in Seattle, Washington, USA. At Harborview Medical Center we have identified, through task analysis and experience, the tasks that, if not done successfully, severely limit an individual's ability to become and remain part of his/her community. This book describes those tasks and how you can put together a community integration program for your facility that will teach the tasks to your patients.

The tasks are combined into modules that concentrate on a patient's interaction with a particular aspect of the community such as a restaurant or bus transportation. We will show you how to pick modules that are appropriate for your patients and combine them together to help your patients learn the skills that they need.

We have used the CIP for patient populations with traumatic brain injury, spinal cord injury, and psychiatric diagnoses. Other facilities have given us feedback on using the CIP for patients with MR/DD, patients in geriatric settings, and pediatric adaptations. The book talks about how to modify the CIP to make it work with each of these populations.

Section 3 of the book contains information on the laws that have been written to help make our communities more accessible for people with disabilities. In the years that we have been running the program, we have seen many changes which have significantly enhanced our chances of integrating patients back into the community. We suggest that you study the relevant laws, which are presented in Section 3, so that you can apply them in your community to help your patients return to lives that are as normal as possible.

# Purpose of the CIP

To some degree, every person who is discharged from a hospital or institution will find that his/her life has changed. If that change is a small one, the individual probably has the ability to adjust to the change without outside help. However, if the change is greater than the individual's coping skills, knowledge, or other resources, there is a problem. Not only does the individual have a problem, but so does his/her support system. If the individual is a parent who now cannot help with homework, or an adult who is no longer able to drive to the store, or an employee who finds the work site inaccessible, or an adolescent anxious to move to a group home, the emotional and financial impact will be felt by many people.

It has been said that "time is money". In the case of an individual making the transition back into the community after a significant change in his/her abilities, the statement is especially true. Instead of learning how to integrate into the community by himself/herself through trial and error, it is more expedient (and usually less expensive) for him/her to be guided by a therapist who understands the process and has the knowledge of how to make that process happen.

The skills needed to successfully live in one's environment are not a closely guarded secret. For almost every skill required, one should be able to find a task analysis of that skill. The mark of a professional is that s/he has a knowledge of the multiple steps required for a given task and how each one of these steps can be modified to help compensate for an individual's disability. Therapy is the ability to identify the modifications that need to be made and then influence either the patient and/or the environment to allow the change to happen.

This book is about the tasks required, not the modifications that you need to make for each patient. Each patient has his/her own combination of skills and disabilities. We leave it to you to determine the best set of modifications, within the broad framework of the CIP, to make for each individual. The CIP provides the framework. The details come from the patient, the therapist, and the rest of the treatment team.

As an example, there are a set of skills which a patient must have to be able to use the bus. Some of them include reading schedules, determining the right bus, and being able to get on the bus and ride safely. The skills are the same for everyone, but your patients may be missing some of the skills. A person with quadriplegia needs to concentrate on the physical aspects of getting on the bus or tying down the wheelchair correctly. A person with a cognitive impairment usually needs to work on keeping track of schedules and selecting the right bus. Your job as a therapist is to figure out which parts of the skills your patients are lacking and making sure that they learn those skills. The CIP should be used to remind you of the required skill sets. Emphasize the skills where the patient is not independent yet. Skip the skills that your patient can do already. Modify it as required to provide your patients with the most effective and efficient treatment that you can.

# History of the CIP

This program is one part of the treatment interventions used by the therapeutic recreation staff at Harborview Medical Center. Harborview Medical Center is a Level I trauma center located in Seattle, Washington, associated with the University of Washington Medical Center. Its mission is to provide quality patient care, educate medical personnel and engage in quality research. The Department of Rehabilitation concentrates its efforts on the rehabilitation of individuals with physical and cognitive disabilities, primarily individuals with spinal cord and brain injury, including strokes.

In 1978, the therapeutic recreation specialists at Harborview Medical Center, Seattle, Washington, in cooperation with the Rehabilitation Treatment Team developed the Community Integration Program for patients who were newly disabled with spinal cord injuries. The program was initiated as a formal treatment protocol after it was determined that a great number of patients admitted to the rehabilitation service were unable to effectively apply the skills they had learned in the hospital setting to the demands of daily community living. In addition, rehabilitation patients readmitted to the hospital expressed similar frustrations with their inability to manage the demands of daily community life and their leisure pursuits. Patients were hesitant to participate in activities that were new, for fear of failure. Integration of the patient with a new spinal cord injury into the community needed to be an integral part of the complete rehabilitation process. Practice outside of the hospital setting gave the patient opportunity to complete the therapy cycle. Realization that skills learned within the hospital were applicable to daily life outside of the hospital, give credibility to the rehabilitation process. It was with this in mind that the Community Integration Program was developed.

By creating an efficient mechanism to measure functional change occurring during therapeutic recreation interventions, the value of the therapeutic recreation services were more easily understood. Since 1979 therapeutic recreation, as the community integration specialist, has played a central role in the rehabilitation program at Harborview Medical Center. The program formally recognized that community integration using recreation and leisure activity was a necessary treatment medium in the rehabilitation process.

After its inception, the program was used with all rehabilitation patients including those with spinal cord injury, traumatic brain injury, and stroke (and more recently, patients with psychiatric diagnosis). These patient groups demonstrate different needs concerning their rehabilitation to the community. Patients with a traumatic brain injury or stroke may require assistance with cognitive deficits and physical deficits. Patients with a spinal cord injury do not require cognitive re-training; rather, consideration is given to their physical, mobility, and problem solving needs. While acknowledging the differences between patient groups, the original goals of the Community Integration Program were focused and written for patients with spinal cord injury. Since then the modules have been adapted for use by patients with traumatic brain injuries, stroke, and psychiatric disorders.

After the first writing, the program was sent to any therapeutic recreation program in the United States and Canada that requested it. We have tried to incorporate all feedback we received into this new document.

The original **Community Integration Program** (1980) was initiated after a significant number of rehabilitation patients reported that they were unable to effectively apply the skills they learned in the clinical setting to the demands of daily community living. In addition, rehabilitation patients re-admitted to the hospital expressed similar frustration with their inability to manage the demands of daily community life and their leisure pursuits. Patients reported that they were hesitant to participate in new activities because they were afraid of failure. While reviewing the rehabilitation program, the members of the Rehabilitation team determined that, while we encouraged constant upgrading of skills and knowledge for our patients, we weren't giving them all the experiences necessary to encourage confidence. To quote one patient, "You gave me the racket and the ball but not the map to the court."

With the encouragement of a physiatrist and a psychologist on the rehabilitation team, three Therapeutic Recreation Specialists revised the way documentation was done to turn the informal reporting process into a structured method of documenting patient changes. The result was the creation of a system that provided evaluation and treatment opportunities in community settings where the patient could develop and apply new or adapted leisure knowledge, skills, and attitudes. Changes were documented in modules that incorporated many normal community based activity. In its original format, the Community Integration Modules were used for pre-test, field trial, and post-test to measure change in the patient's abilities caused by the therapeutic intervention. The desired outcome was successful participation in daily community and leisure based living skills.

The current purpose of the **Community Integration Program** is to provide opportunities and experiences for the patient that promote the development and application of new knowledge, skills, and attitudes necessary for successful participation in daily community living. The goals of the CIP are written with four areas of concentration in mind:

1. application of skills
2. socialization
3. problem solving
4. resource guidance

Keeping those four areas of concentration in mind, the Therapeutic Recreation Specialists developed eleven goals for the CIP. These goals are

1. To provide opportunities for the integration of diverse physical, social, emotional, and cognitive skills.

2. To provide information and related community resources for patient review and use.
3. To provide opportunities for patients to use and evaluate the community resources available.
4. To facilitate and increase patient participation in everyday activities and leisure pursuits.
5. To provide experiences that require the use of independent thinking, problem solving, and organizational skills.
6. To encourage and assist patients in their adjustment to their injury and newly defined physical, cognitive, and emotional limitations.
7. To provide opportunities to perform independently without the assistance of family or therapists.
8. To provide opportunities for the patient to demonstrate the ability to direct others in helping with their care needs.
9. To provide opportunities in new social settings that will increase self-confidence.
10. To provide an atmosphere of acceptance and positive attitude toward patients and their rehabilitation process.
11. To provide opportunities to improve social interaction skills within an atmosphere of <u>fun</u> and <u>good humor</u>.

Successful participation was defined in terms of the independence level attained by the individual patient. Each patient was expected to attain a level of independent functioning necessary for meeting the demands of his/her everyday life. Attention was directed to the development of physical function skills (i.e., wheelchair mobility), the development of independent thinking and problem solving, and the development of skills necessary to direct an attendant or family member to assist if required. Emphasis was placed on solving problems in the present. However, the intent was to teach patients how to anticipate potential problems in future experiences so they could solve them with clear thinking and good organizational abilities. Participants were encouraged to advance beyond the basic needs of daily living. They were encouraged to pursue leisure interests that might require further skill development and to increase their abilities in activities beyond the everyday routine. They were taught that daily leisure and recreation participation are requirements for a healthy lifestyle and a prerequisite for pre-vocational training.

We discovered that the needs of the patient determined the purpose and setting of the community interaction and program plan. The needs of the patient also dictated the role of the therapist. Patients required varying degrees of assistance according to their previously achieved level of independence. Therefore, application of the modules, definition of the therapist's role, and the choice of the community setting were adjusted to meet specific patient needs in integration.

The changing health care environment, the necessity to justify therapy services, a desire to increase efficiency to meet the changed acuity at admission and discharge, decreased length of stay, changes in long term care facilities, changes in regional and federal guidelines, an increase in the number of requests for this material, and a willing publisher pressured the therapists in this facility to update the original document.

As you read through this manual, we hope you will find much that is useful just as we wrote it. We hope that you also recognize that the program's strength and significance is that it was designed to be adapted to your particular situation. There are no right answers, just guided questions. Therapists still have to review the modules to consider their appropriateness given geographical and cultural differences, national and local regulations, individual patient needs, patient diagnoses, and level of family support.

As some of the original authors review the original document, we note that the purpose of the program has not altered. However, changes in the program delivery have occurred. Most significantly, we have enhanced the problem solving and advocacy questions to reflect the changes in patient acuity at most acute care facilities. The changes in treatment focus from inpatient to outpatient has enhanced the value as a treatment modality — patients discharged earlier must be independent in the community with fewer experiences.

The program design continues to encourage the sharing of information with other disciplines, and allows an efficient experiential process to occur in tandem with work by other therapists. It provides structure for students from all disciplines and clearly demarcates the shared roles of the rehabilitation disciplines. Most importantly it continues to offer the patient and their family a valuable tool to ensure their safe integration into the community and leisure lifestyle.

# What's in this Book

This second edition of the **Community Integration Program** has been greatly expanded from the first edition written in 1980. Successes in the fourteen years since the first edition have demonstrated that the modules themselves make a difference to the patient and his/her rehabilitation potential. However, as a book, the authors and editors felt that the second edition needed to be expanded in scope. Hence, the Second Edition of the **Community Integration Program (CIP)** has three main sections: 1. background and pre-use information, 2. treatment protocol modules, and 3. Americans with Disabilities Act information.

Section 1, Background and Pre-Use Information, provides you with information which will help you to decide what part(s) of the program to use, recommendations concerning the type of documentation to use, basic clinical information, and examples of initial screening and discharge tools. A Glossary is available and it may be helpful to refer to it if you have a question about what we mean by certain terms. Many terms from the Americans with Disabilities Act (ADA) can be found in the Glossary and the definitions of some of the terms used in the ADA are not necessarily the same as definitions found in health care dictionaries. (An example would be that an addiction to alcohol is not considered a disability by the Americans with Disabilities Act.)

Section 2 contains the modules which make up the Community Integration Program. While the modules are basically the same as in the first edition, there are four notable changes. The first change is the enhancement of the problem solving and advocacy questions for each module. We found that the patients need this information and related skills to function better after discharge. The second change is that we have added a Field Trial Score Sheet for each module. While we do not always use this form, it is an easy and efficient way to report the patient's demonstrated skill levels on the outing. The third change is the addition of the Flesch Grade Level score to each pre-test/post-test score sheet. (The Flesch Grade Level is an assessment which determines how hard or easy the written material is to read, by giving it a school grade level.) We found that while some of the modules were written at a sixth grade level, others were written at a college sophomore level. This could leave the therapist uncertain as to whether the patient was having trouble due to the reading difficulty, or due to a lack of knowledge. The modules have been re-written so they can be read by someone with about an 8th grade education. The last change is the addition of a module which helps us assess the patient's ability to function if s/he found himself/herself homeless. This module is called 1C Basic Survival Skills.

Section 3 provides the therapist and the patient with some of the basic, practical information on accessibility and the Americans with Disabilities Act (ADA). (Those readers who work outside of the United States will not be directly affected by the ADA, but will still be able to use the information contained in this section.) This section contains many of the measurements and other architectural requirements which help make a building or facility accessible to those who use wheelchairs or other mobility devices. This information is important both because it allows the patient and therapist to educate facility owners as to how to make a building accessible and because it awakens the patient and therapist to the fact that many of the pieces of adapted equipment prescribed by the therapist and used by the patient exceed the measurements required by the ADA. The patient therefore is blocked (legally) from use of the building. At times, the types of equipment needed by the patient will exceed the accessible measurements. However, we as therapists can work with the designers who make the equipment to try to have most of the equipment a size which will fit into the buildings and facilities which already comply with the ADA.

# Scope of Service

The CIP is not the only therapeutic recreation service we offer at Harborview Medical Center. It fits in with three other components to create a balanced set of services designed to meet the needs of our patients after some significant change in their abilities or to provide them with skills that they never learned.

We start by assessing the patient's needs using one of the initial screening tools in Chapter 7. Based on the results of the assessment and our knowledge of the care plan we provide services as required in the following four areas:

1. Functional Activities,
2. Leisure Education,
3. Community Integration, and
4. Recreation Participation

The following shows the activities, treatments, and skills gained in each of the four components of our program.

**Functional Activities**

Activities which will improve social, emotional, cognitive, and functional behaviors as a necessary pre-requisite to future leisure/social involvement.

Treatments might include groups or individual sessions that would include the following skills:

- Self-Esteem
- Social Skills
- Orientation to Self/Surroundings
- Stress/Pain Reduction
- Increased Mobility
- Gross/Fine Motor Coordination
- Aquatics
- Play Therapy
- Ceramics/Art

**Leisure Education**

Activities which will facilitate patient acquisition of knowledge, skills and attitudes needed for adjustment to hospital environment and in preparation for discharge, for responsible decision making and use of free time.

Treatment might include group or individual treatment sessions that would include the following skills:

- Time Management
- Family Education
- Resource Development and Knowledge about Support
- Recognition of Alcohol and Drugs as Deterrent to Positive Leisure
- Age Related Activity
- School Re-Entry
- Pre-Op Teaching
- Support Groups

- Structural Management of Leisure During Recuperation
- Disposition Planning
- Behavior Modification Programs

## Community Integration

Activities which will facilitate transition of patient knowledge, skills, and attitudes from the hospital setting to the community, home, work, and school.

Treatments might include group or individual sessions where these skills are primary and carried out in the hospital setting as well as the Greater Seattle area:

- Adaptations
- Recognition of Architectural and Other Barriers
- Cognitive Re-training (problem solving, orientation, time management, path finding)
- Higher Level Community Skills (transportation, environmental awareness, grocery evaluation)
- Community Resources
- Leisure Opportunities
- Bus Pass
- Family Training
- Disabled Parking
- Disposition Resource
- Community Outings

## Recreation Participation

Activities which will facilitate and improve quality of life, feelings of human dignity, personal social adjustment, and self-expression through leisure choices.

- Performing Arts
- VCR/Videos
- Radio/Tape
- Socialization

Recreation participation may be of a diversional nature and/or it may be an opportunity for the therapists to determine the patient's involvement in leisure, the patient's endurance, tolerance for activity, and social skills.

# 2. Overview

*The Community Integration Program, or CIP, uses recreation and leisure activities as the vehicle for therapy. This chapter explains how to use the CIP as a treatment protocol.*

The CIP works using three basic steps:

1.  **Pre-test** determining the patient's ability to verbally "walk/talk" through the steps required for successful integration back into his/her community,
2.  **Field trial** determining the patient's ability to demonstrate the functional skills necessary for integration into a natural setting, and
3.  **Post-test** determining the patient's ability to remember the problems and solutions encountered on the outing (including awareness, self-evaluation, use of feedback, and anticipation of needs for the next outing).

The CIP is set up in treatment protocol modules. Each module covers a distinct community or leisure experience. Because successful integration back into the community requires a variety of complex skills, the treatment protocols in the CIP call for the completion of 7 - 10 different modules. (An abbreviated length of stay may necessitate the use of only 3 - 5 modules.) Chapter 4 goes into greater detail on how to select modules.

The module structure encourages the development of positive leisure and recreation based activities and incorporates the skills necessary to participate successfully. All modules are intended to meet the needs of the individual's lifestyle, and to incorporate recognition of issues, problem solving techniques, physical skill development and organizational processes into real-life experiences. The CIP provides an experiential process that "tests" those skills while the patient is still under the watchful eye of a trained therapist. It also provides feedback to other therapists who may need to concentrate on specific skills.

The Community Integration Program is based on a leisure continuum, which assumes that recreation can be used both for therapy and as a normal life activity. Interventions using leisure based activity are important assessment and evaluation tools. Intense support and encouragement by the therapist and support by the group process, provide encouragement to the patient so s/he will be confident enough to try independent activities at a later time.

The concept assumes that all therapies build on skills previously learned. For example, a person with a spinal cord injury may learn a transfer in the clinical setting provided by a specific therapist. Community integration provides multiple opportunities to test transfers under different or unique conditions. Should a problem or difficulty occur, the individual can then return to the clinical setting for review or adaptation. Mastery of transfer skills promote confidence to attempt mastery of more difficult skills.

The modules are grouped into six basic domains:

- Community Environment
- Cultural Activity
- Community Activity
- Transportation
- Physical Activity
- Independent Activity

Each module covers a variety of different skills but all of them generally have the same types of questions:

- Pre arrangements: The basic information that the patient should be able to answer prior to embarking on the outing.
- Transportation: How the patient will get to and from the activity.
- Accessibility: What special issues concerning architectural barriers and functional ability the patient will need to know about and problem solve.
- Emergency/Safety: What mobility and health care concerns may come up during the activity.
- Equipment: What equipment the patient will need to bring along.

Some of the modules have other categories added to this format. This was done when we found that activity-specific questions needed to be asked. An example of a module that needed an extra category was banking (Module 3D). To successfully use the bank after discharge, the patient needed to demonstrate the ability to anticipate specific needs concerning banking (e.g., identification required, check cashing policies).

The Community Integration Program is structured to have a pre-test, field trial, and post-test. Because the post-test is used to measure a change in knowledge and problem solving, we use the same form for the pre-test as we do for the post-test. Most of the modules will contain just 2 forms: 1. the pre-test/post-test form, and 2. the field trial form. Some modules also have a chart note form, to show you how we document the module for the patient's chart.

# 3. Why It Works

*The CIP seems to work. The patients, their significant others, and the staff on the treatment team indicate that the CIP program works. But that is not enough. Studies, books, and articles published in the last decade are full of support for this type of program. This chapter contains a general overview of the material supporting the various aspects of the CIP.*

# Usability

The Community Integration Program (CIP) is a structured set of treatment protocols which have been used by therapists throughout North America. Based on the experience of the therapists who have used it, we have identified five elements of the CIP which provide the reasons to use it:

1. basis in leisure skills,
2. expediency,
3. billable status,
4. positive impact on the community as a whole, and
5. popularity.

## Leisure Based

To be able to maintain a healthy, balanced leisure lifestyle a person needs to have many skills. While these skills (deciding between two choices, using a telephone, making change, getting around, etc.) can be learned in an isolated manner in a classroom or clinic, the actual repetitive practice of those skills tends to be more rewarding if it is part of an activity that the person enjoys. This enjoyment enhances the patient's motivation to learn a skill. Once the skill is learned, it should be practiced while immersed in a sensory stimulating environment. This allows the therapist to measure the degree that the stimulation decreases the patient's leisure skill level. The modules in the CIP cover many of the community based leisure skills that an individual needs to integrate into his/her community.

# Expediency

If the therapist does not have a pre-established set of treatment interventions already written, s/he is likely to spend a lot of time writing a treatment protocol for each patient. The therapists providing therapy for individuals will tend to reduce unproductive time by using the CIP. Unproductive time stems from not having a course of treatment already outlined and established. As we said in the introduction, the skills necessary to become a member of one's community are not closely guarded secrets. But it does take time to establish the treatment priorities if the therapists do not have a previously established outline for the community integration skills that may be required. Documenting the patient's demonstrated knowledge and skill level also takes time. The CIP has many of the forms that the therapist will need already thought out and formatted. Because the CIP is an organized set of treatment protocols with most of the necessary documentation forms, it will tend to save time for the therapist who is not using a treatment protocol program.

The CIP may also be used with patients who have a length of stay less than one week (or who will be receiving limited outpatient/home health care services). Based on the patient's previously assessed needs, the physician may request that the therapist use only one or two specific modules (i.e., basic survival skills, transportation, environmental safety). Using the pre-test, field trial, and post-test forms, the therapist should be able to provide the treatment team with important insight into the patient's knowledge and skill level.

Many therapeutic recreation departments conduct a continuous quality assurance program. Because the CIP is an established treatment protocol with specific measurements obtained (not only patient scores, but also the number of hours the therapist was involved providing services related to the CIP interventions), it can easily used to measure quality. The data obtained from the CIP may be used for both continuous quality assurance programs and for efficacy studies.

# Billable Services

Each state has its own set of billing and coverage guidelines for patients who are receiving state or federal assistance to cover the cost of their health care. The format of the CIP is structured in such a manner that it is easily "plugged into" the facilities billing system. The therapeutic recreation specialist and the facility's billing department will need to work with the state and the insurance companies to establish a mechanism for billing. Therapists have received third party reimbursement for interventions based on the CIP modules.

There are some situations where it may not be appropriate to bill for the therapist using the CIP modules with patients. This limitation is not due to the CIP itself, but to state and federal legislation. Endowment legislation (i.e., Medicare, Medicaid, OBRA, or Intermediate Care Facilities for the Mentally Retarded (ICF-MR)) is first and foremost a business contract that the administrators of a facility elect to sign or not to sign. These health care contracts outline the types and quantity of services that the facility will provide to each individual who qualifies for service coverage. In exchange, the state or federal government will reimburse the facility with a pre-established room rate or usage rate.

In some states, Medicare (over 65 years of age) and/or Medicaid (under 65 years with a disability) will not cover any rehabilitation therapy services; in others, the service is covered adequately. In some states specific therapies are excluded from coverage (i.e., occupational therapy, recreational therapy, art therapy). The government is not saying that the excluded therapy is not helpful, and they are not necessarily saying that those services aren't needed by the patient; the government is just saying that the endowment does not cover that kind of health care service.

The federal legislation which covers the contracts with nursing homes and other long term care facilities is called OBRA. The patient's needs related to leisure and activities, under OBRA, are required to be available seven days a week and are paid for through the room rate. However, it is not clear that the therapy services directly related to the assessment, development, and enhancement of skills related to community integration are part of the OBRA contract. In many states these services would be considered billable, but it would be wise to check before submitting a bill. Since OBRA states that services related to leisure activities are already paid for in the room rate, to bill separately for these services may be considered double billing — also known as Medicare Fraud.

In Intermediate Care Facilities for the Mentally Retarded (ICF-MR), the government has again, specifically included leisure and recreation services as required services and pays for those services in the room rate. In addition, the ICF-MR law also states that community integration is a required service, also covered under the room rate. For clients who live in ICF-MR licensed facilities, no direct billing to the government is recommended. The only time that a therapist may bill for those services is if s/he is not an employee of the facility but a consultant. In this case s/he bills the administrator of the facility who pays for the services out of the room rate allowance.

## Community Service

As industrialized nations begin to be more sensitive to the architectural and attitudinal barriers which exist, changes are being made. As the therapist and his/her patients push the frontiers of accessibility in the local community, an awareness will slowly emerge amongst those who are not disabled. With patience, knowledge, and persistence, these barriers may disappear. (See *Food Store Accessibility* later in this chapter.)

## Popularity

As with many of the services that health care providers deliver, a portion of the patients will appreciate the service given. Many patient's have indicated discomfort with having to go into the community after s/he has experienced a loss in skill. Frequently this task is easier with the support of a therapist who is aware of both the patient's feelings and the types of adaptations needed to make the trip successful. Families also tend to appreciate the chance learn how to cope with new limitations and how to make getting back to everyday life a little easier. For some patients, just having the opportunity to get out of the hospital for a short while is beneficial and, therefore, therapeutic. The CIP provides the structure to help facilitate these outings.

One of the strongest reasons for using the CIP with patients is because the interventions do make a difference in the patient's ability. The CIP provides opportunities and experiences for an individual who is newly disabled which promote the development and application of new knowledge, skills, and attitudes necessary for successful participation in daily community living.

# In Support of Community Integration Training

A literature search was conducted to find other studies and reports which lend support to the use of programs similar to the CIP. The table on the following pages provides a summary of some of the material found. We looked at the structure of the CIP, the types of integration experiences covered in the CIP, and the types of therapy interventions (e.g., 1:1 and/or group learning) as we searched the literature.

The studies below confirm the efficacy of programs similar to the CIP. Their overall conclusion is that the patients with disabilities must look at their interactions with the community differently than they did in the past. People do not usually have the resources to make this transition without the help of trained therapists who can help them over the numerous pitfalls and through the many barriers. Without therapeutic intervention, many of these patients would limit themselves unnecessarily in their leisure and lifestyle pursuits.

| Topic | Article Title | Overview | Findings | Reference | Implications |
|---|---|---|---|---|---|
| Accessibility | *Food Store Accessibility*<br><br>L McClain<br>C. Todd | A survey was done to measure the wheelchair accessibility of 20 grocery and convenience stores. A letter was sent to the store managers notifying them of their store's deficiencies. Six months after notification, the surveys were re-done, with 5 out of the 20 stores having made corrections as a result of the letter. | Rural grocery stores did slightly better than urban grocery stores. Convenience stores were significantly less accessible. However, no store was found to be fully accessible. The therapists who conducted the study felt that they had a positive impact on the accessibility in their communities as 25% of the stores increased their level of accessibility after input. | Am Journal of Occupational Therapy 1990 44 p. 487-491 | This study has two implications for the therapist implementing the CIP:<br>1. problem solving of architectural accessibility is an important skill as few buildings are fully accessible, and<br>2. therapist's efforts to educate store managers can make a measurable difference in the number of buildings made accessible. |
| Accessibility | *Restaurant Wheelchair Accessibility*<br><br>L McClain<br>et al | Study to determine how many of restaurants complying with Uniform Federal Accessibility Standards. 120 sites surveyed in 3 midwestern states. | Compliance<br>disabled parking avail...... 53%<br>access isle 60 in wide....... 60%<br>ramps as needed ............... 66%<br>door size........................... 98%<br>restroom accessible........... 60%<br>table knee clearance........... 35%<br>correct toilet height........... 48% | Am. Journal of Occupational Therapy July 93 Vol. 47, #7, p.619-623 | Patients who use a wheelchair will need to be able to demonstrate problem solving and adaptability. |

| Topic | Article Title | Overview | Findings | Reference | Implications |
|-------|---------------|----------|----------|-----------|--------------|
| Community Integration Training | *A Model Therapeutic Recreation Program for the Reintegration of Persons with Disabilities into the Community* C.C. Bullock C.Z. Howe | Description of a model therapeutic recreation program for the integration of persons with disabilities and a preliminary evaluation of the programs results. This program used a model community reintegration program which started as an inpatient service and was continued as an outpatient service. | Improved behavioral functioning, adjustment to disability, autonomy, and enhanced quality of life were evident in the subjects. The authors felt that the preliminary evaluation showed that the program was successful. | Therapeutic Recreation Journal 1991 25 p. 7-17 | The reintegration program in this article is similar to the CIP from Harborview Medical Center. The reader should be able to expect similar results using this program as a basis for integration treatment protocol. |
| Group Learning | *The Contribution of Group Learning to the Rehabilitation of Spinal Cord Injured Adults* J.A. Payne | This study measured attitudes toward group learning and gathered demographic data on 60 adults with SCI, 6 family members, and 8 rehab nurses. | Positive attitudes toward group learning were communicated by all three subject groups. Motivation, sharing of experiences, camaraderie, support from peers, and knowledge that they were not alone were identified as advantage of group learning. | Rehabilitation Nursing 1993 18 p. 375-379 | While the therapist will want to conduct some of the CIP treatment protocols as one-on-one treatment sessions, there is support for, and benefits of, using some of the CIP modules as a group treatment. |

| Topic | Article Title | Overview | Findings | Reference | Implications |
|-------|--------------|----------|----------|-----------|--------------|
| Homelessness | *Therapeutic Recreation and the Homeless: A Clinical Case History* A. Krinksy | This case history describes the therapeutic recreation interventions and functional outcomes as a result of a program to teach cognitive behavioral skills training related to leisure and community survival skills to an adult admitted to a psychiatric treatment program. | This 36 y/o male had been socially disconnected with an isolated life style until he entered the treatment program. The patient increased his social skills, recreation participation (quantity and quality), his coping and problem solving skills, and now is gainfully employed and lives in an apartment. | Therapeutic Recreation Journal 1992 26 p. 53-57 | Community skills training is important to many different patient groups. Receiving some basic social skills and city survival training skills may make the difference between a patient being homeless or having the skills to be gainfully employed. |
| Mobility | *A Mobility Skills Training Program for Adults with Developmental Disabilities* C.A. McInerney M. McInerney | 29 adults with DD were trained to use city buses for leisure outings to local shopping malls. Data were collected for one year after each person left the program and were analyzed with the use of multiple regression procedures. | Participants maintained their mobility skills and utilized them, after receiving training to the level of "independent" in the use of city buses. | Am Journal of Occupational Therapy 1992 Vol. 46, #3 p. 233-239 | Demonstrates effectiveness of teaching specific mobility skills using individualized training sequences for persons with developmental disabilities. |
| Mobility | *National Census of Residential Facilities: A 1982 Profile of Facilities and Residents* F.E. Hauber et al | A national census of all state licensed residential facilities for individuals who are mentally retarded was conducted in 1982. (N Residents = 243,669 N facilities =15,633) Information on characteristics of facilities is presented along with demographic and functional characteristics of the residents. | Lack of transportation skills can limit placements in community-based residences. | Am Journal of Mental Deficiency 1984 89 p. 236-245 | Training in the independent use of public transportation can help facilitate community placement of individuals with developmental disabilities. |

| Topic | Article Title | Overview | Findings | Reference | Implications |
|-------|---------------|----------|----------|-----------|--------------|
| Mobility | *Teaching Supermarket Shopping Skills Using An Adaptive Shopping List* K. Gaule J. Nietupski N. Certo | Three young adults with moderate/severe disabilities were taught to use an adaptive shopping aid in order to a. prepare a shopping list, b. locate and obtain items, and c. purchase items. A multiple probe design was used for validation. | Travel independence is identified as an important prerequisite skill for a variety of community based activities. | Education and Training of the Mentally Retarded 1985 20 p. 53-59 | To help ensure their use of community based leisure and mercantile facilities, adults with a developmental disability also need to learn how to use public transportation. |
| Mobility | *Community Integration of Mentally Retarded Adults Through Leisure Activity* C.L. Salzberg C.A. Langford | The de-institutionalization movement generates considerable interest among service providers regarding provision of more normalized environments. Simply establishing small residences within a neighborhood does not appear to be sufficient to desegregate adults who are mentally retarded. The utilization of age appropriate, commercially available leisure pursuits as a vehicle for facilitating integration within the community is proposed. | Knowledge and skills related to the use of public transportation are an important component in having the skills to utilize public restaurants or movie theaters. | Mental Retardation 1981 19 p. 127-131 | To help ensure their use of community based leisure, restaurants, and movie theaters, adults with a developmental disability also needs to learn how to use public transportation. |

| Topic | Article Title | Overview | Findings | Reference | Implications |
|---|---|---|---|---|---|
| Mobility | **Leisure Programs for Handicapped Persons: Adaptations, Techniques, & Curriculum** P. Wehman S. Schleien | Review of training programs which help break down barriers to leisure participation for adolescents and adults with developmental disabilities. | Ability to use public transportation is an important prerequisite skill to be able to plan recreational outings alone or with others. | **Leisure Programs for Handicapped Persons: Adaptations, Techniques, & Curriculum** Baltimore, University Park Press 1981 | Training in the use of public transportation is an important component of leisure skills training. |
| Mobility | *Teaching Public Transportation Problem Solving Skills to Young Adults with Moderate Handicaps* J. Welch J. Nietupski S. Hare-Nietupski | Six young adults with moderate handicaps were taught to use prosthetic picture-prompt cards to determine if they were on time to catch a city bus to their vocational training site and problem solving procedures to follow in the event that they missed the bus. | Individuals with developmental disabilities can successfully master recovery skills (e.g., what to do if one misses the bus). | Education and Training of the Mentally Retarded 1985  20 p. 287-295 | Because it is likely that recovery skills will need to be used by individuals who use public transportation, it is important to teach the appropriate problem solving skills. The therapist may find that the use of prosthetic picture prompt cards will enhance function of individuals with cognitive impairments. |
| Peer/Family Acceptance of Disability | *Modifying Attitudes Toward Disabled Persons While Socializing SCI Patients* M. Haney B. Rabin | Purpose of study was to identify core problems associated with resocialization of people with a spinal cord injury. | Attitudes of non-disabled college students toward parents with disabilities improved when the student was involved in resocialization program with his/her parent who was disabled. | Archives of Physical Medicine and Rehab. 1984 65  p. 431-435 | By involving family members in the CIP program, negative attitudes toward people with disability should decrease. |

| Topic | Article Title | Overview | Findings | Reference | Implications |
|---|---|---|---|---|---|
| Perceived Freedom | *Therapeutic Recreation Assessment and Intervention with a Patient with Quadriplegia* J.G. Blake | A case study of a 24 y/o male with incomplete transverse SCI readmitted 5 years post injury due to decubitus ulcers. During admission he received leisure education concerning community based leisure activities. Community integration training completed. | Comparison of admission and post treatment scores using the Leisure Diagnostic Battery show an increase in perceived freedom in leisure. Patient's increased motivation in other therapies also noted, as he was interested in being able to immediately engage in his newly learned leisure activities (sports) upon discharge. | Therapeutic Recreation Journal 1991 25 p. 71-75 | This case study of a community integration program similar to the CIP has documented the significant increase in a patient's perceived freedom, measured increase in leisure participation, and measured increase in compliance with other therapies. |
| Quality of Life | *Quality of Life in Quadriplegic Adults: A Focus Group Study* C.A. Bach R.W. McDaniel | This study's purpose was to identify the components of quality of life for individuals with quadriplegia. While small (14), the sample size represented the national population of individuals with quadriplegia in terms of age and gender. | Eight categories related to quality of life were identified: 1. relationships, 2. job & productivity, 3. dependence vs. independence, 4. finances, 5. health, 6. inner strength and survival, 7. assertiveness, and 8. level of activity. | Rehabilitation Nursing 1993 18 p. 364-367 | Increased mobility skills and greater options for leisure activities were noted as important elements to increase a patient's quality of life. These skills and knowledge can be obtained through the CIP program. |
| Quality of Life | *Quality of Life: The Physician's Dilemma* M. Freed | Academy Presidential Address by Murray M. Freed, MD, Boston University Medical Center. | Identification of the fact that over the last 40 years the length of life expectancy has increased and institutionalization has decreased for individuals with SCI. "Now that we have added years to peoples lives, it is also our responsibility to add life to their years" (p. 109) | Archives of Physical Medicine and Rehab. 1984 65 p. 109-111 | Identifying need to address quality of life in patients with SCI. |

| Topic | Article Title | Overview | Findings | Reference | Implications |
|---|---|---|---|---|---|
| Return to Premorbid School Environments | *Returning to School After a Spinal Cord Injury: Perspective From Four Adolescents* M.J. Mulcahey | Explores impact of returning to premorbid environment on social interactions, role change, self-image, coping strategies, accessibility, and feelings. | All four adolescents found major changes in: 1. their friends, 2. roles identity (including social identity in school), 3. self-image, 4. coping skills including social withdrawal, 5. ability to reach basic spaces such as the lunchroom or library, and 6. feelings. (The up and down emotions associated with adolescence were significantly increased.) | Am. Journal of Occupational Therapy April 1992  Vol. 46 #4 p. 305-312 | All four subjects had an extremely difficult time returning to school. Having a supportive staff to help problem solve barriers and help educate school staff and peers may have made the transition easier. |
| "Revolving Door" Syndrome with Psychiatric Patients | *Leisure Education: Meeting the Challenge of Independence of Residents in Psychiatric Transitional Facilities* J.K. Dunn | This article describes the importance of leisure education programs to facilitate the independent leisure functioning of residents in transitional facilities. Leisure education goals, objectives, and program processes are outlined. Implementation ideas are suggested. | A program of leisure education in a transitional facility has tremendous potential to contribute to the independent functioning and quality of life for patients residing in that facility. | Therapeutic Recreation Journal 1981 15  p. 17-23 | The use of a structured treatment protocol to help patients with psychiatric diagnoses can help facilitate the development of community survival skills and enhance the patient's constructive use of leisure time. |

| Topic | Article Title | Overview | Findings | Reference | Implications |
|---|---|---|---|---|---|
| Self Concept | *The Effects of Wheelchair Competition on Self-Concept and Acceptance of Disability in Novice Athletes* <br><br> G.D. Patrick | 10 novice athletes who were mobility impaired were measured prior to and 5 month post involvement in wheelchair sports and compared to veteran athletes and non-athletes on self-concept and acceptance of disability. Acceptance of Disability Scale and Tennessee Self Concept Scale were used. | Participation in wheelchair sports has a positive influence upon their self-concept and acceptance of disability. A public and dramatic activity such as wheelchair athletic competition has important qualities for improving self-concept and acceptance of disability. | Therapeutic Recreation Journal 1986 20 p. 61-71 | The involvement in wheelchair athletic programs seems to improve the individual's self-image. Introducing a patient to his/her opportunities in the area of wheelchair sports may help the patient improve his/her self-concept and adjustment to disability. |

# Smith-Armstrong Study

S. Harold Smith of Brigham Young University and Missy Armstrong conducted a formal review of the outcomes of the CIP itself in 1985. They reviewed patient records from 1980 through 1985 with particular attention being given to completed CIP forms and their related progress notes. They hoped that completed CIP forms would provide raw data that could be organized to perform a statistical analysis. Unfortunately the review of the CIP forms indicated that staff had not provided complete or consistent information on the great majority of the forms. Therefore a descriptive analysis of the 24 forms with sufficient data was all that could be made. (For those of you interested in demonstrating the efficacy of your treatment programs, this points out the need to keep complete and accurate records of all treatments performed.)

The review also indicated few, if any, common denominators among patients other than their basic disability classification. Because of this, the original 24 patients were subdivided into two disability groups, spinal cord injury (10) and brain injury (14) for the purposes of this study.

Interestingly, a review of related progress notes and demographic information indicated that the patients with a spinal cord injury were, generally, treated early in the program (1980 - 1982) while those patients with brain injuries were treated later (1982-1985). This followed a pattern that had been recognized by the Harborview staff regarding the types of patients being treated over the five year period. During the early 1980's the majority of their patients had moderate to severely involved spinal cord injuries. For the next two years the majority of patients had severe brain injuries. Medical and trauma care advances in the treatment of both spinal cord injuries (SCI) and traumatic brain injuries (TBI) led to this change in basic patient populations. As an example, the use of steroids significantly reduced the number of patients with a complete spinal cord injury.

Since the CIP was originally developed for use with patients who had sustained a spinal cord injury and was later implemented with patients who had sustained a traumatic brain injury, a review of these two groups was deemed important to determine whether the CIP was appropriate for the new population.

Tables 1 and 2 presented the data and findings for the two disability groups. It is interesting to note that in the majority of cases (8 of 10) patients with a spinal cord injury achieved lower scores on the field trials than in their pre-test. Just the opposite was the case with patients with a traumatic brain injury where the majority (13 of 14) achieved higher scores on the field trial than on the pre-test. A close review of related progress notes shows that the therapeutic recreation staff felt that the CIP was just as helpful for patients with a spinal cord injury as it was patients with a traumatic brain injury.

**Table 1 Summary CIP Results - SCI** Differences Between Pre-test Percentage Scores and Field-Trial Percentage Scores on the CIP - Spinal Cord Injury

| Patient # | High Diff. | Low Diff. | Ave. Diff. | Total Items | CIP Items Reported by Name |
|---|---|---|---|---|---|
| S-1 | -2.0 | -18.0 | -7.7 | 7 | Movies, Restaurant, Airport, City Bus, Downtown, Grocery Store |
| S-2 | -12.0 | -32.0 | -25.8 | 4 | Sporting Event, Swimming, Airport, Grocery Store |
| S-3 | -27.0 | -46.0 | -34.8 | 5 | Restaurant, Swimming, City Bus, Laundromat, Grocery Store |
| S-4 | +17.0 | -7.0 | -0.6 | 5 | Movies, Restaurant, City Bus, Grocery Store, Shopping Mall |
| S-5 | 0 | -13.0 | -5.2 | 5 | Swimming, City Bus, Laundromat, Downtown, Grocery Store |
| S-6 | -8.0 | -40.0 | -22.0 | 5 | Restaurant, Wheelchair Sport, Airport, Downtown, Grocery Store |
| S-7 | -4.0 | -28.0 | -15.8 | 9 | Movies, Restaurant, Swimming, Airport, Bus Station, Bank, Laundromat, Downtown, Grocery Store |
| S-8 | +5.0 | -15.0 | -4.7 | 7 | Restaurant, City Bus, Bank, Laundromat, Downtown, Grocery Store, Shopping Mall |
| S-9 | +10.0 | -8.0 | +1.6 | 9 | Movies, Restaurant, Swimming, City Bus, Train Station, Personal Travel, Downtown, Grocery Store, Shopping Mall |
| S-10 | +15.0 | -5.0 | +10.0 | 4 | Swimming, Personal Travel, Grocery Store, Shopping Mall |

To explain why the groups showed different patterns of scores, the authors looked at the problems that the patients were trying to solve. The first community integration problem for patients with spinal cord injuries is physical accessibility. For individuals with a traumatic brain injury the first major community integration problem is related to cognition and cognitive reasoning ability.

Because of these differences, the CIP was used with patients who had spinal cord injuries to help them overcome personal physical limitations and physical barriers in the community. In the majority of cases it was found that the patient could do better in the pre-test situation because it was conducted in a more protective environment. The actual situation during the field trial in the community was usually more difficult, so the field trial scores were not as good.

In the case of patients with a traumatic brain injury, the CIP was used more as a training and cognitive learning tool. For these patients, the actual experience in the community, where the patient was dealing with a real situation, appeared to be easier for the patient than the more abstract pre-test situation in the hospital. They generally made higher scores in the concrete field trial than in the more abstract pre-test situation.

An interesting sidelight was that therapeutic recreation staff reported that the CIP was a more accurate indicator of community integration skill development for patients with spinal cord injuries than for patients with traumatic brain injuries. The primary reason for this, again, had to do with the types of problems the two groups of patients were trying to solve. The patient with a traumatic brain injury was working to regain the necessary cognitive skills through the CIP experience. However, the loss of judgment skills which typically accompanies this type of injury combined with the variability in the level of stress during any particular community outing made it difficult to translate the skills learned in the relatively calm hospital setting to the more variable and stimulus-intensive community setting. The patients with spinal cord injuries, on the other hand, were not affected by the variability of the community setting as much. Their problems were more straight forward ones and easier to predict: getting around in the community is simply harder than getting around in the hospital.

**Table 2 Summary CIP Results - TBI** Difference Between Pre-test Percentage Scores and Field-Trial
Percentage Scores on the CIP - Traumatic Brain Injury

| Patient # | High Diff. | Low Diff. | Ave. Diff. | Total Items | CIP Items Reported by Name |
|---|---|---|---|---|---|
| B-1 | +7.0 | -10.0 | +3.4 | 7 | Movies, Restaurant, Swimming, Bus Station, Laundromat, Grocery Store |
| B-2 | +7.0 | +4.0 | +5.1 | 7 | Sporting Event, Restaurant, Swimming, City Bus, Laundromat, Downtown, Grocery Store |
| B-3 | +2.0 | +6.0 | +12.8 | 6 | Movies, Restaurant, Swimming, City Bus, Downtown, Shopping Mall |
| B-4 | +29.0 | +4.0 | +13.8 | 5 | Sporting Event, Swimming, City Bus, Downtown, Grocery Store |
| B-5 | +50.0 | +14.0 | +29.0 | 6 | Sporting Event, Restaurant, Swimming, City Bus, Downtown, Grocery Store |
| B-6 | +39.0 | +12.0 | +21.8 | 5 | Movies, Swimming, City Bus, Laundromat, Grocery Store |
| B-7 | +20.0 | -17.0 | +6.2 | 9 | Movies, Sporting Event, Restaurant, Swimming, Wheelchair Sport, City Bus, Downtown, Grocery Store, Shopping Mall |
| B-8 | +10.0 | -13.0 | +0.25 | 4 | Movies, Swimming, City Bus, Grocery Store |
| B-9 | +10.0 | -10.0 | +1.7 | 7 | Movies, Restaurant, Bus Station, Bank, Downtown, Grocery Store, Shopping Mall |
| B-10 | +30.0 | -15.0 | +3.4 | 5 | Restaurant, City Bus, Downtown, Grocery Store, Shopping Mall |
| B-11 | +15.0 | +6.0 | +10.0 | 4 | Sporting Event, Bus Station, Downtown, Grocery Store |
| B-12 | +20.0 | +6.0 | +11.3 | 6 | Sporting Event, Restaurant, Swimming, City Bus, Grocery Store, Shopping Mall |
| B-13 | +16.0 | -41.0 | -9.6 | 5 | Movies, Swimming, Bus Station, Downtown, Grocery Store |
| B-14 | +29.0 | +14.0 | +16.0 | 5 | Restaurant, Swimming, Bus Station, Downtown, Grocery Store |

Table 3 listed each of the seventeen possible CIP activity items and indicated which of these items were used by the therapeutic recreation staff with each population group. They found that six of the seventeen items were used with a majority of both patient groups. It appeared that these six items were the most effective in teaching the necessary skills for these patients. It was interesting to note that these six items included a representative of each of the four general activity areas used in the CIP. Cultural Activities were represented by movies/theater and restaurant, Physical Activities by swimming, Transportation Activities by city bus and Community Living Activities by downtown and grocery store. While other activity items were used, these six appeared to be the most effective in the CIP process.

**Conclusions and Recommendations**

Even though objective data is extremely limited, subjective information strongly supports the continued use and refinement of the Community Integration Program. It is evident that the CIP is used by the therapeutic recreation staff as a consistent means of teaching and evaluating the community integration skills with their patients. It appears that use of the six identified activity items provide sufficient information and training for successful community integration skills.

It is also recommended that further research be done on the use of the CIP. The treatment team at Harborview Medical Center are interested in working with individuals and agencies who wish to use the CIP as part of their research. It is by working together and compiling data that the field of therapeutic recreation will be able to further refine the treatment that we deliver.

**Table 3 Cumulative Frequency of CIP Activities** This chart shows the frequency of each CIP activity that was reviewed for this study listed by diagnostic group.

| Activity Item | Spinal Cord Injury | Traumatic Brain Injury |
|---|---|---|
| Library | 0 | 0 |
| Movies* | 5 | 7 |
| Sporting Events | 1 | 6 |
| Restaurant* | 7 | 9 |
| Swimming* | 7 | 11 |
| Wheelchair Sports | 1 | 1 |
| Airport | 5 | 1 |
| City Bus* | 6 | 9 |
| Bus Station | 1 | 4 |
| Train Station | 1 | 0 |
| Personal Travel | 2 | 1 |
| Bank | 2 | 1 |
| Laundromat | 4 | 4 |
| Downtown* | 7 | 10 |
| Grocery Store* | 10 | 13 |
| Shopping Mall | 3 | 5 |

*Those items rated/used most frequently

Lastly, it is also strongly recommended that the therapeutic recreation staff continue to use the CIP in the total rehabilitation process with its patients. Care should be given in keeping accurate data, maintaining accurate progress notes and in using the CIP program both as an effective teaching as well as evaluation tool.

*Sample Module from the original version of the Community Integration Program*

This module may apply to the following community setting:

      A. Bank
      B. Laundromat
      C. Downtown
     **\*D. Grocery Store**
      E. Shopping Mall

**********************************************************************************

Therapist Statement:
You are making your weekly grocery list, and plan to shop this afternoon. Consider the following questions while planning your outing.

**********************************************************************

A. Pre-arrangements
    1.  Which grocery store will you choose? Why?
    2.  Will you plan to take a grocery list with you?
    3.  How will you plan to pay for your groceries?

B. Transportation
    1.  How will you get to and from the store?
    2.  How will you transfer in and out of the vehicle?
    3.  Where is the store located?
    4.  Where will you park?

C. Accessibility
    1.  Where will you enter the store?
    2.  Is the store accessible?
    3.  How will you get in and out through turnstile entrances?
    4.  How will you reach items on the top shelf?
    5.  How will you reach items from the cold storage section?
    6.  How will you carry your groceries while shopping?
    7.  How will you check out, if the cashier's aisle is too narrow for your wheelchair?
    8.  How will you carry the grocery bags to your car, bus, or taxi?

D. Emergency
    1.  As you are checking out, you learn that you do not have enough money for all that you've chosen. What will you do?
    2.  What will you do if you've to cath yourself or go to the bathroom while you are shopping?

E. Equipment
    1.  What medical equipment will you require for your trip?
    2.  What special equipment or supplies will you take to make your shopping more convenient?

# 4. Program Management

*The information in this chapter will help guide the therapist to implement the Community Integration Program. Included in this chapter is help for the therapist and patient in selecting the most appropriate modules, selecting the process to follow when running modules, and modifying the CIP for different patient populations.*

The CIP was developed to be flexible. There is little sense in working through a module with a patient if s/he will not be using those skills upon discharge. The information in this chapter will help the therapist and the patient to outline a community integration plan. It is recommended that each patient complete seven to ten modules, but again, each patient's specific needs and length of stay will have a big influence on the final decision.

The most successful utilization of the program includes:

1. a formal assessment to determine the needs of the patient and family.
2. a plan agreed to by the therapist, patient, and family which should be reviewed with the rest of the therapy team. The plan includes the activities to be done and an anticipated time frame for completion of each activity.
3. at least two one on one evaluations with the therapist: one to measure the patient's environmental skills of path finding, mobility, safety, and problem solving in high stimulus situations; the second to measure transportation options using personal and/or public transportation. These should be stressed because lack of these skills is reported to be the biggest barrier to active participation.
4. group community outings supported/directed by therapy staff to ensure specific skill development, and opportunities for generalizing experience.
5. at least one patient directed activity.

# Modules to Use

Determination of module selection should come during the initial assessment and evaluation of the patient. Particular attention should be paid to the following:

- physical, cognitive, and emotional capabilities, especially in high stimulus situations
- previous life style and experiences
- language, financial, and cultural issues

- social skills
- attitudes towards leisure and readiness for reintegration
- proposed discharge plan and future geographic location

| Modules | Suggested Participation Requirement |
|---|---|
| **Community Environment**<br>    Environmental Safety<br><br>    Emergency Preparation<br><br>    Basic Survival Skills | Environmental Safety - strongly recommended for each patient<br>Emergency Preparation - review formally or informally with each patient<br>Basic Survival - recommend for patients who are discharged to a less-than-stable residential environment (including those who may experience homelessness) |
| **Cultural Activity**<br>    Theater<br>    Restaurant<br>    Library<br>    Sporting Event | At least one of these |
| **Community Activity**<br>    Shopping Mall<br>    Grocery Store<br>    Downtown<br>    Bank<br>    Laundromat<br>    Community Skills | At least one of these |
| **Transportation**<br>    Personal Travel<br>    Taxi<br>    Train<br>    Air Travel<br>    City Bus<br>    Bus Station | At least one of these |
| **Physical Activity**<br>    Aquatics<br>    Wheelchair Sports<br>    Physical Leisure Activity | Only one activity is required; however, it is suggested that the patient attend the activity at least twice.<br>Wheelchair Sports is an introduction to possible future participation in the activity |
| **Individual Plan**<br>    Leisure Activity | At least one group and one patient directed |

Individuals should also be assessed in regard to their problem solving and organizational skills. This enables the therapist to assess the patient's needs and current independence level so that future training can be adjusted to suit the particular patient.

The information can be gathered from interviews, chart documentation, multidisciplinary team meetings, and the family. The ongoing collection of information, especially about physical abilities may alter particular aspects of the plan. Using this information, a skilled therapist should be able to determine when the patient is ready to participate in the Community Integration Program.

Our experience has shown that individuals should participate in some in-house activity to determine behavior, social skills, medical concerns (i.e., reaction to high stimulus, tolerance to activity, wheelchair use, pain management, intellectual and memory capabilities, and ultimately patient readiness) prior to the start of the Community Integration Program.

The program should be run in tandem with leisure education, behavior modification (if necessary), and the development of community resources. At Harborview the patient is not given clearance to leave the facility until s/he is cleared in the community by a Certified Therapeutic Recreation Specialist to determine the degree of support required, ensure patient safety and compliance with medical precautions and, if necessary, to facilitate family education and comfort level.

Patients have reported that the most successful plans have included at least one transportation module (usually the functional use of the city bus) and the environmental awareness evaluation. These can be completed on a one to one basis with a therapist or incorporated into another evaluation like the grocery store.

We promote physical activity at least once a week with an aquatics evaluation and treatment, a bias suggested by our geographical area. We also require at least one event in which the patient assumes responsibility for arrangements, transportation, community resources, and medical concerns for themselves and all other participants of a group outing.

The strength of the program has proven to be its ability to be adapted to meet the unique needs of an institution's varied population. How each facility uses the program and selected modules will be dependent on the type of population, length of stay, and diagnosis.

# Approaches To Follow

The approaches a therapist may follow are divided in two ways. The therapist needs to decide on the size of group s/he wants to observe and s/he needs to decide how actively s/he wants to participate in the process of the outing.

## Individual or Group

A module may be run one on one with the therapist and the patient or the therapist may choose to use a module for a group outing. The decision depends on the patient diagnoses, the needs of the individuals, and the specific module being used. We recommend a combination of individual and group evaluations because it encourages patients to learn from each other. However, some modules, particularly those that monitor safety and environmental awareness, are best done individually, because the distractions or leading by other patients influence decisions of the patient being evaluated. This is particularly true with those who are cognitively impaired. Modules which are best run individually are the ones in the Community Environment and Transportation categories.

All approaches require the documentation of observed behaviors; physical, emotional and cognitive abilities and/or limitations; patient's perception and/or stated learning curve; and additional goals to be met before discharge from treatment.

Acceptable answers to pre-test planning questions will need to be agreed upon by the staff and may have to be altered depending on the patient diagnosis, capabilities, and mobility status. There are also geographical references which need to be modified to meet each patient's situation.

## Formal, Informal, or Independent

Part of the treatment plan agreed to by the patient, therapist, and team describes the formality of the planned outings. For each outing, the team must decide which of the three approaches (formal, informal, or independent) will best meet the patient's need. The primary difference between the approaches is the role of the therapist. In the formal approach the therapist acts as an observer who is evaluating the patient's skills and abilities. This is most appropriate for evaluating an individual's abilities in environmental awareness and transportation. In the informal approach the therapist is an active participant in the process. In the independent approach the therapist may only participate to check on the patient's perceived degree of success.

### Formal Approach

The formal approach is usually done on a one on one basis. First the pre-test planning guide is reviewed with the patient. The patients are asked to respond either in writing or during an interview process with the therapist. All answers are written down and scored for correctness. If an investigative process is suggested (i.e., calling the bus station to select times for trips), this can occur at this time.

Shortly before the field trial the therapist can check with support staff to determine if the patient is ready for the trial. If it is clear the patient has forgotten, it is appropriate for the therapist to remind the patient. The therapist should also note on the field trial score sheet that the patient was not getting ready for the outing at the appropriate time.

The therapist's role in the formal approach is to act as a trained observer only. S/he only steps in if the person being evaluated demonstrates an unsafe behavior. The patient should be reminded of the therapist's role with the following instructions: follow verbal directions exactly, make safe choices, and seek outside resources to find answers (i.e., ask the bus driver for information rather than therapist). Conversation is appropriate during the evaluation process to both normalize the situation and to determine the patient's ability to perform with multiple stimuli. This is often an opportunity to explore with the patients their ability to transfer knowledge to reality and ultimately to their leisure lifestyle.

The therapist is responsible for observing and counting errors, unsafe physical actions, and requests for therapist assistance. Field trial forms are provided for each of the modules. A formal check list can be disruptive to the patient so the therapist may decide to keep a mental note of errors and document all observations on the field trial form after the trial is complete.

After the field trial, the patient is asked to complete the same set of questions s/he filled out during the pre-test. The therapist should score the post-test evaluation and share the results of the pre-test, field trial, and post-test evaluations with the patient. This feedback is vital for tying the activity to positive leisure and for helping the patient see where s/he was successful and where s/he could be more efficient. It gives the therapist a chance to help the patient work through the frustrations and problems so that future outings will be more successful. The therapist should be especially careful to note safety errors and to reinforce successful problem solving behavior.

Comparing the pre- and post-test scores will provide one indication of the amount of learning which took place on the outing. However, some patient populations, especially those with spinal cord injuries, score much better on the pre-test than they do in the field. The difference in their pre- and post-test scores would not necessarily be a good measure of their learning. Since the goal is to measure the ability of the patients to succeed in community outings, the only valid test for the efficacy of the program is to measure the difference in score between the first time a patient does an outing and the second time the patient does the same outing. Time restrictions and lack of patient willingness to go on the same outing twice mean that, for most cases, the therapist needs to use his/her best judgment to decide how fast the patient is progressing. Scoring and changes in knowledge should be noted on progress notes or individualized assessments to track the patient's progress.

## Informal Approach

In the informal approach the planning guides are used by the therapist and patient to generate discussion during either individual or group processes. Group discussion can identify concerns, establish a plan to include the collection of information (i.e., ticket prices, accessibility, location, fears) and the areas of emphasis to be monitored by the therapist during the community activity.

These outings should not be formally scored. In fact, the therapist should take a very active role in promoting the learning process: encouraging peer interaction, promoting socialization, processing fears and concerns in non-clinical settings, and addressing mobility and safety issues.

This is the approach that best addresses family education. Since the therapist takes the leadership role, the patient and family have the opportunity to interact and learn through experience, training, and guidance of trained staff.

Although this isn't a formally scored procedure, all observations, skill levels, and interactions should be documented.

## Independent Approach

The planning guides can be distributed to patient and/or family members as review documents prior to a therapist directed outing or an independent venture. Follow up by the therapist is used to check the patient's perception of success.

The therapist may want to send a few of the module pre-test sheets home with the patient. They can be used by his/her family and significant others or through an outpatient service to help continue the integration training and awareness.

# Documenting the CIP

One of the key elements of the CIP is documentation. This includes but is not limited to the following:

- patient functional skill level and ability
- family education and training
- patient's perception of progress
- therapist's clinical judgment
- establishment of the course of treatment, goals, and objectives

Without documentation neither you nor anyone else (including your patients) will be sure that the program is working as planned.

## Documentation of Patient Functional Skill Level and Ability

Documenting a patient's functional skill level and ability is usually done in several phases. It starts with the initial screening or assessment. Later, progress is documented to show the level of integration that the patient has achieved through chart notes and the results of the modules. Finally a discharge and follow-up plan describes what should happen when the patient leaves the hospital. Post discharge reports are useful to monitor the patient's success after leaving the hospital. These reports are excellent references for team members during out-patient clinic visits to determine the level of function at discharge and progress with community integration. (Examples of the forms used by the staff at Harborview e.g., an initial screening tool, chart notes, and discharge form, may be found in Section 2 of this book.)

The first documentation that a therapist writes on a patient usually comes from an initial screening or an intake assessment. (The screening is usually a much quicker procedure than the assessment.) The initial screening helps the therapist determine if his/her services are required to help the patient meet recovery goals, to determine the scope and intensity of involvement from the therapeutic recreation service, and to help identify safety issues. An intake assessment is done when it is clear that the patient requires therapeutic recreation service and information is being gathered to define the specific service required.

The next set of documentation comes when the patient is reviewing his/her treatment plan. For each module run as a formal procedure, the patient chart should include a record of the pre-test, field trial, and post-test evaluations. Modules run with informal procedures should document if the patient met the level of achievement required. Included in this set of documentation should be the patient's perception of his/her performance on the module(s) completed.

The final set of documentation during the hospital stay is the discharge documentation. This documentation should include a review of assessments and evaluations, patient abilities, patient perceptions, family education and training, and goals for continued improvement.

If it is possible, documentation should be added to the patient's records even after discharge to record how well the patient is doing in the community. In our facility patients are routinely monitored with routine out-patient evaluations during clinic visits. This is useful for modifying the CIP and establishing the usefulness of the program as discussed below in the efficacy section.

## Establishment of The Course of Treatment

Treatment should be carefully planned so that the patient receives all of the training s/he needs to return to the community successfully. The community integration training was developed as a standardized treatment program with distinct modules. Each module stresses a particular skill or functional ability. By carefully documenting the plan of treatment the therapist and the rest of the therapy team can be sure that the patient will receive all of the training s/he needs to be successful when s/he is discharged back into the community.

Having the treatment clearly outlined at the start of the program sets up clear goals for treatment and helps the patient measure his/her progress toward those goals. Family and friends who are working with the patient will also be able to see progress. At least some of the frustration at the often slow pace of recovery can be alleviated by seeing that some real progress is being made.

## Establishment of a Data Base for Efficacy Studies

One of the biggest advantages of careful documentation is that the therapeutic recreation staff and the rest of the treatment team can measure the impact of treatment. This type of measurement makes the third party payers and the survey teams happy.

Even more important, though, is that it helps to clearly define the specific skills that a patient newly discharged from a rehabilitation setting needs. Community integration is an evolving process. As the needs of the patients change, the requirements of the program change, too. Accurate documentation changes therapy from being exercises done in a vacuum (or hospital) and makes it the basis for survival once the patient is discharged from the hospital. By documenting the specific skills required, keeping records of how different patients performed, and receiving patient success reports after discharge, we (all therapists) can continue to modify the Community Integration Program so that it meets future needs.

## Standardizing Documentation

Documentation works best when it is standardized. For the CIP there are two major aspects to standardizing the documentation:
- consistency in the use of words and abbreviations
- consistency in the method used to score the pre-tests, field trials, and post-tests

The use of agency wide definitions of words and abbreviations helps provide a more consistent delivery of care for the patient. The reader will be able to turn to the Glossary to find definitions of many of the treatment related words throughout this book, but even then be sure that the definitions are consistent with the definitions that your agency uses.

The second aspect of consistency is in the method used to score patient skills. Two different types of keys are presented in this book. The therapeutic recreation department may have their own which they choose to use instead. It is not important which method of coding is used, as long as one type of coding is used by the entire department consistently. This unified coding will enable the other members of the health care team understand what they are reading, and will help facilitate efficacy of treatment evaluations.

The first system presented here, the Plus Minus System, requires the therapist to make a determination whether the patient does or does not possess a particular skill at the required level of performance. The second system, the Functional Independence Measure, grades the patient on his/her level of independence in performing the skill. It is possible to use one or the other (or even both together) and have useful documentation of a patient's progress in the CIP.

**Plus Minus System**

At Harborview we use a four symbol system for documenting on our assessments and CIP forms. If the patient has demonstrated the ability to independently demonstrate a functional skill or required piece of knowledge a "+" is written in the appropriate location on the form. If a patient is not able to independently demonstrate a functional skill or required knowledge, a "-" is written in the appropriate location on the form. Our forms all have spaces for a written description of important details. This system of documentation allows us to provide a detailed note on the patient's functional ability without spending much time on documentation. The four symbol system used by the Therapeutic Recreation Department at Harborview is listed below.

---

**Harborview Medical Center CIP Documentation Key**
Therapeutic Recreation Department, Seattle, WA

Key:　　　(+) = independent function, affirmative response, or demonstrates appropriate knowledge
　　　　　(-) = patient needs assistance, negative response, or the lack of appropriate knowledge
　　　　　(N/A) = not applicable
　　　　　(N/T) = not tested

---

**Functional Independence Measure**

One of the most common coding systems used in assessment and charting on rehabilitation units is the Functional Independence Measure, or the "FIM". The FIM is a seven point scale which is divided into two basic levels of ability.

The first level of ability in the FIM scale is called "Independent." If a patient is able to start, work through, and end an activity by himself/herself, s/he is considered to be independent in that activity. If the patient requires the use of some adapted equipment, but is able to access the equipment, use it, and replace it on his/her own, then the patient is still considered to be independent. The key to this level of the FIM scale is that the patient is able to engage in the selected activity without the assistance of another person. To distinguish the difference between the patient who does not require adapted equipment versus the patient who does, the "Independent" level of the FIM is divided into two sections. *Complete Independence*, represented by the number "7", indicates that the patient does not require adapted equipment. *Modified Independence*, represented by the number "6", indicates that the patient requires the use of adapted equipment and yet is still able to independently engage in the activity.

The second level of ability in the FIM scale is called "Dependent". The term "Dependent" indicates that the patient is unable to engage in the activity without the assistance of another person. Obviously there can be a great degree of difference in the amount of help required from one patient to the next. For that reason, this part of the FIM scale is divided further into two subsections. The first section, *Modified Dependence*, indicates that while the patient requires the assistance of another person to engage in the activity, that assistance consists primarily of verbal cueing, equipment setup, or just moderate touching and little physical help from the other person. The second section, *Complete Dependence*, indicates that the patient requires another person to complete most of the activity for him/her.

---

# Functional Independence Measure (FIM)
© Copyright 1987 Research Foundation - State University of New York

**Independent** - Another person is not required for the activity (No Helper)

7    **Complete Independence** All of the tasks described as making up the activity are typically performed safely without modification, assistive devices, or aids, and within reasonable time.

6    **Modified Independence** Activity requires any one or more than one of the following: an assistive device, more than reasonable time, or there are safety (risk) considerations.

**Dependent** - Another person is required for either supervision or physical assistance in order for the activity to be performed, or it is not performed (Requires Helper).

   **Modified Dependence** The subject expends half (50%) or more of the effort. the levels of assistance required are:

5    **Supervision or Setup** Subject requires no more help than standby, cueing or coaxing, without physical contact. Or, helper sets up needed items or applies orthoses.

4    **Minimal Contact Assistance** With physical contact the subject requires no more help than touching, and subject expends 75% or more of the effort.

3    **Moderate Assistance** Subject requires more help than touching, or expends half (50%) or more (up to 75%) of the effort.

   **Complete Dependence** - The subject expends less than half (less than 50%) of the effort. Maximal or total assistance is required, or the activity is not performed. The level of assistance required are:

2    **Maximal Assistance** Subject expends less than 50% of the effort, but at least 25%.

1    **Total Assistance** Subject expends less than 25% of the effort.

Modified Dependence, while indicating that the minimal to moderate assistance of another person is required, has been further divided into 3 levels to allow better clarification of the actual skill level of the patient.

For the patient who requires only standby assistance from the therapist or limited cueing to carry out a task, the term Supervision or Standby assistance has been used. The FIM scale indicates Supervision or Standby assistance with the number "5".

Some patients are able to complete most of an activity by themselves but, for some parts of the activity, they actually require some physical contact from the therapist. An example would be an elderly patient who can slowly walk to the bus stop with his walker but requires physical assistance from the therapist or bus driver for balance as he takes the large step up into the bus. This type of assistance would be considered to be a Minimal Contact Assistance and is coded with a number "4".

The patient who is able to independently complete half of the task to three fourths of the task but requires more then just a little physical assistance is said to require Moderate Assistance. The patient who is at a restaurant and is able to feed herself after the therapist sets up her plates, gives her the adapted silverware, puts a straw in her drink, and cuts up her food is considered to need Moderate Assistance. Moderate assistance is scored with the number "3".

Patients who are not able to do at least half of a task should be considered to be completely dependent. One of the key criteria that divides Dependence and Complete Dependence is the degree of hands on, more-than-touching assistance from the therapist. Any time that the patient requires more than just touching assistance to complete a task, that patient is considered to be completely dependent in that task. The category of Complete Dependence is divided into two sub categories: Maximal Assistance and Total Assistance.

When ever possible the therapist should allow the patient opportunity to complete as much of a task as realistically possible. If a patient is able to complete between 25% and 50% of the task himself/herself, and the therapist is required to provide considerable physical assistance or the task is not done, that patient requires Maximal Assistance. Maximal Assistance is scored with the number "2".

The patient who is not able to complete a task without extensive effort from the therapist (the patient is able to complete less then 25% of the task independently) is considered to be Completely Dependent. Complete Dependence is scored with the number "1".

# Adapting the CIP

"When do I use the pre-test, field trial, post-test combination and when do I not?" is a question frequently asked by therapists using the CIP for the first time. The answer will need to be individualized for each patient. Determining what type of information the treatment team and the patient need, as well as what kind of skills the patient needs to develop may help the therapist determine how best to modify the CIP. The information in this section is intended only as examples to help the therapist's decision making process.

Patients who have a spinal cord injury (SCI) tend to have few problems with cognition.[1] The therapist may want to ask a patient with a SCI the questions on the pre-test prior to the outing. Our experience has shown that these patients usually score well on formal pre-tests but have significant difficulty performing

---

[1] A percentage of patients with an SCI received their SCI as a result of engaging in a high risk activity without taking appropriate precautions. If this is a possibility, the therapist may need to look for that pre-morbid behavior showing up during outings.

as well on the field trial. The therapist may want to mark the patient's demonstrated skill level on the field trial sheet. If the therapist wants to measure the patient's increased ability to anticipate and solve problems after an outing, then time should be made to administer the post-test. With patients with SCI the pre-test and post-test scores will likely be fairly similar. Since most patients with a SCI will go on more than one community integration outing, the use of the post-test after each outing is not always indicated. Unless the therapist has some reason to believe that the patient with a SCI will have a lower score on the post-test then on the pre-test, s/he may not need to administer the post-test in many situations.

- The therapist receives a physician's order to evaluate a patient's bus riding skills, as he will need to use the bus to attend daily outpatient therapy appointments. The patient is a 24 y/o male 2 months post GSW (gun shot wound) with a T5 incomplete injury to his spine. This patient scores poorly on his first pre-test for using the city bus, as he has never before had to ride the bus while being ambulatory, let alone while using a wheelchair. The therapist runs the first field trial using the city bus using a formal approach. (Adolescents tend to deny that they will have problems. By running outings formally the full impact of their disability tends to "wake them up.") One more outing using the city bus (and one more city bus field trial form) show a marked improvement in the patient's demonstrated skill level. The last evaluation showed that he was able to independently use the bus from his home to his outpatient therapy sessions. The therapist administered the post-test to measure the improvement in being able to verbally problem solve and to demonstrate an increased knowledge about using the bus system. The patient's scores on the last field trial demonstrated that he was able to function independently while using the city bus.

It is hard to make generalizations about the type of modifications to the CIP program for patient's admitted to a psychiatric or drug and alcohol service. Generally, the therapist using the Community Integration Program with this population will want to measure three basic competencies: 1. the ability to be oriented to one's environment, 2. the ability to correctly interpret events in the environment, and 3. the ability to demonstrate socially appropriate skills. Individuals with physical disabilities are not immune from mental illness, so, at times, the therapist will also need to evaluate the patient's ability to problem solve architectural barriers. If the treatment team is trying to determine which psychotropic medication is best for the patient, the therapist may find himself/herself running modules using the formal method. The purpose would be to measure the patient's demonstrated level of coping and community survival skills while on different doses of medications. The informal approach may be taken if the therapy session's primary purpose is either for exercise or for social skills training.

- The therapist is part of a treatment team treating a veteran with a primary diagnosis of Post Traumatic Stress Syndrome. The patient has 3 days until discharge and the environment that he will be discharged to is less than stable. The physician writes a prescription for the therapist to evaluate the patient using the Basic Survival Skills module. The therapist administers the pre-test questions and notes that the patient missed approximately one third of the questions. The therapist then spends time with the patient going over the correct answers. Not sure that the patient was able to grasp all of the information (due, in part, to his diagnosis) the therapist consults with the unit's social worker. The social worker and the therapist meet and write up a discharge "book" which provides the patient with both the questions and the answers. The patient receives instruction from the social worker in how to use the book. The therapeutic recreation specialist takes that patient on one outing into the community using the Basic Survival Skills Module. The patient is discharged with the book in hand. The therapist feels that a narrative note is called for each time he writes in the patient's medical chart. The only form from the CIP to go into the chart is the pre-test questionnaire.

Individuals with traumatic brain injury or other kinds of brain injury tend to do poorly on the pre-test, especially if they have word finding problems. As long as the patient has had a good night's rest and does not decompensate with extra stimuli, the therapist might be able to expect the patient with a brain injury to do better on the field trial then on the pre-test. However, probably one of the greatest challenges to the therapist is the fact that you cannot comfortably predict how a patient will do when impacted by the multiple stimulatory inputs from the community. At some point during the patient's early rehabilitation admission, and at some point near the end of the admission, the therapist may want to run one of the modules formally. This helps establish a baseline and a measured change at discharge. The therapist may want to run the rest of the modules informally to reduce the patient's stress and to promote good learning opportunities.

- A 67 y/o female has experienced a right cerebral vascular accident (CVA - stroke) and as a result has noted weakness on her left side (+3 UE - upper extremity and +3 LE lower extremity) with a dense, left sided visual neglect. The patient did not appear to have any notable problems with cognitive orientation. When asked the questions on the pre-test for the grocery store module, she scored near perfect. However, due to her visual neglect, she was not able to get half of the items on her grocery list (the ones on the left side of the paper), was not able to manage mobility skills without bumping into objects, and was not able to locate many of the items that she knew that she was to get because of the visual neglect. The therapist also noticed that she had difficulty doing two things at once - she could not talk with the therapist and walk at the same time, nor could she push the cart and scan the food items at the same time. The therapist wrote a narrative note in the chart indicating how well she had done on the pre-test questions, used the field trial form to record the patient's demonstrated skill level while on the outing, and completed the "Assessment of Skills in a Grocery Store" progress note to place in the chart.

It is not unusual for children and adolescents who are ill or disabled to be treated in a facility separate from adults. This separation makes sense, as the staffs need to take more of a developmental approach to treatment as well as needing to have different sized equipment (smaller). One of the major challenges for the therapist to make when working with children and youth is to modify the questions for age appropriateness. Most six year olds do not know how to make change for a dollar, and yet that is not considered to be a disability for someone of that age - it is normal development. Also, most younger children would not be expected to self-medicate. Another modification is the inclusion of the parents in many of the outings, as they, and not the child, will be responsible for transportation and shopping. The therapist will find that s/he seldom uses the formal version of the CIP with patients in a children's hospital unless the patients are over the age of 12. For those over the age of 12, a formal evaluation is often called for if the team is going to recommend community integration training through the special education program at the school. The formal CIP assessment then would become part of the child's IEP (Individual Education Program).

- The therapist had followed a 5 y/o male with a C1 complete spinal injury for the last 12 months of his stay at the children's hospital. The child was now going to be discharged to his parent's home with 24 hour nursing care (due to his ventilator dependency). The patient's wheelchair was a full 20" longer than the accessibility guidelines called for, and the protocol for his equipment called for it to be plugged in (not on battery) if they were stationary for any length of time. The plugs required an outlet that would take two 3 pronged plugs. Staff also had to take along a portable suctioning machine and extra cathing supplies. The therapist conducted inservice training to the entire home nursing staff, using the CIP manual as the course outline. The therapist also provided the nursing staff with a map indicating locations of commercial/recreation oriented businesses which could accommodate the patient's wheelchair and supplies. The therapeutic recreation specialist also worked with school staff on accessibility issues as well as developmentally appropriate ways to inform the patient's classmates about his equipment.

When using the CIP with adults who have a developmental disability, the therapist may find that the questions and the field trial forms are not detailed enough. Frequently, adults with developmental disabilities have significant impairments in memory and learning ability. Complicating the situation is the frequency of mental illness among those with a developmental disability (thought to be as high as 30%). In these situations, the therapist runs the CIP modules formally, interjecting cues as needed for safety. The number and types of cues are noted. After the outing the therapist analyzes the client's score on the pre-test *and* post-test, as well as the demonstrated skill level. These findings are taken to the IDT (Interdisciplinary Team) and the team decides if a training goal is indicated. If the team decides a training goal is indicated, the client's IPP (Individual Program Plan) is modified to include the new goal. The therapist then writes up a training program based on a detailed task analysis of the skill needing to be learned. The CIP is still valuable when working with adults with developmental disabilities. It helps remind the therapist about the "big picture" of skills that still need to be learned. Also, for some clients who live in the community, the CIP will contain enough detail.

- The recreation consultant (a CTRS) for a group of group homes used the CIP on a regular basis to measure the clients capabilities related to community integration. All of the clients in one of the group homes were diagnosed as having Prader-Willi Syndrome with IQ's ranging from the mid 80's to the mid 50's. The primary disabilities for the therapist to address with this population are that they are compulsive eaters (stealing food, scrounging trash cans, etc.) and that they tend to be very argumentative. It is critical that these clients do not gorge themselves with food and gain weight. It appears that the more weight they gain, the lower their IQ drops. They do not regain the IQ points lost if they then loose the extra weight that they gained. While all six of the clients in this one group home demonstrated the ability to ride the city bus, only one of them was allowed to. It seems that the others aggressively stole any food that other riders were carrying when staff were not on the bus, and then they would argue and argue about their right to do so until, frequently, it ended with fisticuffs and the police being called. Originally the city bus module was used (in a formal manner) to measure each client's skill level. This story is told to show that at times, the CIP modules need to be further adapted to meet the patients' (or, in this case, clients') needs. It was because of this situation that the Bus Utilization Skills Assessment (Idyll Arbor) was written — to function as an extended field trial form of the **CIP** City Bus Module.

In summary, as you use each module, you will find that some questions on the pre-test form do not seem appropriate for the actual situation. This situation usually happens when you have a patient who will not have a problem with some of the concerns presented. It is appropriate for you to skip some of the topics and only use the ones that you find appropriate. The score sheets are set up for this to happen by allowing you to write in the number of questions asked as well as the number of questions answered correctly.

One warning may be in order though. To be sure of the change resulting from the activity, you do need to ask the same questions on the post-test as you asked on the pre-test. Write down any changes that you make on the pre-test form and use the same form for the post-test.

# 5. Clinical Information

*The purpose of this chapter is to provide the therapist with a rudimentary review of some of the clinical information needed to take patients into the community safely. We also recommend that the therapist review Section 3 for information on accessibility.*

This chapter serves two purposes. One is to discuss how the CTRSs at Harborview Medical Center function as team members. The other is to provide the therapist with a rudimentary review of some of the clinical information needed to take patients into the community safely. We caution that this is rudimentary. Experience, mentorships, and continuing education are still required to meet the standards of the field.

The selection of articles and other information in this chapter are used at Harborview as background information for therapists who are responsible for community integration outings. The topics include skin care (including recognition and treatment of pressure sores), the latest classification standards for spinal cord injuries, the importance of executive function in patients with traumatic brain injuries, body jackets, quad coughing and other respiratory issues, bladder control, and autonomic dysreflexia.

These issues are important. For example, not understanding the issues surrounding skin integrity can lead to pressure sores or shearing which can result in weeks or months of time being added to the patient's hospitalization. Autonomic dysreflexia can lead to death.

Other issues are important for knowing what your patients will be able to accomplish during their community integration outings. You need to know the physical and mental limitations caused by the patient's injuries. You also need to know what normal is before you set your level of expectations too high.

We understand that this set of information is not complete and welcome feedback from you telling us other information you want or areas that you need to have clarified.

# Team Membership

The trend in health care is to work as a team in treating a patient. Each member of the team works mainly in his/her area of specialization, but the goal is to help the patient in the most efficient way possible. Team members are valued for the information they bring to the team and their abilities in helping their patients. Therapeutic recreation is valued when the information communicated to the team describes functional skill development and educational value. The team doesn't need to know that the patient played Bingo. They need to know that the patient was able to tolerate a group for more than an hour, maintained behavioral control, engaged in positive socialization, manipulated objects, and met time commitments.

No information is valuable unless the therapist is competent. Excellent patient care is based on sound clinical reasoning and grounded in therapeutic recreation theory and practice. The modules presented are basic guidelines and should be used with your common sense. Do your homework, read charts, be involved in team meetings, observe therapy sessions, review protocols regularly and update your skills with the other disciplines.

Safety of the patient is an important consideration for the team in potentially risky situations such as community outings. A CTRS must learn about and demonstrate understanding of issues like mobility, bowel and bladder, nutritional status, behavior, and cognitive function. The therapist has to know the capabilities of the patient so as to not expect standards that cannot be met. This requires that the schedule allow for regular participation in patient care planning meetings, as your safe management of the patient depends on your understanding of the whole treatment plan.

We aren't saying that the CTRS must do everything including all the teaching of a specific skill (for example, ADLs). What we do is report back the functional skill level that we observed in a practical setting. The report is based on our knowledge of the patient's current functional level and our understanding of the goals of the care plan. We do not feel it is necessary to regularly include other disciplines to evaluate functional skills. With our clinical knowledge and ability to document, we provide the team with information about what the patient can do in the real world.

On the following two pages is one of the checklists used at Harborview by the senior therapist or the internship supervisor to determine whether a therapist or a student intern in therapeutic recreation has obtained the minimum clinical knowledge and skills necessary to conduct community integration outings.

There is a separate checklist for each therapist. For each of the specific knowledge areas, the senior therapist notes the dates when orientation, demonstration of the skill, and the six month review took place. You can use this form as a guideline to develop a proficiency checklist of skills required by your facility.

# Proficiency Checklist

Harborview Medical Center, Seattle, WA

| Area of Knowledge | Specific Topic | Orient to Procedure | Demonstrate Skill and Explain Rationale | 6 Month Review |
|---|---|---|---|---|
| **Knowledge** | Spinal Cord Injury | | | |
| | Brain Injury | | | |
| | Medical Terminology | | | |
| | Skin Protocol | | | |
| | | | | |
| **Evaluation and Assessment** | Individual Patient Plan and Assessment | | | |
| | Community Integration | | | |
| | Environmental Awareness | | | |
| | Transportation: Bus | | | |
| | Grocery Store | | | |
| | Cultural | | | |
| | Downtown | | | |
| | Independent Patient Plan | | | |
| | | | | |
| **Documentation** | Standards | | | |
| | Assessment | | | |
| | Progress Notes | | | |
| | Community Skills Notes | | | |
| | Environmental Awareness | | | |
| | Community | | | |
| | Metro (City Bus) | | | |
| | Kardex | | | |
| | FIM Scores | | | |
| | | | | |
| **Procedures** | Age Related Activity | | | |
| | Leisure Education | | | |
| | Stress/Pain Reduction | | | |
| | Exercise and Relaxation | | | |
| | Orientation | | | |
| | Family Education/Training | | | |
| | Time Management | | | |
| | Chemical Dependency | | | |
| | Community Resources | | | |
| | Ventilation Review Orders | | | |
| | Van Breakdown | | | |
| | Alternative Transportation | | | |

| Area of Knowledge | Specific Topic | Orient to Procedure | Demonstrate Skill/Explain Rationale | 6 Month Review |
|---|---|---|---|---|
| **Precautions** | Tilt Back/Pressure Releases | | | |
| | Catheterization | | | |
| | Nutrition Status | | | |
| | Diet Restrictions | | | |
| | Dysreflexia | | | |
| | Hypotension | | | |
| | Skin/Sheering | | | |
| | Sitting Time | | | |
| | Ace Wraps | | | |
| | Pressure Garments | | | |
| | Orthotics | | | |
| | | | | |
| **Transfers** | wheelchair to bench van seat | | | |
| | wheelchair to floor | | | |
| | wheelchair to toilet seat | | | |
| | | | | |
| **Safety** | Security | | | |
| | Show of Force | | | |
| | Transfer Belt/Restraints | | | |
| | Incident Reports | | | |
| | Patient Security System | | | |
| | Seizure Precautions | | | |
| | Fire | | | |
| | Code | | | |
| | Disaster | | | |
| | | | | |
| **Systems** | Van | | | |
| |    wheelchair lift | | | |
| |    wheelchair restraint system | | | |
| |    child restraint | | | |
| | Safe driving techniques | | | |
| | Cellular Phone | | | |
| | | | | |
| **Procedures** | Universal cuff | | | |
| | Wrist cock-up | | | |
| | Wheelchair takedown | | | |
| | Electric wheelchair takedown | | | |
| | | | | |

# Basic Goals of Good Skin Care

The Certified Therapeutic Recreation Specialist should have a basic understanding of the principles of good skin care. While inactivity (such as prolonged bedrest or watching too much television) may cause a pressure sore, excessive activity may also damage the integrity of the skin.

**Each Therapist Should Be Able To :**
- Identify what healthy skin looks like.
- Be able to explain or show how to correctly position patients in bed.
- Know how to maintain good skin care by diet and fluids.
- Know how to prevent skin breakdown.
- Know signs of skin breakdown, what to look for.
- Know the pressure points and bony areas which cause skin breakdowns.
- Describe how to treat a minor skin breakdown (pressure sore).

**Assessment of Good Skin Appearance**
- The patient's skin should be clean and dry, not moist (wet) because moisture causes bacterial growth which can cause skin breakdown, especially in the groin area.
- The patient's skin should not be red or discolored.
- The patient's skin should not be dry and flaky. This can cause cracks in the patient's skin which lead to skin breakdown.
- The patient's skin should be supple and soft; check bony areas for hardness, lumps, increased warmth and redness. Be sure to check especially carefully during exposure to extreme weather elements while out on a community integration outing.

**General Skin Care**
- Prevent long periods of pressure on any area of the skin, especially bony areas.
- Good nutrition from a daily diet which includes whole grain breads and cereals, meats, poultry, fish, milk products, fruits, and vegetables promotes healthy skin.
- Maintain proper body weight for body build.
- Bathe to remove dirt, bacteria, and dead skin cells. Washing increases circulation which increases the nutrition and oxygen supply to the skin. Be sure to remove all soap to avoid drying the skin.
- Use lotions and bath oil for especially dry skin.
- Keep toenails trimmed straight. Ingrown toenails cause irritation which can increase muscle spasms and the risk of infection.

**Positioning**
- Use as many different positions as possible; abdomen, back, sides and sitting, standing if possible (use braces or standing table if needed).
- After each change of position, check for redness over bony areas.
- Skin tolerance in bed: The patient will usually start out with 2 hour turns on both sides and on his/her back. Turn times are usually increased at 30 minute intervals as his/her skin tolerates the added time to a maximum of 4 hours per side or up to 8 hours prone (on his/her abdomen).
- Allow a rest period of at least 60 minutes before resuming the same position. Only resume the same position for the same length of time if the patient's skin faded to normal color within 15 minutes.

# Pressure Sores

A **pressure sore** is a wound which develops when constant pressure is applied to an area for too long a period. Pressure blocks the blood flow. This leads to dead tissue.

**Skin tolerance** is the amount of time a patient can lie or sit in a certain position without damage to his/her skin.
- Wheelchair skin tolerance usually starts out at 15 minutes the first time up.
- The second time up may be increased another 15 minutes provided that the patient's skin tolerated the first 15 minutes.
- The patient's wheelchair time can increase either 15 minutes each time (or per day depending on physician preference) until the patient has reached between 5-6 hours of "up" time.
- Once the "up" time goal has been reached, the patient is usually up "ad-lib" as long as s/he does pressure releases and does not have any problems with redness or skin breakdown.
- The patient should follow established skin tolerances for each position. When sitting, the patient will probably need to do a pressure release every 15-20 minutes.
- The patient has established a "good" tolerance when s/he has no reddened areas over bony prominences (red areas fade in 15 minutes or less).
- If the patient or therapist notices reddened areas which persist longer than 15 minutes, up time or turn time should be decreased by 30 minutes.

## Signs of a Pressure Sore
- hot/warm area to touch due to irritation leading to hyperemia
- whiteness of skin due to interrupted blood flow
- hard area/lump due to subcutaneous injury
- red area that doesn't fade in 15 minutes or less, which indicates damaged tissue

## Factors in Developing a Pressure Sore
- Weight of the patient: it is important for the patient to keep his/her weight within normal limits for his/her body build. Too much weight causes increased pressure and increases the danger of breakdown of the skin. Too little weight causes decreased sub-cutaneous tissue over bony areas which makes the patient more prone to skin breakdown.
- Foreign objects or wrinkles: sitting or lying on wrinkles or foreign objects causes small sites of concentrated pressure.
- Trauma: bumping into his/her wheelchair when transferring; running into door with his/her feet
- Tight clothing or coarse materials
- Friction: in transfers or sliding around in bed. This is especially bad if the patient has a fragile area on his/her skin.
- Wetness: the patient should not sit on or lie on wet or soiled areas. Change the patient into dry clothes and be certain that the patient's skin is washed and dried well.
- Burns: sunburns, hot coffee or hot water spills, tap water over 110 °F
- Shearing: caused by sitting up in bed or a wheelchair and sliding down.

## Contributing Factors
- Illness: increased temperature leads to increased metabolism. The patient needs to turn on schedule even if s/he doesn't feel like it.
- Dryness: when the patient's skin is dry it can lead to cracking. These openings admit bacteria and lead to further breakdown.
- Maceration: softening of skin due to moisture. The patient's skin will break down more easily.
- Patients with diabetes must be especially careful to watch their diets and check their skin thoroughly and frequently. They often have decreased circulation from both the paralysis resulting from their injury and from the diabetes. The skin breaks down more easily and can be more difficult to heal.

# Treatment of Pressure Sores[2]

Pressure sores (ulcers) are a common affliction in two clinical situations: when people are immobilized, as in paralysis, coma, dementia, and forced bed rest; and when they must wear artificial devices, such as casts, splints, braces and prostheses. It is not surprising, therefore, that pressure ulcers frequently occur after spinal cord injury. In such cases they usually involve the ischial areas, or, less often, the sacral and trochanteric regions.

The etiology of pressure ulceration is multifactorial. Blood pressure at the arterial end of the capillary loop is approximately 30 mm of mercury. Since pressure over bony prominences have been measured at between 40-150 mm of mercury, it seems clear that ischemic necrosis [cell death from lack of blood] is the probable pathologic event. But there are other contributory causes as well: shearing injuries and other trauma; increased temperature, as with fever; moisture, including sweat and urine; poor nutrition; denervation and infection all increase the skin's sensitivity to ischemia.

The length of time necessary for ischemia to produce ulceration varies with each person and situation, but is not long in any case. Generally, it is believed that two hours of pressure-induced ischemia is sufficient to begin the process of skin ulceration.

Most pressure ulcers begin as a red area of skin. Given the magnitude of the problems that arise when such areas are allowed to progress to ulceration, this early stage should be considered a medical emergency. The pressure on the area should be relieved quickly and should not be reapplied until the skin has recovered, even if this requires hospitalization. A hospital stay of a few days, to heal this type of pressure problem, is preferable to the longer stay required after their skin and underlying tissues are actually destroyed.

Without proper care, the early stage proceeds to actual ulceration. If this ulceration involves only a small area of skin or a partial thickness skin loss, the sore may still be treated non surgically. Again, it is a medical emergency requiring relief of pressure, and if hospitalization is necessary to accomplish this, it should be done. If not treated successfully, the sore develops into a grade 3 or 4 pressure ulcer, involving breakdown of fat or bone tissue (see the next page for stages of pressure ulcer development). These rarely heal without operative closure unless the area of skin loss and the zone of undermining are both very small.

The management of these deep ulcers cannot stop with skin flap closure by the plastic surgeon. It must also include additional training in skin care, transfers, etc. by the physiatrist or primary care physician. Skin flaps are never as durable as the original skin cover. If the patient's skin care habits permitted his original skin to break down, flaps have little to no chance without a change in behavior. Once the physiatrist or primary care physician is convinced that the patient is better able to care for his skin, ulcer closure, usually with flap tissue, is indicated. If the patient or his support system cannot be educated in skin care, then closure of the ulcer is not possible, and open wound care must be provided for the remainder of the patient's life.

Care of deep ulcers at the University of Washington is provided on the Rehabilitation Service, as for other problems related to spinal cord injury. The first step is evaluation by the physiatrist. If it is decided that the patient and/or his family can learn and execute adequate skin care, further training is instituted and plans are made for surgical closure of the wound.

---

[2]Engrav, Loren H. "Treatment of Pressure Ulcers" *Rehabilitation Spinal Cord Injury Update* Vol. 2, No. 4 Fall/92

Preoperative care includes sharp debridement, hydrotherapy, and wet to dry dressing changes. Actual osteomyelitis is not common, so a workup for this diagnosis is rarely indicated. Spasms must be relieved with oral Dantrium, Valium or baclofen, or intrathecal baclofen, or with surgery. Bladder infections are controlled. Bowel control is achieved, although enemas are not used, since they may produce intraoperative evacuation. The postoperative immobilization plans made and rehearsed.

Operative closure nearly always involves removal of the ulcer, trimming of the underlying bony prominence, and coverage with local flap tissue. Perioperative broad-spectrum antibiotics are administered. These operations commonly last 3 to 4 hours, and require one or two units of blood.

The postoperative plan involves three weeks of immobilization on some type of air bed. There should be no motion of the operative site. The surgical wounds are quite large, and involve large areas of undermining, and therefore will not tolerate motion too early. Two weeks may be adequate; one of the ongoing studies at the University of Washington is designed to test this possibility.

This treatment is lengthy and expensive, sometimes involving six or more weeks of inpatient care. Prevention should therefore be a primary goal in the skin care. Turning the patient every two hours is fundamental, but proper hygiene and nutrition are also required. Proper pads for sitting are essential. Foam cushions and sheepskin are effective in the prevention of shearing and maceration, and are also inexpensive. Most importantly, quick and thorough treatment is vital in the early stages of redness, before actual ulceration occurs.

Loren H. Engrav, MD

*Note: The Certified Therapeutic Recreation Specialist plays a vital role in the education of good skin care during leisure activities and in the modification of the patient's everyday habits.*

Stage One: Skin is unbroken, but red or discolored. Redness does not fade within 30 minutes after pressure is removed.

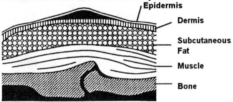

Stage Two: The epidermis is broken, creating a shallow open sore. Drainage may or may not be present.

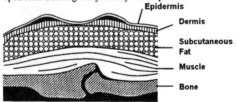

Stage Four: The breakdown extends into the muscle. Dead tissue and drainage are usually present.

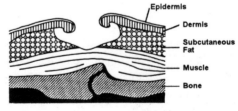

Stage Three: The break in the skin extends through the dermis into the subcutaneous fat tissue.

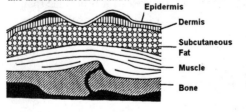

Stage Four: The breakdown may extend to the bone.

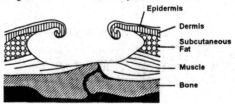

# Severity of Tissue Injury

Tissue injury, damage to any part of the body from impact, pulling, etc., is divided into three degrees of severity. Patients with tissue injury must be treated in a way appropriate to the severity of the injury.

### First Degree   Grade 1

The onset of mild pain within 24 hours of an impact with another object or excessive pulling of tissue. Some tissue damage is evidenced by mild swelling and local tenderness. Pain may be evident with direct pressure or when the tissue is stressed through movement. Redness of skin is noted.

### Second Degree   Grade 2

Moderate pain which increases significantly during palpation or movement. The pain is significant enough to cause most patients to stop activity. If ligaments are involved in the injured sections, the patient may experience a decrease in stability because the torn ligaments allow an increase in joint mobility.

### Third Degree   Grade 3

Over 50% of the tissue involved is torn or avulsed. Severe pain is experienced even without movement; movement of effected part does not significantly increase pain. Significant joint instability may be noted if tendons or ligaments are involved.

# New ASIA Standards for Classifying SCI[3]

An individual's progress after spinal cord injury can be assessed by looking at the success of vertebral column stabilization, spinal cord recovery (or lack thereof), and the re-establishment of daily life activities. Recent pharmacological advances and likely future ones, designed to reduce secondary pathology in spinal cord injury (SCI), and various vertebral column surgical techniques presumed to protect the spinal cord, have made it increasingly imperative that quantitative assessment of spinal cord function be serially performed.

In 1969, H. L. Frankel, MD introduced the 5-point scale (A through E) for delineating sensory and motor function that bears his name.[4] Refinements in the scale have since occurred under the aegis of the American Spinal Injury Association (ASIA), adding increasingly precise scoring of sensory and motor function. The first *Standards for Neurological and Functional Classification of Spinal Cord Injury* appeared in 1982, and subsequent revisions were published in 1987 and 1990. However, an unequivocal adoption of these standards eluded the field, leading ASIA to seek a broader array of inputs.

The new Standards, published this year by ASIA with the assistance of the American Paralysis Association, were the result of a series of meetings with experts from the fields of orthopedic surgery, neurosurgery, physical medicine and rehabilitation (PM&R) and epidemiology; representatives from the Model Spinal Cord Injury Care Study (NASCIS), the International Medical Society of Paraplegia and the 12 major national organizations in neurological surgery, orthopedic surgery, PM&R and trauma.

The committees dealt in depth with defining "complete" and "incomplete" injuries, sensory and motor neurological level and the zone of partial preservation (ZPP), and precise methods of scoring sensory and motor function. As these definitions were refined, so were the definitions of the 5-point scale. In the resulting new scale, called the ASIA Impairment Scale (modified from Frankel) or AIS, change is most evident in the definitions of an incomplete lesion.

## Complete or Incomplete

The prior definition of incomplete, the presence of some sensory or motor function in more than three levels directly caudal to the normal level, produced peculiar classifications as recovery occurred.[5] For example, if a patient had normal C5 sensory function and also had a ZPP that included C6, C7, C8 and T1, the patient was labeled as Frankel B: C5 Sensory Incomplete. Or, in a case of motor function with the same ZPP, Frankel C: C5 Motor Incomplete. Such a patient might improve his C6 function over time to normal, but without an increase in the ZPP, he would change to Frankel B: C6 Complete in the case of sensory function, or Frankel C: C6 Complete in the case of motor function. Thus, an improving patient would paradoxically change from incomplete to complete.

The new definition of an incomplete lesion eliminates this paradox. To be sensory incomplete, a patient must actually perceive sacral sensation, which is tested by insertion of the examiner's finger into the anal opening. Sensory incomplete, therefore, means preservation of enough fiber tracts in the spinal cord to

---

[3]This article is reprinted with permission from *Rehabilitation Spinal Cord Injury Update* Fall/92 Vol. 2, No. 4 published by the University of Washington. Walter C. Stolov, MD is the author of the article. Information about this publication may be obtained by writing to the University of Washington, Rehabilitation Medicine RJ-30, ATTN: SCI Update, Seattle, WA 98195.

[4] Frankel, HL, Hancock DO, Hyslop G, et al. The value of postural reduction in the initial management of closed injuries of the spine with paraplegia and tetraplegis. Paraplegia 1969; 7(3):179-92.

[5]Waters RL, Adkins, RH, Yakura, JS. Definition of complete spinal cord injury. Paraplegia 1991;29(9):573-81.

perceive sacral sensation through the site of injury. Similarly, a patient is considered motor incomplete only if there is voluntary anal sphincter function.

Under this new definition of incomplete, the patient cited above would change from C5 Complete with four levels of ZPP to C6 Complete with three levels of ZPP, assuming no sacral sensory or motor function was present.

The five levels in the new AIS are as follows:

**A: Complete.** No sensory or motor function is preserved in the sacral segments S4-S5.

**B: Incomplete.** Sensory and/or motor function is preserved below the sensory neurological level and extends through the sacral segments S4-S5.

**C: Incomplete.** Sensory and/or motor function is preserved in the S4-S5 segment and some motor function below the neurological motor level is present. The majority of the key muscles in those [muscles] with some function below the neurological level have a muscle grade less than 3.

**D: Incomplete.** Sensory and/or motor function is present in the sacral S4-S5 segments, motor function below the neurological level is present, and the majority of the key muscles below the neurological motor level have a muscle grade greater than or equal to 3.

**E: Normal.** Sensory and motor function is normal. (A persistent hyperflexia does not negate this classification.)

## Neurological Level, Sensory

Two modalities, light touch and pin prick, must be tested. For each dermatome, therefore, four tests are made - two on the right side and two on the left. The neurological sensory level is defined as the most caudal segment in which sensory function is normal (light touch and pin prick are preserved) and all the proximal segments are also normal. For example, if the T4 segment has normal sensation, the T3 segment has absent sensation and the T2 segment and all proximal ones have normal sensation, then the neurological sensory level is T2, not T4. For there to be uniformity among examiners, the sensory test must always be made on the same places on the skin (see Figure 1 and Sensory Scores).

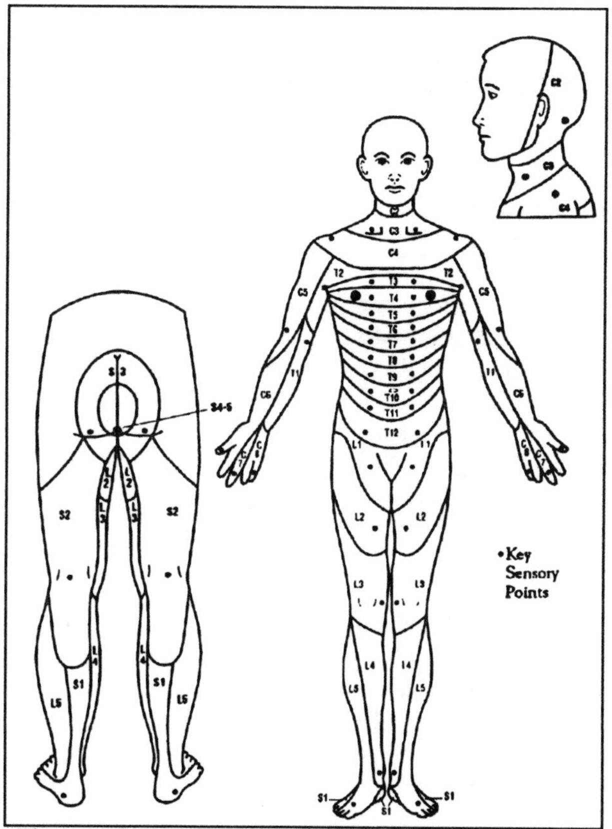

## Neurological Level Motor

The neurological sensory level requires that the most caudal segment have normal function with all proximal segments also normal, but the requirement for the neurological motor level is less stringent, due to the multiple innervations of the various muscles, Most of the muscles selected for scoring

*Figure 1*. Location of the key sensory points for each of the dermatomes. (Graphic provided by the American Spinal Injury Association.)

purposes have only two levels of innervation, so the requirement for defining a motor level is that the most caudal muscle have a grade of at least 3, the next most proximal muscle have a grade of at least 4, and all proximal ones be fully normal. If a muscle is at least grade 3, it is presumed that its more proximal nerve root is normal, while the more distal root may not be functioning. Again, for uniformity among examiners, the same muscles would have to be used in making motor level determinations (see Motor Scores, below).

## Sensory Scores

The Standard identifies 28 sites for testing the 28 dermatomes, beginning with C2 and ending with S4-S5, which are considered together as a group. Each of the precise locations is identified (e.g., C2 is at the occipital protuberance, T10 is at the level of the umbilicus in the mid-clavicular line, and L4 is at the medial malleolus). At each of these 28 levels, the score is (0) if sensation is absent: (1) if it is impaired, via either hypo- or hyperesthesia; and (2) if it is normal. This is done separately for light touch and for pin prick, so the maximum score for someone who is Frankel E (normal) is 56 each for light touch and pin prick on the right and left sides, or 224.

## Motor Scores

Available muscles with predominantly two root innervations that are suitable for examinations in an emergency room do not yield the breadth that exists in the sensory scoring. The Standard identifies only 10 levels and specific muscles for testing:

C5: elbow flexors
C6: radial wrist extensors
C7: elbow extensors
C8: flexor digitorum profundus (middle finger)
T1: small finger abduction (abductor digiti minimi)
L2: hip flexors
L3: knee extensors
L4: ankle dorsiflexion
L5: long toe extensors
S1: ankle plantar flexors

As far as motor innervation is concerned, the thoracic levels T2 to T12 are not precisely testable. One therefore defines levels in the thoracic area primarily on sensory function. Motor scores for each of these 10 levels are graded on the traditional 6-point scale (0 through 5). If a patient is normal on both sides, his maximum motor score will be 100. A patient with grade 3 antigravity triceps, at least grade 4 radial wrist extension and grade 5 elbow flexors, and no sacral sensory or motor function, would have a classification of AIS A: C7 Complete. Similarly, a patient with grade 3 quadriceps function and grade 4 or 5 hip flexion with normal motor function in all proximal segments and no sensory or motor function in the sacral area would be classifies as AIS A: L3 Complete.

## Skeletal Level

One must always be careful to not attribute to the neurological level the vertebral location of the bone or ligamentous disruption. Skeletal levels refers only to the level at which, by radiographic examination, the greatest vertebral damage is found. More likely than not, skeletal level will not be equal to neurological level and the two must not be confused.

# Thoracic Lumbar Sacral Orthosis (TLSO) Body Jacket Protocol

A Thoracic Lumbar Sacral Orthosis, also called a "body jacket" is a support made of plastic that fits over the chest, belly, and lower back. It is designed to support an unstable or recently fused spine. It is not unusual for the Certified Therapeutic Recreation Specialist to have one or two patients at a time who use this type of orthosis, so an understanding of the treatment protocols for body jackets is important. An inappropriate activity, or activity duration, can cause serious skin breakdowns. Part of a patient's prescriptive leisure education will need to be the understanding of how to adapt activities and how to understand the limitations with the use of a body jacket.

- Do not raise the head of the bed even with a body jacket on. If the patient has swallowing problems, respiratory difficulties, or is on NG feeding, the head of the bed may be raised by putting the bed in a reverse trendelenburg.

- No independent rolling by the patient unless the body jacket is on. When the body jacket is off, the patient must be log rolled by staff.

- The patient needs a tight fitting under-garment (a T-shirt 1 size smaller than usual, or size "small" stockinette). The stockinette should be cut 1 1/2 to 2 times longer than the patient's torso.

- Observe the correct way to put the body jacket on: Put on the back piece first, then apply top (front) by strapping one side then the other. This method avoids pinching which can occur if the front is applied in one step.

- A typical body jacket wearing schedule is:

    1. Begin with 2 hours on, then do a skin check. If skin is OK put the body jacket back on.

    2. Increase wearing time by 30 minutes each time worn, until body jacket is on 11 hours straight.

    3. At this point, the patient is to have the body jacket on 24 hours per day except for skin airings BID (off about 1 hour BID). If red marks develop beneath the jacket, problem solve (i.e., wrinkled shirt, needs refitting). If refitting is indicated, patient needs to be up in a wheelchair with the body jacket on. A weight change of 10 pounds requires the body jacket to be re-evaluated by the fitter.

- Specific restrictions may be ordered by the physician, i.e., no asymmetrical movements.

- An X-ray is usually done at approximately the 2 month mark to determine if the patient can be cleared for asymmetrical activities. Any clearance *requires* a written medical order.

- Proper positioning during activities is critical. Too much pressure along any edge due to patients straining to reach an activity or equipment can quickly lead to pressure sores.

# Quad Coughing

The patient with quadriplegia is not able to generate enough backward airflow to dislodge thick secretions which may block his/her trachea. By assisting the patient with a "Quad Cough," the therapist may help avoid the need to suction the patient. A quad cough is an external application of force that is applied by the therapist to help clear the respiratory tract of secretions.

**Position of Patient:**

1. When in bed, the patient is positioned flat on his/her back.

2. When in a wheelchair, the patient's spine should be straight. The wheelchair should be placed against a wall or firm object with the wheelchair brakes on, to prevent the wheelchair from tipping back.

**Position of Therapist:**

1. Place one hand flat just below the ribcage with the upper part of the hand (the fingers) fitting into the space just below the sternum. Caution: No pressure should be placed on the ribs or the sternum themselves.

2. The patient should take three deep breaths and on the third exhalation, s/he should attempt to cough.

3. The therapist at the same time gives a quick, forceful inward and upward sustained thrust with the attempted cough.

4. Repeat until the patient gets relief.

# Types of Contractures

| Type | Pathology | Intervention |
|---|---|---|
| Myostatic Contracture | ROM is decreased through inactivity: no pathological structures evident. | A myostatic contracture responds to a set of leisure activities which promote gentle stretching of the effected area multiple times a day. Also referred to as a "tight" muscle . |
| Scar Tissue Adhesions | The presence of scar tissue between healthy tissue will decrease ROM through adherence of the scar tissue to surrounding healthy tissue. Type of tissues which may be involved are: skin, muscles, tendons, and/or the joint capsules themselves. | The primary intervention in recreational therapy for scar tissue adhesions is prevention. The adhesions may be prevented or reduced through enjoyable leisure activities which promote the use of the affected area through its complete range of motion. Some "burning" or "stretching" may be experienced by the patient; discourage painful ranging during leisure activities. |
| Fibrotic Adhesions | When a patient experiences chronic inflammation as with arthritis the soft tissues involved tend to become more fibrotic. These changes cause tissues to adhere to each other, significantly reducing ROM. | Fibrotic adhesions are extremely difficult, if not impossible, to reduce through leisure activity. |
| Irreversible Contracture | Soft tissue and connective tissue structures are replaced by tissue such as bone or fibrotic tissue which does not stretch. | Irreversible Contractures are not amenable to treatment short of surgery. The Certified Therapeutic Recreation Specialist must take precautions not to stress the irreversible contracture beyond comfort, as serious tearing may result. |
| Pseudomyostatic Contracture | With certain kinds of neurological disorders (e.g., hypertonicity due to cerebral palsy), the muscle may be held in contraction without any tissue damage evident. | The decrease of hypertonicity may be achieved through various types of leisure activities, most notably therapeutic swimming in a pool with the correct water temperature. |
| Contraction and contracture are NOT synonymous and should not be used interchangeably. | | |

# Terms of Movement

**Active**    movement voluntarily done through the patient's use of his/her own muscles

**Angular**    movement which changes the angle of two bones joined together by a common joint

**Associated**    movement of body parts which normally would move together, e.g., the eyes

**Athetoid**    movement which is marked by slow, continuous, writhing movements, especially in the hands

**Automatic**    movement caused by the patient's own muscles, but not a voluntary movement, e.g., knee reflex, a muscle spasm

**Choreic Choreiform**    involuntary jerky and irregular movements of a muscle or group of muscles

**Contralateral Associated**    movement of a paralyzed body part which is caused by a voluntary active movement on the non paralyzed side

**Dystonic**    movement which is a slow, gross motor movement with athetoid characteristics

**Frenkel's**    movement exercises prescribed for patients with ataxia to help restore functional ability

**Passive**    movement of a body part caused by another person or a machine

**Reflex**    movement which is caused by an external stimulus which produces a reliably consistent response. A "knee jerk" is an example of a reflex; patients with spinal cord injuries or nerve damage may have increased, diminished or absent reflexes.

**Spontaneous**    movement which is initiated by the patient without any cueing.

**Synkinetic**    small, involuntary movements which naturally accompany larger, voluntary movements. An example might be when a patient pushes hard, his/her facial expression contorts.

# Range of Motion

Range of Motion refers to the amount of measurable movement of two parts of the body connected by a joint.

*Range of Motion – Active* The movement of two connected body parts caused by the active (patient initiated) contraction of muscles across the joint.

*Range of Motion – Passive* The movement of two connected body parts caused by external forces

The Certified Therapeutic Recreation Specialist should to be aware that there is not a nationally set standard for measuring ROM. There are four major systems of measuring and recording the measured Range of Motion (ROM). The most widely used system was first described by D. Silver in 1923 and published in the Journal of Bone and Joint Surgery[6]. This system measures movement with a 0 degree to 180 degree numbering system, "0" being the anatomical position. (Pronation and supination are not included.) All movement away from the anatomical position proceeds toward 180.

The ROM in degrees listed below is from Daniels and Worthingham, 1972. In parentheses next to the ROM degree is the range of "normal" ROM according to the 12 other primary ROM tables (Rothstein et al 1990, page 62 - 66).

| Range of Motion for Joints | | | |
|---|---|---|---|
| **Shoulder** | | | |
| Flexion | (130 - 180) | Extension | 50 (30 - 80) |
| Abduction | (150 - 184) | Internal Rotation | 90(55 - 95) |
| External Rotation | 90 (40 - 104) | Horizontal Abduction | (30 - 45) |
| Horizontal Adduction | (135 - 140) | | |
| **Elbow** | | | |
| Flexion | 160 (143 - 160) | | |
| **Radioulnar** | | | |
| Pronation | 90 (75 - 90) | Supination | 90 (70 - 90) |
| **Wrist** | | | |
| Flexion | 90 (60 - 85) | Extension | 90 (60 - 85) |
| Radial Deviation | 25 (15 - 35) | Ulnar Deviation | 65 (30 - 75) |
| **Hip** | | | |
| Flexion | 125 (100 - 130) | Extension | 15 (10 - 45) |
| Abduction | 45 (30 - 55) | Adduction | 0 (0 - 45) |
| Internal Rotation | 45 (20 - 47) | External Rotation | 45 (36 - 60) |
| **Knee** | | | |
| Flexion | 130 (135 - 160) | | |
| **Ankle** | | | |
| Plantar Flexion | 45 (45 - 65) | Dorsiflexion | (10 - 30) |
| **Subtalar Joint** | | | |
| Inversion | (30 - 52) | Eversion | (15 - 30) |

---

[6]The other three systems are: 1. 180 to 0 system by Clark (1920), 2. the 360 Degree system by West (1945), and 3. the SFTR System of Recording ROM Values by Gerhardt and Russe (1975).

# Muscle Strength

A standardized rating scale was developed by Daniels and Worthingham to indicate the degree of strength demonstrated by the patient.

---

**Muscle Strength**

(From Daniels and Worthingham. (1972) **Muscle Testing Techniques of Manual Evaluation by Comparison** (Ed. 3). Philadelphia: WB Saunders Company).

**Manual Muscle Evaluation**          **Strength**

| | | | | |
|---|---|---|---|---|
| 100% | 5 | N | Normal | Complete ROM against gravity with full resistance |
| 75% | 4 | G | Good | Complete ROM against gravity with some resistance |
| 50% | 3 | F | Fair | Complete ROM against gravity |
| 25% | 2 | P | Poor | Complete ROM with gravity eliminated |
| 10% | 1 | T | Trace | Evidence of contractility |
| 0% | 0 | 0 | Zero | No evidence of contractility |
| S | | | Spasm | |
| C | | | Contracture | If spasm or contracture exists, place S or C after the grade of a movement incomplete for this reason. |

---

# Sensation

Sensation refers to a message carried by the nerves as a result of some action or event.

**Terms of Sensation**

| | |
|---|---|
| **Absent** | lack of awareness of contact |
| **Articular** | awareness of the contact and movement of joints |
| **Cutaneous** | awareness of contact with the dermis (skin) |
| **Delayed** | awareness which happens some time after the initial contact |
| **Diminished** | a subnormal awareness of contact |
| **Epigastric** | referring to "that sinking feeling" produced by worry or fear; felt in the stomach |
| **Hyper** | an abnormal increased awareness of contact |
| **Internal** | awareness of sensations to the body not caused by an external event |
| **Negative** | lack of awareness of contact because the contact/stimulation is below the threshold of the nerves involved |
| **Objective** | a cognitive awareness of an event through the use of multiple senses |
| **Proprioceptive** | awareness of the movement and position of the body from nerves chiefly in the muscles, tendons, and inner ear |
| **Vascular** | awareness of a change in the tone of the surface capillaries e.g., blushing |

# The Bladder After Spinal Cord Injury

At the time of injury the spinal cord goes into shock. The bladder is unable to empty normally. The time that the bladder remains this way and how much recovery there will be varies with the individual and the level of the spinal cord injury.

An indwelling Foley catheter is usually placed in the bladder soon after injury and throughout the acute phase of medical care to continually empty the bladder.

The normal bladder empties almost completely when it contracts. If it doesn't empty completely, the remaining urine allows bacteria that remain in the bladder to grow and cause infections (UTIs).

In a normal urinary tract, there are small valves that prevent urine from flowing from the bladder back up toward the kidneys. Damage to these valves can result from over distention (too full of a bladder) and infection. If the valves are not working properly, urine can flow back up the urethers, sometimes into the kidneys. This is called reflux. This is dangerous if there are bacteria in the urine, which can cause kidney infections.

There are two types of bladders that are common after spinal cord injury: *upper motor neuron* or spastic bladder and *lower motor neuron* or flaccid bladder.

When a spinal cord injury is above T12, the bladder reflex center is still intact. The voluntary control for the bladder has been lost because the brain can't get the message down the spinal cord. Since the reflex is still intact, it will cause the bladder to empty when it gets full. A person with this kind of bladder may need to wear an external collection (condom cath) device because the bladder will often empty on its own.

The flaccid (limp) bladder occurs when the injury is below T12. The nerves to the bladder are usually damaged. The reflex for the full bladder doesn't work, and the bladder will not automatically empty. Instead, the bladder is flaccid and will continue to fill until it is emptied. This bladder can become damaged if the urine volumes get too big and can cause urine to back up into the kidneys - causing kidney damage.

## Intermittent Catheterization

Intermittent catheterization is the manual emptying of a patient's bladder. While the Certified Therapeutic Recreation Specialist will seldom have to "cath" a patient, it may be required while on a community integration trip. The information presented here on intermittent catheterization is meant only as an introduction. Each therapist who takes patients with spinal cord injuries out into the community should receive training from the nursing staff about the actual technique. If the therapist is with a patient who has a spinal cord injury at the 7th thoracic level or above, this knowledge should be required, as a sudden onset of autonomic dysreflexia may prove to be life threatening before help can arrive. (The next topic in this set is autonomic dysreflexia.)

There are two primary purposes of intermittent catheterization:

- To keep the bladder filling and emptying as normally as possible, and
- To reduce the problem of infection that generally results from indwelling catheters.

## Fluid Intake

The patient should normally drink up to three quarts of fluid a day. However, when s/he is first starting or getting ready for ICP (Intermittent Catheterization Program), s/he will be put on a fluid restriction of around 150 cc/hour with 150 cc for the entire night shift. The goal is to have 500 cc or less in the bladder every four to six hours. The patient will eventually learn how much fluid s/he can drink and still stay within the allowed bladder volumes.

A patient who has an indwelling catheter (Foley) in place is usually monitored for 48 hours or more prior to removal of the catheter. Before the catheter is removed urine output must be 500 cc or less every four hours before the catheter can be removed. Fluids are usually restricted to 150 cc/hour during the day and only 150 cc for the an entire night shift (about 12 hours). When the urine output is less than 500 cc every four hours for 48 hours the Foley can be removed. After the Foley is removed, the patient will usually be started on an every four hour cathing schedule until his/her urine volumes are low enough to be cathed every six hours.

If any patient's total urine output at catheterization is 550 cc or above (referred to as "dump") s/he will usually be catheterized every three hours if on a every four hours schedule; or cathed every fours hours if on a every six hours schedule for 48-72 hours.

Leisure activities and extreme weather conditions can effect the patient's fluid retention. It is very important for the Certified Therapeutic Recreation Specialist to help the newly injured patient monitor his/her fluid intake and output during the various community integration outings. This will help the medical staff modify the patient's cathing schedule to help him/her avoid embarrassing leaking and dumping.

# Autonomic Dysreflexia

Autonomic dysreflexia is a serious medical problem that can occur in individuals with a spinal cord injury above the 7th thoracic level. Autonomic dysreflexia can be caused by many type of noxious stimuli below the level of the spinal cord injury, and its symptoms may be mild or severe. Severe autonomic dysreflexia is a *medical emergency* which if not properly treated can result in cerebral vascular hemorrhage (stroke).

**Causes** (*from most to least common*):
1. Full or spastic bladder -urinary retention, UTI, stone
2. Full rectum
3. Abdominal pathology - kidney stone, bowel impaction, acute abdomen, etc.
4. Pressure sore, ingrown toenails
5. Tight or irritating clothing
6. Fracture or other undiscovered painful stimulus

**Signs and Symptoms:**
1. Sudden severe high blood pressure (as high as 250/150)
2. Slowed pulse rate after initial tachycardia
3. Pounding headache
4. Flushing of skin and sweating above level of injury
5. Apprehension/anxiety
6. Nasal stuffiness
7. Vision changes - blurring, spots before the eyes
8. "Goose bumps"

**What to Do First:**
Goal: reduce severity of symptoms and identify triggering source
1. Place patient in sitting position
2. Drain the bladder
   - If catheter in place, check for kinking. If catheter is plugged, do not try to irrigate. Change Foley using Xylocaine jelly for lubrication.
   - If no catheter is present, insert a catheter using Xylocaine jelly for lubrication. Do not push on the bladder.
3. If emptying the bladder has not lowered the blood pressure, check for stool in the rectum. Apply Xylocaine jelly to the anal sphincter and wait 3 minutes. Then, using Xylocaine-lubricated gloved finger, gently remove stool from the rectum.

**Medical Treatment**
1. If the autonomic dysreflexia episode is not resolving after the above measures, medical treatment is necessary. If the patient does not have his/her own supply of autonomic dysreflexia medication, transport him/her to an emergency room.
2. If the autonomic dysreflexia episode is not resolving and/or the blood pressure reaches 160 systolic, give the patient Nifedipine 10 mg sublingual. Instruct patient to bite through the capsule and hold it beneath the tongue. May be repeated after 15 minutes if blood pressure has not responded.
3. Continue to look for causes of autonomic dysreflexia by checking the patient's entire body.
4. Blood pressure may be safely lowered to 90/60, which is typical of quadriplegics in sitting position. Because autonomic dysreflexia episodes may recur, patient's blood pressure should be checked every 30-60 minutes for the next 4-5 hours

# Traumatic Brain Injury[7]

## Epidemiology of Traumatic Brain Injury

Traumatic brain injury (TBI) has a high incidence compared to other neurologic disorders and other traumatic injuries. The overall incidence of TBI in the United States is about 180 per 100,000 population per year and 80% of all TBI is mild TBI. Approximately 50% of all TBI is caused by motor vehicle or motorcycle accidents and alcohol is involved at least 50% of the time. Since traumatic injuries generally occur in otherwise healthy young individuals, it has an significant cost to society not just in acute medical care but lost productivity and long-term care.

## Definition of TBI

Traumatic brain injury is caused by trauma to the head in the form of direct impact or can also be caused by rapid acceleration/deceleration to the head without any head impact. It can be classified as mild, moderate, or severe depending on a Glasgow Coma Scale (GCS) score, duration of loss of consciousness (LOC), and duration of post-traumatic amnesia (PTA). The Glasgow Coma Scale is a 15 point scale measuring a person's ability to respond to stimuli with eye opening, verbalizations, and movement. Post-traumatic amnesia is the time between injury and the recovery of continuous memory. A severe TBI is characterized by a GCS of < 8, LOC > 6 hours and a PTA of weeks. A moderate TBI is characterized by a GCS of 8 - 12, LOC between 30 minutes and 6 hours, and PTA of days. A Mild TBI is usually defined as an injury with a GCS of 13-15, LOC < 30 minutes and PTA< 24 hours. A mild TBI can occur without a LOC and a traumatic injury with transient confusion or amnesia is classified as a mild TBI.

## Pathology of Brain Injury

Traumatic brain injury can result in focal or diffuse brain damage. Focal damage can be caused by a penetrating injury or focal contusion can occur. Contusions typically occur in the anterior temporal and frontal region of the brain. This is caused by the brain impacting the interior of the skull in those regions during an acceleration/deceleration injury. Focal injuries can also result from hemorrhages within the brain tissue or in the layers of tissue covering the brain (subdural and epidural hematoma).

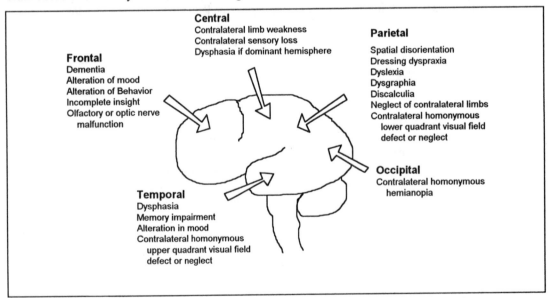

---

[7]Peter Esselman, MD, Harborview Medical Center

High velocity acceleration/deceleration forces to the brain do diffuse brain injury. This results in the tearing of axons and is called diffuse axonal injury. This injury is more prominent in certain areas of the brain such as the brainstem.

## Neurobehavioral Sequelae of Traumatic Brain Injury

Focal brain injuries, as shown in the figure, cause typical deficits depending on the area of brain damaged. An example of this is the hemiparesis caused by damage to the parietal lobe on the side opposite to the weakness. Less obvious are the deficits caused by frontal and temporal contusions and diffuse axonal injury. These injuries result in significant deficits in memory, attention, and concentration. The patient will also have problems with behavioral and impulse control as a result of the brain injury. Balance problems are also commonly seen after TBI. These problems improve with time, but may persist and be significant barriers to return to pre-injury activities and work.

## Rehabilitation After TBI

Rehabilitation after TBI is a multi-disciplinary approach to emphasize not only mobility and activity of daily living training, but also to increase the patient's cognitive abilities and train the person in ways to compensate for deficits. The ultimate goal of rehabilitation has to be to return the person as much as possible to a productive lifestyle including leisure activities and vocational activities.

# Executive Function

"Deficits in executive functions, perhaps more than any other cognitive process, determine the extent of social and vocational recovery." (Sohlberg and Mateer, 1989). Executive functions include planning, problem solving, goal selection, self monitoring, and time management. In order to do well at these tasks the frontal lobes must be functioning properly, as they are responsible for integrating and monitoring information from the rest of the brain.

Due to the location of the frontal lobes in the cranium they are extremely susceptible to damage when a traumatic brain injury (TBI) occurs. Thus a high percentage of patients with a TBI demonstrate deficits in executive functions.

Deficits in executive functions are common even in patients who score above average on IQ and other tests of intellectual abilities and seem to be functioning well in daily living skills. Such patients can do complex tasks well. They only have problems when they have to decide which tasks to do first, or how long to spend on a task, etc.

To give an example, most ten-year-old children have the skills needed to watch TV for 30 minutes, put away their toys, feed the dog, take a bath and go to bed. However, it is not likely this will happen unless a parent is nearby. The job of the parent is to: 1. monitor the passage of time and tell the child to stop watching TV, 2. initiate putting away the toys, 3. monitor quality control in putting the toys away, and 4. realize that it is getting late and ask another family member to feed the dog.

Our executive functions perform the role of the parent, first helping us make goals, then change them if new information requires it. For the patient who held a complex job and had a busy social life, even a small decrease in executive functions can be devastating, because a high percentage of the day was spent in an environment that required those skills.

If memory is impaired, executive functions will be impaired as well, because they depend on a relatively intact memory or memory compensation system. As an analogy, if vision is impaired, reading will be impaired. It is just as inappropriate to evaluate executive functions with memory deficits as it is to test reading without correcting vision. Some examples of appropriate memory compensation are: alarm watches for time management and "To Do" lists for goal selection and prioritizing.

All members of the rehabilitation team provide information about different aspects of the patient's executive functions. For example: Psychology uses tests such as the Halstead Category Test, the Wisconsin Card-Sort Test, the Porteus Maze Test, the Tower of London (moving rings on three pegs) or the Tinkertoy Test (analyzing initiation and planning in construction).

The speech pathologist might evaluate verbal problem solving and the ability to use an organized approach in a task such as finding a hidden word on the Herald's Hark computer program. This problem is too complex to solve without using compensatory strategies, e.g., writing down information and reorganizing it.

The occupational therapist observes meal planning and preparation. Often a patient with impaired executive functions can prepare one item such as a salad without difficulty. However, when the patient tries to make two or three items simultaneously, problems occur.

Therapeutic recreation specialists evaluate executive functions in real-world settings. Many patients are able to show up for daily inpatient therapy session on time because they are used to the routine. It requires higher level skills to plan ahead for a therapeutic recreation outing. The patient must plan for medication and cathing times and select clothing according to the weather. On a trip to the grocery store many executive functions are evaluated: remembering to take a list of items needed, organizing them by location in the store and crossing them off, judging traffic for safe street crossing, knowing when to ask for assistance, etc.

All members of the team share their information. This allows the group to decide how much structure the patient needs as the plan for therapy is developed. Both internal and external structure may be needed. Internal structure therapy might be teaching the patient to improve time estimation, and take on fewer tasks at the same time. Examples of external structure are alarms for time management and having a supervisor review work.

Rehabilitation units provide a supportive structure for patients and an understanding of deficits in executive functions. This is not the case outside the hospital setting. Thus it is important for each team member to start preparing the patient and family before discharge. The more firmly a therapy program and support structures are in place, the easier the transition will be.

# 6. Equipment and Supply List

The following is a suggested equipment and supply list to be reviewed by the therapist to meet needs of patients going into the community.

1. Medications
2. Catheter kit
3. Sliding board
4. Backpack
5. Sidepack
6. Velcro straps (small, medium, or long)
7. Reachers
8. Gloves (regular)
9. Gloves (rubber palmed)
10. Lapboard
11. Leg braces
12. Eating Utensils
13. Universal cuff
14. Cup holder
15. Ratchet hand splint
16. Wooden wedges (for theater outings)
17. Emergency phone numbers including the hospital and an appropriate contact person
18. Picture identification
19. Schedules
20. Money
21. Sports Equipment
22. Tickets

# *Section 2*

# *CIP Modules*

**Success is important but ...**

> *A young male with paraplegia was on a group outing to a University of Washington football game. Anxious to get seated before kick-off, one patient was upset that the van was stuck in traffic, needing to cross three lanes of cars to reach an accessible entrance to the stadium. He leaned out the window, attracting the attention of the first car, and yelled, "We have a patient with autonomic dysreflexia". The driver in the car leapt out of his car, cleared a path for the van, and the group traveled forward, parked, unloaded, and reached their seats just as the game began. This provided a great opportunity to talk with the whole group about appropriate problem solving and different ways to promote a positive, strong image of people with disabilities.*

# 7. Related Forms

*A Therapeutic Recreation Assessment helps the therapist determine when and/or if his/her services are required to help the patient meet recovery goals, to determine the scope and intensity of involvement from the therapeutic recreation service, and to help identify safety issues. Discharge summaries describe what was done by the therapeutic recreation group as part of the treatment team.*

This chapter presents two of the types of forms that we have found necessary in running the CIP successfully. The first set show therapeutic recreation assessment forms which the different departments at Harborview use when they get referrals for community evaluation and training from other members of the treatment team. The second set is a discharge form that we use to summarize the therapeutic recreation treatment that the patient has received while at Harborview. You will need to have forms like these as part of your way of interacting professionally with the other members of your treatment team.

# Initial Screening and Initial Assessment

At Harborview Medical Center, therapeutic recreation services are initiated after receiving a consultation request for services from the medical staff. These consultation requests are sent to all rehabilitation team members. We have found that it is important to be included in this process for two primary reasons:
1. to assist the therapeutic recreation personnel to quickly and efficiently initiate services and
2. to provide on-going educational opportunities for rehabilitation residents to understand the purpose and need for including therapeutic recreation in the rehabilitation process.

Patients are treated using a problem list approach versus a discipline specific approach (i.e., decreased ability to ambulate is a problem oriented approach, PT is a discipline specific approach). The "problem" which therapeutic recreation specifically addresses is community integration. Although we address other areas (i.e., mobility, psychosocial adjustment, ADLs), community integration is our primary focus. Having therapeutic recreation services on a consultant only basis, means that community integration is included on all patient problem lists. Since we are required to answer the consult request or medical order within 72 hours (the standard length of time across most of the nation) an initial screening note was developed to expedite the initial documentation process.

Once the consult request is received, the Certified Therapeutic Recreation Specialist must review the chart to determine the patient's readiness for treatment and intensity of services. During the chart review certain factors can be found which help to make decisions on potential needs.

Once the patient has been accepted to the therapeutic recreation service, a more formal assessment is completed using one of the two therapeutic recreation assessment forms. After the chart review, the therapist spends time with the patient and, if possible, with his/her significant others. It is during this time that the therapist can ask about premorbid leisure lifestyle. The information found at this time will help the therapist plan the types of activities the patient will want to participate in. This information can also be shared with the rest of the treatment team. The types of leisure activities that the patient enjoyed prior to his/her injury can help the entire team know how active the patient was, and if s/he enjoyed taking risks. We have one example where the information turned out to be very valuable:

> A patient with a head injury was being evaluated for transfer from the acute care service to the rehabilitation service. The Certified Therapeutic Recreation Specialist saw the patient for an environmental assessment and leisure education during his recuperative period. Medical management told the patient that he could return to normal activity when he left the hospital. During the therapeutic recreation evaluation, the patient informed the therapist that one of his normal activities was a weekly deep sea dive. (This is an activity which is almost never recommended for patients recuperating from a brain injury.) The medical team was informed at the rehabilitation team meeting and the return to activity order was "clarified".

One initial screening tool and one therapeutic recreation assessment tool developed by the Certified Therapeutic Recreation Specialists at Harborview Medical Center are on the following pages. The initial screening tool is used by the therapists on the rehabilitation medicine unit. The *Therapeutic Recreation Initial Screen* is used to determine if a patient is ready to received therapeutic recreation services after the initial referral is received. Most of material used in this assessment is obtained from the medical chart, consulting with other team members, and a short interview with the patient and/or family. Using his/her clinical judgment, the therapist decides if therapeutic intervention is needed and what type of intervention is indicated.

The *Therapeutic Recreation Assessment* used by Harborview Medical Center is used by the therapists who work on rehabilitation medicine team. This assessment is a report form instead of a standardized testing tool (like the Idyll Arbor Leisure Battery). The material used to complete this form comes from the medical chart, an interview with the patient and/or significant others, and input from other team members. The therapist uses his/her knowledge of the functional skills required to engage in leisure activities and to be part of one's community as s/he determines the patient's actual skill levels. The therapists translate the patient's skill level into one of the seven levels of the FIM scale (discussed in a previous chapter). This FIM Score is then placed in the appropriate boxes on the Therapeutic Recreation Assessment. In the box next to the Admit FIM Score is a second box for the therapist's prediction of which FIM level the patient will likely achieve by discharge. To be able to predict a discharge FIM score takes experience, knowledge, and solid clinical skills.

The Certified Therapeutic Recreation Specialists who work on the various psychiatric units have an assessment tool which is shared with the occupational therapists. Either the therapeutic recreation specialist or the occupational therapist complete the assessment form after a chart review and an interview with the patient and/or significant others. The therapeutic recreation specialist then takes the information from the combined assessment tool and after conferring with the patient, outlines a treatment plan. The *Therapeutic Recreation Treatment Plan for Psychiatry* is also included in this chapter.

The therapists on the psychiatric medicine units have a more consistently used set of TR goals and interventions so they have them on the form to be checked off as required. The rehab team's form leaves more room for flexibility in planning interventions. You may notice that there is no place for a patient name on some of these forms. Harborview Medical Center uses a name stamp to put the patient name in the lower left hand corner of many forms before they are placed in the patient's chart.

We use the boxes on both the Therapeutic Recreation Assessment and the Discharge Summary to indicate the date(s) and length of time that the therapist spent with the patient. This information can be used for billing purposes, for quality control, and to help determine the average amount of therapist time normally scheduled for patients with similar FIM Scores.

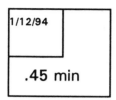

As with all of the forms in this book, the department or therapist who purchased the CIP may make copies for use with his/her patients. You may be able to use one of these forms as it is. Probably, though, you will need to create a similar form appropriate for your situation using pieces of the forms shown here. Please feel free to do so.

# Therapeutic Recreation:  Initial Screen

Key:        (+) = independent function, affirmative response, or demonstrates appropriate knowledge
                (-) = patient needs assistance, negative response, or the lack of appropriate knowledge
                (N/A) = not applicable
                (N/T) = not tested


Pt is a _____ admitted on _____ with a diagnosis
of _____.
Pt. is referred by medical staff for treatment and evaluation in the following areas:
Community Skills _____, Functional Leisure Skills _____, Participation _____,
Leisure Education/Behaviors _____, Family Education _____, Cognitive _____,
Emotional _____.
**Information obtained:** interview _____, chart review _____, family resource _____,
observation _____, other _____.


**Barriers to Leisure**     Social _____, Financial _____, Physical _____, Lifestyle _____,
          Transportation _____, Language _____, Attitudinal _____, Leisure Skills _____.


Pt. determined to be:
_____ **Appropriate for Therapeutic Recreation Assessment. Treatment will include:**
     _____ Community living skills training
     _____ Functional leisure development
     _____ Physical skills development
     _____ Cognitive skills development
     _____ Social skills development
     _____ Leisure education
     _____ Emotional/behavioral adaptation
     _____ Family education
     _____ Community resources/packet
     _____ Leisure education

_____ **Inappropriate for treatment at this time due to:**
     _____ Medical issues
     _____ Decreased tolerance to activity/endurance
     _____ Unwillingness/Non Compliance
     _____ Pt. will be monitored through weekly team rounds. Assessment process to begin
           when condition has changed enough to benefit from treatment.


**Targeted Equipment/Information:**
     _____ Bus pass
     _____ Parking Permit
     _____ Community Resource
     _____ Van Service/Taxi Scrip
     _____ Adapted Leisure Equipment
     _____ Other (please describe)


Therapist Signature _____ Date _____

# Therapeutic Recreation Assessment

Pt. is a _____ admitted on _____ with a diagnosis of _____.
Pt. is referred by medical staff for treatment and evaluation in the following areas:
      ☐ Community Skills, ☐ Functional Leisure Skills, ☐ Leisure Education/Behaviors,
      ☐ Participation, ☐ Family Education
Information obtained: ☐ interview, ☐ chart review, ☐ family resource, ☐ observation, ☐ other: _____

## Precautions for Treatment:


## Barriers to Leisure:
    ☐ Social, ☐ Financial, ☐ Physical, ☐ Lifestyle, ☐ Transportation,
    ☐ Language, ☐ Attitudinal, ☐ Leisure Skills


## Functional:
Cognitive/Affective:

### FIM Score

| Admit | Target D/C |
|-------|------------|
|       |            |


Social:



Physical:



## Leisure Education Behaviors:
Attitude/Awareness/Participation:

### FIM Score

| Admit | Target D/C |
|-------|------------|
|       |            |

**Community Skills:**
Transportation:

**FIM Score**

| Admit | Target D/C |
|-------|------------|
|       |            |

Knowledge of Community:

**Assessment:**

**Plan/Goals for Discharge:**

This treatment plan has been discussed with the patient: ☐ Yes ☐ No

**Targeted Equipment/Information Distributed:**

_____ Bus pass
_____ Parking Permit
_____ Community Resource
_____ Van Service/Taxi Script
_____ Adapted Leisure Equipment
_____ Other (please describe)

**Summary of Treatment in 15 minute units per week/month:**

| | | | | | | |
|--|--|--|--|--|--|--|
| | | | | | | |

Therapist Signature _____ Date _____

78

# Therapeutic Recreation Treatment Plan for Psychiatry

Date: _____   Diagnosis _____

Pt. is referred by medical staff for evaluation and treatment in the following areas:

**Community Skills**                                                      Goal Completed: _____
Goals:
_____ ↑ activity level by participating          **Approach:**
_____ Evaluate safety and judgment in the community          ☐ Patient will attend 30 min. walk x3
_____ Provide an appropriate outlet for energy          ☐ Bus Evaluation
_____ Engages in physical activity          Community Outings:
_____ ↑ socialization by participating in a group activity
_____ ↓ anxiety and stress through exercise

**Functional Leisure Skill Development**                          Goal Completed: _____
Goals:
_____ ↑ fine/gross motor skills through the use of task projects          **Approach:**
_____ ↑ concentration by focusing on an activity for one hour          ☐ Attend art groups, group projects,
_____ ↑ leisure skills by attending new activities                  cooking activities x3
_____ ↓ anxiety by providing appropriate outlets for expression of feelings
_____ ↑ socialization
_____ ↑ self-esteem through activities that will help pt. recognize strengths
_____ Project completion

**Leisure Education**                                                      Goal Completed: _____
Goals:
_____ ↑ leisure awareness to develop a healthy lifestyle          **Approach:**
_____ Improve or acquire social interaction skills          ☐ Attend x 2, leisure education groups
_____ Acquire knowledge of community recreation resources          ☐ which will inform pt. on appropriate
_____ ↓ substance abuse by educating pt. on drug-free activities                  community resources
          ☐ help pt. identify personal values

**Recreation Participation**                                          Goal Completed: _____
Goals:
_____ ↑ motivation and activity level through participation          **Approach:**
_____ ↑ social skills          ☐ Offer pt. a variety of rec. options
_____ ↑ self-esteem through activities that help pt. ID strengths          ☐ Allow pt. to control nature of involvement
_____ ↑ sense of autonomy by choosing his/her level of participation          ☐ Social skills training
_____ ↓ anxiety by providing an appropriate outlet for expression of feelings/energy

Information obtained by: ☐ observation  ☐ chart review  ☐ family resource  ☐ other: _____

Treatment plan discussed with patient? ☐ yes ☐ no  Date: _____

Barriers to leisure:     ☐ social          ☐ financial          ☐ physical          ☐ lifestyle
          ☐ transportation ☐ language          ☐ attitudinal          ☐ leisure skills

**Precautions:**



**Comments:**



**Treatment Plan:**



Therapist: _____   Date: _____

# Discharge Summary

A discharge summary is a report that the therapist writes when s/he will no longer be treating the patient. This report may be seen by another health care professional the same day that the report is written, or it may be reviewed by a health care professional years later. To help make the discharge summary useful and easy to understand, we recommend that:

- Whenever possible, refer to the specific instead of the general; be concrete instead of abstract.
- Take care with what you say, and how you say it. Avoid fancy or obscure words, abbreviations, or words which overstate. Avoid qualifiers such as "rather, very, little, pretty."
- When you write be clear, document sequentially; be brief but do not take short cuts and leave out key information.
- Whenever possible, write your statements in the positive, e.g., "patient was able to ambulate 45 feet between stores before needing to rest" versus "patient was not able to ambulate 45 feet between stores before needing to rest". The second sentence also leaves the reader wondering if the patient could not ambulate at all or if the atient actually went 43 feet before needing a rest – two very different cases. While being positive, do not be reluctant to provide realistic or negative findings.
- If the treatment was as a result of a referral, make sure that all issues addressed in the referral are answered in the discharge summary.
- It will not be helpful to future readers of the discharge summary if you include just raw data from your assessments. Include a concise interpretation of all data presented.
- Whenever you make a recommendation, make sure that the justification for that recommendation can be found in your discharge summary.
- Without being long winded, include an alternative recommendation or an alternative course of action, if it is appropriate for the situation.
- Make your recommendations realistic for the patient, his/her cultural, social, and economic background, and for his/her discharge destination.
- Remember that the discharge summary is just that, a summary. All of the information presented should be brought together in a way that presents the entire picture of all the pertinent information.

The discharge summary form used by the Certified Therapeutic Recreation Specialists at Harborview Medical Center was developed to help facilitate writing discharge notes. The primary areas addressed by the therapeutic recreation staff are outlined on the summary. The therapeutic recreation specialists at Harborview Medical Center provide more services then just community integration The scope of our practice is reflected on the discharge summary. Each therapist will need to modify the discharge summary to meet their own needs and scope of service.

As with our other chart notes, this summary uses the "+" and "-" method of documentation. In addition, spaces for pertinent information are placed throughout the document to help guide the therapist as s/he completes the summary.

# Therapeutic Recreation: Discharge Summary

**Key:** (+) = independent function, affirmative response, or demonstrates appropriate knowledge
(-) = patient needs assistance, negative response, or the lack of appropriate knowledge
(N/A) = not applicable
(N/T) = not tested

Patient is a _____ with a diagnosis of _____
seen on _____ to assess the following skills:

## I. Lifestyle Prior to Hospitalization:
Residence: _____
Social Support: _____
Vocation: _____
Leisure: _____
_____
Transportation: _____
**Comments:**

## II. Discharge Plans:
Residence: _____
Social Support: _____
Vocation: _____
Leisure: _____
_____
Transportation: _____
**Comments:**

## III. Barriers to Leisure:

| _____ Social | _____ Financial | _____ Physical |
| _____ Lifestyle | _____ Transportation | _____ Language |
| _____ Attitudinal | _____ Leisure Skills | _____ Other |

**Comments:**

## IV. Evaluations Completed/Level of Function:

| _____ Bus (_____) | _____ Community Skills Training (_____) |
| _____ Grocery (_____) | _____ Leisure Educ/Awareness (_____) |
| _____ Aquatics (_____) | _____ Other (_____) |

Continued on next page

## V. Community Skills:

_____ Demonstrates willingness to venture out into community
_____ Demonstrates appropriate and realistic comfort level in community
_____ Demonstrates ability to safely: maneuver w/c _____ power _____ manual
        ambulate with _____ , or ambulate independently in community over a variety of terrains
_____ Demonstrates knowledge and ability to problem solve common problems in the community
        (i.e., physical barriers, emergency situations, finding assistance when needed)
_____ Demonstrates ability to interact positively in the community
_____ Demonstrates ability to carryover clinical ADL skills in community (i.e., manage skin care,
        grooming, bowel/bladder, eating)
        **Comments:**

## VI. Leisure Functioning/Education:

_____ Demonstrates knowledge of transportation options
_____ Demonstrates ability to problem solve barriers, emergency situations and precautionary procedures
_____ Demonstrates ability to direct others in assisting with needs
_____ Family and friends demonstrate ability to safely assist patient when necessary
_____ Family and friends demonstrate ability to problem solve barriers, emergency situations,
        precautionary procedures
        **Comments:**

## VII. Equipment/Information Distributed:

_____ Bus pass                _____ Bus routes/schedules
_____ Parking permit       _____ Community recreation resources
_____ Van service/taxi script   _____ Adapted leisure equipment
_____ Other (describe)

## VIII. Recommendations:

**Summary of Treatment in 15 minute units per week/month:**

FIM Score

                                        Admit            D/C

**Therapist Signature:** _____    **Date:** _____

# 8. Community Environment

Fifteen years of experience working with individuals with brain injuries have demonstrated that we must test each patient's ability to manage the community environment. It is common to have patients who do not use common street signs for guidance or pay attention to street lights and signs. They may become confused in high stimulus situations and lack the endurance to complete an activity, or for that matter, to even find their way home. Without these modules we could not reasonably expect any patient to manage their leisure lifestyle safely and independently if it involved community participation.

There are three modules in this section:
- Environmental Safety which tests the patient's ability to move around in the community safely.
- Emergency Preparedness which asks the client to solve hypothetical emergency situations in a way that will allow him/her to get through the emergency as safely as possible.
- Basic Survival Skills which should be used when there is the possibility that the patient will find him/herself without shelter or food.

Some form of the Environmental Safety module is used with every patient. The Emergency Preparedness module is typically incorporated into all of the other modules. (When the client is on any outing, it is a good idea to ask what s/he would do if a particular emergency came up.) You should decide if the third module is appropriate for any particular patient.

**Environmental Safety**

The environmental safety module should include path finding, safety awareness, and mobility in high stimulus situations. At Harborview Medical Center this evaluation is completed by the therapeutic recreation staff on a one-on-one basis. It is a diagnostic tool used to evaluate the need for continued rehabilitation or to define the amount of supervision needed by the individual. The results are used to establish goals and objectives for future treatment if it's deemed necessary.

This module is the most commonly requested evaluation by our out-patient services, neurology and neurosurgery services and is required before we use one of our transportation modules. It is used for adults and children.

The module clearly defines a patient's ability with regard to memory (and compensating memory strategies), knowledge of community resources, and need for supervision. It can assist the team in determining if a patient needs to continue his/her inpatient stay for further training in safety issues or if the patient can be safely transferred to outpatient status.

Because the advisability of releasing the patient back into the community is the question we are trying to answer, we feel that these evaluations should be completed in a community setting, rather than a clinical setting. The additional variables encountered in the community are a significant factor which may strongly influence (both positively and negatively) the patient's ability to transfer skills from the clinical setting to the community. For example, we complete an entire trip on the bus, rather than simply evaluating the ability to get on and off the bus.

When completing the Environmental Awareness evaluation we suggest using the same route for all patients with a fixed script for the therapist and patient to follow. The route should include, but not be limited to, marked and unmarked cross walks, a high stimulus environment, use of street signs, directional sense (North, South, East, West), and map reading. This can be achieved by using a standardized set of one to five directions that can be given in either written or verbal form depending on the patient diagnosis. Knowledge of patient's ability to process information is imperative in order to get a fair picture of capabilities (i.e. patients with aphasia may require gestures with verbal cues). Members of the speech therapy team will be able to tell you the best way to provide the directions.

To help standardize their Community Environmental Awareness evaluation, the therapeutic recreation specialists' wrote a specific five step set of instructions for the environmental safety module. These are handed to the patient after s/he and the therapist have stepped outside the door of the hospital building and are on the sidewalk. Since Harborview Medical Center has more than one building, the instructions clearly indicate which door the patient is to start from.

> When directed by the therapist with you, follow the written directions below.
>
> 1. From the Emergency entrance of the hospital, go North on 9th, crossing Jefferson and James. Then stop.
>
> 2. On the corner of James and 9th, facing East, cross the street and turn left. Stop.
>
> 3. Proceed three blocks, turn right, and walk two blocks. Stop
>
> 4. Cross Boren, turn right, and proceed to James. Stop
>
> 5. Cross Boren again, and proceed back to the hospital.

The standardized instructions usually work but for some patients it will not provide an accurate assessment of the patient's abilities. For example...

> *The CTRS had a young male patient with a brain injury from a self inflicted gun shot wound to the head during a gang initiation rite. This patient had noted right upper extremity weakness and some impaired auditory processing ability. During the environmental evaluation the patient did poorly, being so distracted by cars, people, traffic, etc. that he failed miserably. During the post outing discussion with the therapist, the patient said he was scared about being "out of territory". The therapist scheduled a second environmental evaluation for the patient, this time in his own gang territory. The patient was able to stay on task, follow directions, problem solve bus routes, and arrive at the desired location. One of the therapist's conclusion was that the patient was safe and independent on his home turf. (One question that the therapist needs to consider in this situation: Should the therapist allow the patient to wear his gangs "colors" while out on the evaluation? Our answer is no. Any showing any colors puts the patient and therapist more at risk.)*

and

> *The therapeutic recreation department was asked to complete an environmental assessment on an elderly male who was to be discharged soon. The patient failed miserably on the environmental assessment and the discharge orders were changed to placement in a nursing home. Using her clinical judgment, the therapist took the patient out on a second environmental assessment in his home environment. Within the 12 blocks surrounding his apartment, he was successful in pathfinding: to his home, the store, the senior center, and a restaurant where he met with others every day for socialization. In each store, the owners or managers greeted him by name and expressed concern about his whereabouts. He was introduced to the senior center for exercise, and they agreed to monitor his health and notify Harborview Medical Center about concerns. The therapist made an argument for home discharge with monitoring which was accepted by the rest of the therapy team.*

Because of our professional experience, we feel capable of making informed decisions about a patient's functional skills in the community. Often, even though pathfinding is not a problem, a patient may not seem able to cross streets safely. Sometimes the patient lacks the cognitive ability to understand the dangers because of his/her injury. Sometimes the patient is crossing the street the same way they always crossed the street (pre-morbid bad habits). You must do your best to figure out which type of problem you are facing, because your job is to find the intervention which will teach the patient to cross streets safely.

Sometimes using the formal mode for the Environmental Awareness evaluation creates stress that alters the patient's judgment and performance. If you think that the patient would do better in an informal trial and the treatment plan allows it, you can conduct this module again informally.

Most of the items you will be looking for are relatively obvious. The most significant behavior that is not as obvious is the clothing that the patient chooses for the outing. If the patient can't figure out what clothes to wear, it is impossible for him/her to be safe on his/her own in the community.

You must be sure to inform other members of your staff that you are conducting a evaluation that includes clothing. The staff must not help the patient get dressed so you can assess how well your patient understands dressing appropriately for the weather and activity. If you or any other member of the staff needs to help the patient choose the proper clothes, be sure to note that deficit on the field trial score sheet and in the summary on the post-test form.

In addition to the pre-test and trial forms, Harborview Medical Center has developed two styles of chart notes to go with the Environmental Awareness module. They can be found after the field trial score sheet. The first form (titled Therapeutic Recreation: Community Integration Evaluation, Assessment of Environmental Awareness Skills - Rehabilitation) is the one used by the rehab unit. The second form (titled Therapeutic Recreation: Community Integration Evaluation, Assessment of Environmental Awareness Skills - Psychiatry) is used by Psych. You should use the one that fits the reporting needs of the patient or a combination that meets the needs of your patients.

The other chart note (titled Therapeutic Recreation: Community Integration Evaluation, Assessment of Community Skills) is used to describe the patient's leisure attributes. If you were able to conduct an informal discussion of leisure opportunities and barriers while you were on the outing, you can use this chart note to describe the patient's skills in the community.

**Emergency Preparedness**

The purpose of this module is to determine how ready the patient is to deal with the inevitable unexpected event. This module, different from all of the other modules in the CIP, incorporates all potential emergency situations to be considered. Many are addressed in the modules themselves.

There are four primary skill and knowledge areas that this module addresses:

1. specific awareness of personal needs/safety,
2. specific awareness of options when faced with money shortages,
3. specific awareness of transportation and mobility options in emergency situations, and
4. specific awareness of how to handle the breakdown/failure of adaptive equipment.

Just as every patient needs to demonstrate the skills necessary to safely complete day to day tasks in the community, the patient also needs to demonstrate what s/he would do in unusual, emergency situations. It is just as important for the patient to demonstrate the ability to function independently in emergency situations as it is to function day to day situations. Adaptive strategies and equipment need to be developed to compensate for deficits in this area.

One real-life situation was ...

> *A male friend of both authors was attending a wedding and reception which two of the CTRSs from Harborview were also attending. The friend was well known to the two therapists because of his weekly participation in their outpatient swim program and because they often marveled at the changes he has made to his electric wheelchair to enhance his positioning and the speed it travels. However, the modifications were unique to his chair. At the end of the reception the gentleman, traveling by bus, left to catch his ride home. The two therapists left with their families about half an hour later. While driving out they found their friend stuck in his electric wheelchair on a steep incline and in the middle of the road. Realizing the he had blown a fuse, one husband was sent for a replacement, and the remaining three pushed their friend back into the building, and dismantled the wheelchair with the friend's verbal guidance and makeshift tools. This proved to be no slight task, since the fuse was now located on the bottom of the wheelchair, under the battery and drive mechanism. The fuse was replaced and the friend was on his way. (After this experience the friend moved his fuse box to an accessible location.)*
>
> *Learning opportunity: Be sure that patients understand the mechanics of their wheelchairs even though physical limitations may not allow them to participate and or view the upkeep and maintenance.*

The Environmental Preparedness Module has two forms - the pre-test/post-test form and the field trial form. In most cases the therapist tests the patient's skills and knowledge concerning emergency situations while running another module. The therapist will usually record all of the pertinent information from the Emergency Preparedness Module on the form for the other module being run. However, if the patient has had significant difficulty being independent in emergency situations, we recommend that the therapist document the patient's specific deficits on the Emergency Preparedness Form(s).

The emergency statements and questions are examples that have been developed for use by therapists during the field trial. The patient with a spinal cord injury must be aware of special conditions and limitations that affect his/her ability to respond in emergency situations. One way of developing this awareness is to catch the patient off guard during a field trial. Deliver the emergency question, and consider the speed, effectiveness, possibility of success, awareness of consequences, etc. as guidelines for evaluating the patient's awareness level.

## Basic Survival Skills

The purpose of this module is to ensure that the patient has the knowledge and skills needed to survive "on the street." The basic knowledge and skill areas that this module addresses:

1. shelter,
2. food,
3. architectural barriers,
4. transportation options, and
5. other basic needs.

Many of the patients seen by the therapeutic recreation specialist will experience situations which increase a person's chances of becoming homeless.[8] Some of the highest risk situations are

- unemployment
- single female with two or more children
- history of residential instability
- no supportive relationships
- no discernible economic resources
- limited social ties/social skills
- serious and chronic mental illness
- alcohol/drug abuse
- criminal involvement
- physical disability

The Seattle Times carried the following statistics in a story from the Associated Press:

**Facts on 46 Million**[9]

Some facts from the Census Bureau about the 46 million Americans aged 15 and older with disabilities:

- Use wheelchairs: 1.5 million
- Use cane, crutches, or walker: 4 million
- Have difficulty reading a newspaper with glasses: 9.7 million
- Can't see the letters at all: 1.6 million
- Find it hard to hear a normal conversation: 10.9 million
- Can't hear a normal conversation at all: 924,000
- Have difficulty making speech understood: 2.3 million
- Can't speak understandably at all: 237,000
- Can't lift 10 pounds: 7.7 million
- Can't climb stairs without resting: 9.1 million
- Can't walk three city blocks: 9 million

---

[8]Schutt, R.K., & Garrett, G.R.. (1992) Responding to the Homeless: Policy and Practice. New York, Plenum Press. This book is a good resource for therapists who find themselves working with patients who have the potential to become homeless. It presents practical advice on how to provide services to individuals at risk, as well as barriers and problems they typically experience.

[9]Bovee, T. (1994, January 28). Many disabled who want to work can't afford to. **Associated Press Article in the Seattle Times** pp. A3

# Module 1A Environmental Safety

☐ pre-test    ☐ post-test

**A. Pre-arrangements**
1. Do you know how to get to your destination?
2. Do you have a map?
3. If someone has given you directions, how will you remember them?
4. Are you carrying enough money to call for assistance?
5. Do you have adequate clothes to be prepared for the weather?
6. Have you allowed enough time to meet appointments or obligations?

**B. Transportation**
1. How will you reach your destination?
2. Have you reviewed the transportation planning guide?
3. Do you know the cost of public transportation?

**C. Accessibility**
1. Can you negotiate curbs, curb cuts, ramps, and doorways?
2. Are the bathrooms accessible?
3. Who will provide assistance for transfers, toileting, or dressing?
4. Can you direct others to safely assist you?
5. How long can you walk, or sit in your wheelchair without a rest? If you tire out, where will you rest?
6. Are you fast enough to cross a street before the light changes?
7. Can you see the street signs, lights, stop signs, curb cuts?
8. Can you read a map?
9. If you can not locate your destination, what will you do?
10. If you need to ask for directions, how will you remember them?

**D. Emergency/Safety**
1. What will you do if you get tired, or begin to feel ill?
2. Will the extreme heat or cold affect you?
3. If someone confronts you with questions or asks for money, what will you do?
4. If your wheelchair or equipment breaks down, what will you do?
5. Will you need to bring any medications so that you don't miss your next dose?
6. Do you recognize the symptoms of concern for your diagnosis, i.e., dysreflexia, diabetes, seizures?

**E. Equipment**
1. What equipment will you need to meet your medical needs?
2. What equipment will you need to help you carry items you have purchased or received?
3. Are you carrying picture identification? Money?
4. Do you carry information on special medical conditions i.e., autonomic dysreflexia?

Flesch Grade Level: 7.8

Score: _____ out of _____ appropriate questions

Patient: _____ Therapist: _____ Date: _____

# Community Integration - Environmental Safety
### Field Trial Score Sheet

| A. Pre arrangements | score | cues | unable | N/A |
|---|---|---|---|---|
| Upon being asked to plan a trip, the patient demonstrated the ability to plan ahead for the trip by: | | | | |
| 1. identifying its location (address and route) | | | | |
| 2. being able to recount directions | | | | |
| 3. selecting appropriate clothing | | | | |
| 4. considering financial needs of the trip | | | | |
| 5. allocating adequate time | | | | |
| **B. Transportation** | | | | |
| Upon learning the address and location, the patient demonstrated the ability to arrange transportation by: | | | | |
| 1. considering all transportation alternatives and choosing one | | | | |
| 2. obtaining fare and schedule information, if needed | | | | |
| 3. making a reservation, if needed | | | | |
| 4. considering parking arrangements, if needed | | | | |
| 5. knowing emergency transportation options | | | | |
| **C. Accessibility** | | | | |
| The patient compensated for accessibility barriers by: | | | | |
| 1. negotiating architectural barriers | | | | |
| 2. managing personal care needs | | | | |
| 3. utilizing visual cues (street signs, maps, etc.) | | | | |
| 4. demonstrating adequate speed for carrying out required activities | | | | |
| 5. interacting appropriately with others to solve problems | | | | |
| **D. Emergency/Safety** | | | | |
| When presented with a hypothetical emergency situation, the patient demonstrated the ability to respond appropriately by: | | | | |
| 1. recognizing personal needs | | | | |
| 2. showing awareness of and consideration for the options available | | | | |
| 3. choosing the safest and most reasonable option with regard to the situation at hand | | | | |
| **E. Equipment** | | | | |
| The patient demonstrated the ability to anticipate the types of equipment and supplies that s/he needed by: | | | | |
| 1. having the necessary equipment throughout the trip | | | | |
| 2. having the necessary medical supplies throughout the trip | | | | |

**Summary**

Score: _____ out of _____ appropriate questions

Patient: _____ Therapist: _____ Date: _____

# Therapeutic Recreation: Community Integration Evaluation

**Assessment of Environmental Awareness Skills - Rehabilitation**

Key:    (+) = independent function, affirmative response, or demonstrates appropriate knowledge
        (-) = patient needs assistance, negative response, or the lack of appropriate knowledge
        (N/A) = not applicable
        (N/T) = not tested

Patient is a _____ with a diagnosis of _____
seen on _____ to assess the following skills:

## I. Preplan Phase

### A. Demonstrates orientation, knowledge, or memory of:

_____ purpose of evaluation (awareness)
_____ date and time of evaluation (orientation)
_____ appropriate dress and grooming needed for weather (anticipation)

**Comments:**

## II. Future Leisure Phase:

_____ Demonstrates knowledge of accessible recreation/leisure sites or
facilities appropriate to discharge site

**Comments:**

## III. Problem Solving Phase:

_____ Demonstrates ability to successfully anticipate problems/solutions
related to health issues
_____ Demonstrates ability to anticipate and solve potential problems
related to weather
_____ Demonstrates the ability to problem solve equipment breakdown issues
_____ Demonstrates the ability to anticipate transportation/mobility problems
_____ Demonstrates an appropriate awareness of personal safety and
awareness in the community

**Comments:**

## IV. Management Phase

### A. Functional Behaviors: Demonstrates:

_____ ability to negotiate architectural barriers; curb, curb cuts, ramps, and
doorways (mobility/wheelchair skills)
_____ ability to tolerate activity
_____ speed adequate to safely cross street, monitor traffic
_____ ability to scan or locate road signs, curb cuts, etc.

**Comments:**

**B. Cognitive Behaviors: Demonstrates ability to:**
_____ pathfind selected spots
_____ remain task oriented
_____ read maps, follow verbal directions
_____ remember destination, medical needs, information
_____ utilize directional sense
_____ follow verbal directions
_____ solve emergency contingencies if lost
**Comments:**

**C. Social Behaviors: Demonstrates:**
_____ consistently positive social interactions
_____ appropriate and realistic comfort level in community setting
_____ appropriate response to authority or conflict
**Comments:**

**Assessment:**

**Recommendations:**

**Therapist:** _____ **Date:** _____ **Time Spent:** _____

# Recreation Therapy: Community Integration Evaluation
## Assessment of Environmental Awareness Skills - Psychiatry

**Key:**        (+) = independent function, affirmative response, or demonstrates appropriate knowledge
(-) = patient needs assistance, negative response, or the lack of appropriate knowledge
(N/A) = not applicable
(N/T) = not tested

Patient is a _____ with a diagnosis of _____
seen on _____ to assess the following skills:

## I. Pre-plan phase
### A. Demonstrates orientation/knowledge or memory of:
_____ purpose of evaluation
_____ date and time of evaluation
_____ appropriate dress and grooming needed for weather
**Comments**

## II. Management Phase
### A. Functional Behaviors: Demonstrates:
_____ ability to stay with group, adapting pace
_____ ability to tolerate activity, stimulation of environment
_____ speed adequate to safely cross street, monitor traffic
_____ ability to scan or locate road signs, traffic, lights
_____ demonstrates coordination, balance and physical stamina
**Comments**

### B. Cognitive Behaviors: Demonstrates ability to:
_____ remain oriented to surroundings
_____ monitor traffic, use pedestrian signs (mobility)
_____ demonstrate good judgment concerning personal safety
_____ process information
_____ tolerate activity
**Comments:**

**C. Social Behaviors: Demonstrates:**
_____ appropriate social interactions
_____ appropriate and realistic comfort level in community setting
_____ appropriate response to authority or rules and limits on walk
_____ ability to initiate interactions
_____ ability to respond to interactions
_____ communicates appropriately
**Comments:**

**D. Affective Behaviors: Demonstrates:**
_____ change in affect: positive, negative, no change
_____ changes as demonstrated by:
**Comments:**

**Assessment:**

**Recommendations:**

**Therapist** _____ **Date** _____ **Time Spent** _____

# Therapeutic Recreation: Community Integration Evaluation

## Assessment of Community Skills

Key:    (+) = independent function, affirmative response, or demonstrates appropriate knowledge
        (-) = patient needs assistance, negative response, or the lack of appropriate knowledge
        (N/A) = not applicable
        (N/T) = not tested

Patient is a _____ with a diagnosis of _____
seen on _____ to assess the following skills:

## I. Pre-Plan Phase

### A. Demonstrates orientation, knowledge, or memory of:
_____ date and time of evaluation
_____ appropriate dress and grooming needed for weather
_____ medical necessities (i.e., pressure releases, medications, splints/braces)
**Comments:**

## II. Community Skills

### A. Demonstrates ability to maneuver: w/c _____ power _____ manual, ambulate with _____
_____ on level surfaces (i.e., side walks)
_____ rough terrain (bumps, slanted or uneven pathways, grass, gravel)
_____ curb cuts, ramps, inclines
_____ up/down 2,4,6 inch curb (circle measurement)
_____ adequate speed to cross streets safely
**Comments:**

### B. Safety/Judgment: Demonstrates knowledge/ability to:
_____ problem solve emergency situations
_____ problem solve/adapt to barriers in community
_____ locate accessible/appropriate pathways (i.e., curb cuts, crosswalks)
_____ initiate assistance when needed
_____ direct family or staff assisting with patient needs
**Comments:**

### C. Social Behaviors: Demonstrates:
_____ willingness to venture into community
_____ appropriate and realistic comfort level in community
_____ positive social interactions
_____ appropriate response to authority or conflict
**Comments:**

**D. Clinical ADL carryover in community: Demonstrates ability to:**
_____ eat independently
_____ manage skin care
_____ consider medical needs (i.e., pressure releases, bowel/bladder)
**Comments:**

**III. Leisure Functioning/Education:**
    **A. Demonstrates ability to:**
_____ identify leisure activities in community
_____ knowledge of transportation
_____ knowledge of accessibility issues/barriers
**Comments:**

    **B. Family/Friend demonstrates ability to:**
_____ safely assist patient when necessary
_____ know about problem solving barriers, emergency/precautionary
        procedures
**Comments:**

**Assessment:**

**Recommendations/Plan:**

Therapist: _____ Date: _____ Time Spent: _____

# Module 1B: Emergency Preparedness

☐ pre-test    ☐ post-test

The therapist may set up a mock situation or integrate this module with any of the other modules.

## A. Guidelines for Evaluating Emergency Preparedness

1. Is the patient unwilling or unable to recognize this as an emergency?
2. Does the patient respond immediately, or does the patient hesitate?
3. Is the patient aware of alternative courses of action?
4. Is the patient able to produce a reasonable solution?
5. Does the patient appear confident with his/her response?
6. Does the patient seem unsure about his/her response?

## B. Statements and Questions

These statements are presented as samples only. Therapists must use their own judgment as to what sort of emergency statement and question will be most appropriate for the individual patient. To help ensure that a variety of situations or problems are addressed, the situations are divided into categories. The therapist is not required to go over all categories with the patient.

### Personal Safety and Health Emergencies

1. You have spasmed out of your chair, and some people have offered to help you get back into it. Give a detailed description of how you will tell them to assist you.
2. You are in a theater, and your chair has been stored away from you. Suddenly, the guests in the theater are asked to quickly exit the theater. What do you do? What pre-arrangements might have you made?
3. You get to your selected activity only to find that the activity is canceled or the store is closed. What do you do?
4. The weather changes suddenly and now you find yourself in a downpour with no umbrella or coat. You are very wet. What do you do?

### Money Emergencies

1. You have gone to the bank, and placed the money in your backpack. Someone walks up behind you, pulls that backpack off your chair, and runs. What are your options?
2. You get to the theater only to find that you left your wallet back home. What do you do?

### Transportation Emergencies

1. You are driving and run out of gas. What do you plan to do?
2. Your attendant/driver is intoxicated at a party, and it is obvious that he/she will be unable to drive you home. What are your alternatives?

### Mobility and Equipment Emergencies

1. You are going up a sidewalk on a hill when the fuse on your electric wheelchair blows. What do you do?
2. You run over broken glass in the parking lot on the way into the store and, as a result, get a flat tire. What do you do?
3. You have been looking for place you are going to for a long time and you now realize that you are completely lost. What do you do?

Flesch Grade Level: 7.3

Score: _____ out of _____ applicable questions

Patient: _____ Therapist: _____ Date: _____

# Community Integration - Emergency Preparedness
## Field Trial Score Sheet

| A. General Preparedness | score | cues | unable | N/A |
|---|---|---|---|---|
| When the need arose, the patient demonstrated the ability to be prepared for emergency situations by: | | | | |
| 1. identifying that a problem/emergency existed | | | | |
| 2. responding in a timely manner with little hesitation | | | | |
| 3. producing reasonable options for courses of action | | | | |
| 4. having an awareness of the consequences of his/her choice | | | | |
| 5. knowing the amount of assistance s/he would require | | | | |
| **B. Personal Safety and Health Emergencies** | | | | |
| When confronted with a problem related to personal safety or health emergency, the patient demonstrated the ability to handle the problem by: | | | | |
| 1. explaining his/her needs to others who were needed to assist | | | | |
| 2. anticipating or problem solving emergencies related to the emergency exit | | | | |
| 3. being flexible in planning and in actions | | | | |
| 4. anticipating climatic conditions and being prepared for changes | | | | |
| **C. Money Emergencies** | | | | |
| When confronted with a problem related to money, the patient demonstrated preparation by: | | | | |
| 1. using safe methods of carrying money | | | | |
| 2. being aware of potential robbery/mugging situations | | | | |
| 3. problem solving when a shortage of money arose | | | | |
| **D. Transportation Emergencies** | | | | |
| When confronted with a problem related to transportation, the patient demonstrated the ability to handle the situation by: | | | | |
| 1. knowing emergency transportation options | | | | |
| 2. directing others to assist as needed | | | | |
| **E. Mobility and Equipment Emergencies** | | | | |
| When confronted with a problem related to mobility or equipment, the patient demonstrated the ability to handle the situation by: | | | | |
| 1. trouble shooting problems related to his/her adaptive and mobility equipment | | | | |
| 2. instructing others how to assist in the repair, modification, or stowing away of his/her equipment | | | | |
| 3. selecting alternative ways to function without the equipment | | | | |

**Summary:**




Score: _____ out of _____ appropriate questions.

Patient: _____ Therapist: _____ Date: _____

97

# Module 1C  Basic Survival Skills

☐ pre-test    ☐ post-test

You find that you do not have enough money to pay the rent at your rooming house and your landlord has locked you out.

**A. Pre-arrangements**
1. Do you know how to find a local shelter? If the shelters are full, what will you do?
2. If someone has given you directions, how will you remember them?
3. Do you know where to go to get help?
4. Do you have adequate clothing to be prepared for all weather?

**B. Transportation**
1. How will you reach your destination?
2. Do you know the cost of public transportation?
3. Do you know of any discounts you are eligible for as far as public transportation goes? Bus? Taxi?

**C. Accessibility**
1. Can you negotiate curbs, curb cuts, doorways?
2. Do you know which emergency shelters are wheelchair accessible?
3. Are there personnel to assist you with transfers, toileting, or dressing?
4. How long can you walk, or sit in your wheelchair without a rest? If you tire, where can you rest?
5. Are you fast enough to cross the street before the light changes?
6. Do you know where the public accessible bathrooms are?

**D. Survival Skills and Community Resources**
1. Do you know where the food banks are located? Are they accessible?
2. If you need medical assistance and/or supplies, do you know where the free clinic is?
3. Are you aware of places to wash your clothes, or obtain dry and/or additional clothes?
4. What services are available to obtain messages? Mail? Job referral services? Storage of additional medical equipment?
5. If you receive government checks, do you know where to cash them?
6. Do you know where the local AA, NA, CA meetings are held? Is the building accessible?
7. If you are on a drug maintenance program, is the building accessible? Do you know where the clean needle exchange is?

**E. Emergency Safety**
1. Will the extreme cold or heat affect you?
2. If someone attempts to rob you, what will you do?
3. If your wheelchair or equipment breaks down, what will you do?
4. Where will you keep your medications? How will you know what time to take them?
5. What effect does alcohol have on you with your medications?

**F. Equipment**
1. What equipment will you need to meet your medical needs?
2. What equipment will you need to carry items?
3. Do you have a picture identification?
4. Do you know where to obtain an identification?
5. Do you recognize the symptoms of concern for your diagnosis, i.e., dysreflexia, diabetes, seizures?
6. Do you have a safe place to keep your money that is easy for you to reach?

Flesch Grade Level: 7.3

Score: _____ out of _____ applicable questions

Patient: _____   Therapist: _____   Date: _____

# Community Integration - Basic Survival Skills
## Field Trial Score Sheet

| A. Pre arrangements | score | cues | unable | N/A |
|---|---|---|---|---|
| The patient demonstrated the ability to be prepared for homelessness by: | | | | |
| 1. being able to recount directions | | | | |
| 2. being able to identify and locate shelter(s) | | | | |
| 3. being able to identify and locate clothing needed | | | | |
| 4. allowing adequate time | | | | |
| **B. Transportation** | | | | |
| Upon learning the address and location, the patient demonstrated the ability to arrange transportation by: | | | | |
| 1. considering all transportation alternatives and choosing one | | | | |
| 2. obtaining fare and schedule information, if needed | | | | |
| 3. making a reservation, if needed | | | | |
| 4. knowing emergency transportation options | | | | |
| **C. Accessibility** | | | | |
| The patient compensated for architectural barriers by: | | | | |
| 1. negotiating architectural barriers | | | | |
| 2. managing personal care needs | | | | |
| 3. utilizing visual cues (street signs, maps, etc.) | | | | |
| 4. demonstrating adequate speed for carrying out required activities | | | | |
| 5. interacting appropriately with others to solve problems | | | | |
| **D. Survival Skills and Community Resources** | | | | |
| The patient was able to demonstrate the skills and knowledge required to survive while homeless by: | | | | |
| 1. being able to identify and find the location of foodbank(s) | | | | |
| 2. being able to identify and find the location of health care clinic(s) | | | | |
| 3. being able to identify and find the location of place(s) to wash shelf and clothing | | | | |
| 4. being able to identify and find the location of place(s) to leave and receive messages | | | | |
| 5. being able to identify and find the location of place(s) to receive and to cash checks | | | | |
| 6. being able to identify and find the location of support group meeting(s) | | | | |
| **E. Emergency/Safety** | | | | |
| When presented with a hypothetical emergency situation, the patient demonstrated the ability to respond appropriately by: | | | | |
| 1. recognizing personal needs | | | | |
| 2. showing awareness of and consideration for the options available | | | | |
| 3. choosing the safest and most reasonable option with regard to the situation at hand | | | | |
| **F. Equipment** | | | | |
| The patient demonstrated the ability to anticipate the types of equipment and supplies that s/he needed by: | | | | |
| 1. having the necessary equipment available | | | | |
| 2. having the necessary medical supplies available | | | | |

**Summary**

Score: _____ out of _____ appropriate questions

Patient: _____ Therapist: _____ Date: _____

# 9. Cultural Activities

Many therapists utilize community group outings as opportunities for learning or reinforcing skills learned in the clinical setting. The cultural activity modules provide a strong first introduction to life after hospitalization for the following reasons:

- The outings can easily absorb family members, providing a forum for teaching in a relaxed atmosphere,

- The outings can be low stimulus depending on the diagnosis of the patient,

- The outings are usually successful (although as any Certified Therapeutic Recreation Specialist can tell you, despite the best efforts to plan, something always goes wrong), and

- Evaluations allow the patient to demonstrate independence either through personal function or by directing others to assist him/her

The therapist may want to include a site with some barriers. We use restaurants and theaters that have architectural barriers: inconvenient bathrooms, small steps or sharp corners, problematical or inaccessible ticket counters. By using these semi-accessible buildings, we are able to introduce the need to problem solve. The patient has the benefit of having the therapist who is experienced in solving these problems along with him/her. Appropriate role-modeling along with a few well-timed cues, helps make a potential disaster into a positive learning experience.

One obstacle to accessibility that we have found in Seattle (and probably everywhere else as well) is the public's lack of knowledge of what "accessible" means. More than once both the therapist and patient used the phone to be sure that a building was accessible, to find, in reality, that the building staff did not know what accessible meant. Despite the best efforts of the Americans with Disabilities Act, architectural accessibility and functional accessibility can be different. For example ...

> *A large group of young men, all of whom were in halo vests, were desperate to see the new movie with its unique sound system. Patient planning included talking to the manager about wheelchair access. The patients were assured that the theater was wheelchair accessible. The group arrived at the theater, unloaded from the van, and purchased their tickets. Where is the access? "Right here." says the manager as he pointed to two large male attendants, "These guys just lift the wheelchairs up the eight stairs into the wheelchair section of the theater."*

*The staff at Children's Hospital (which is part of the University of Washington) also had memorable experiences at the same theater. The therapist arrived at the theater with two teenagers in wheelchairs and two on gurneys. One of the teens in a wheelchair was a patient not on the rehab unit but on the adolescent medicine unit. The medical resident pleaded, begged, bribed the therapist into taking this young man along on the outing. This patient had been admitted two months prior, secondary to attempted suicide. He was so excited about leaving the hospital for the first time in two months that he gulped down his meal so that he would be ready to go. That same meal was deposited in the form of vomit all over the uniform of the usher as he was carrying the patient and wheelchair up the eight steps. A little while later, undaunted and now cleaned up, the usher approached the therapist to say "You get paid to go to the movies and do this, cool!". It takes all kinds.*

The selection of at least two of these cultural activities also provides an opportunity to reinforce healthy leisure patterns. The development and maintenance of a positive attitude toward leisure requires three elements: 1. cognitive attitude, 2. affective attitude, and 3. behavioral attitude.

Dr. Ragheb and Dr. Beard have done extensive research into the attitudinal components of leisure enjoyment. They have further defined leisure attitude as:[10]

The *cognitive* component of leisure attitude consists of the following areas:
1.　general knowledge and beliefs about leisure,
2.　beliefs about leisure's relation to other concepts such as health, happiness, and work, and
3.　beliefs about the qualities, virtues, characteristics, and benefits of leisure to individuals such as: developing friendship, renewing energy, helping one to relax, meeting needs, and self improvement.

The *affective* component of leisure attitude consists of the following areas:
1.　the individual's perception of his/her leisure experiences and activities,
2.　the individual's perceived degree of satisfaction of those experiences and activities, and
3.　the individual's immediate and direct feelings toward leisure experiences and activities.
The affective component of leisure generally reflects the individual's like or dislike of leisure activities.

The *behavioral* component of leisure attitude is based on the individual's verbalized behavior intentions toward leisure choices and activities and on self reports of current and past participation.

---

[10]Ragheb and Beard have developed a short testing tool called the Leisure Attitude Measurement which measures the degree to which the individual has a positive attitude/experience in each of the three areas related to leisure. This assessment is available through Idyll Arbor, Inc.

# Module 2A  Theater

☐ pre-test  ☐ post-test

Your favorite musical has come to town. You need to consider these things prior to your departure.

## A. Pre-arrangements
1. How can you learn about scheduled performances and reservations?
2. Will you need to make arrangements for special wheelchair seating?
3. How would you do this?
4. Will you need to pick up tickets in advance?
5. How will you pay for your tickets?
6. Does the theater have equipment to help you hear? (Hearing impaired)
7. Will you need appropriate dress for this event?

## B. Transportation
1. How will you plan to get to and from the theater?
2. Will you need to allow extra time?
3. Is there special parking available?
4. Do you have a disabled parking permit?
5. If the program gets out late at night, will you still be able to get back?

## C. Accessibility
1. Is the theater accessible?
2. Will you need to transfer to a regular seat?
3. If so, where will your wheelchair be placed?
4. How will you get from one floor to another?
5. How will you get through turnstile entrances?
6. How can you determine if the bathrooms are accessible?
7. Does the theater make special accommodations for those with hearing impairments?

## D. Emergency/Safety
1. If you are seated in a theater seat, and your chair is moved away, will you be able to get out quickly in an emergency?
2. Do you recognize the symptoms of concern for your diagnosis?
3. Do you have all necessary supplies to deal with those symptoms?
4. How would you explain to someone the type of help that you need?
5. Do you carry a medical identification card?
6. Will you need to bring any medications so that you don't miss your next dose?
7. Are the bathrooms accessible?
8. How will you communicate with your attendant/friend? (If you have a voice generating communication system or a picture board?)

## E. Equipment
1. What medical equipment will you require for the trip?

Flesch Grade Level: 8.6

Score: _____ out of _____ applicable questions

Patient: _____  Therapist: _____  Date: _____

# Community Integration - Theater
### Field Trial Score Sheet

| | score | cues | unable | N/A |
|---|---|---|---|---|
| **A. Pre arrangements** | | | | |
| Upon being asked to plan a trip to the theater, the patient demonstrated the ability to plan ahead for the trip by: | | | | |
| 1.  obtaining schedules/reservations (if needed) | | | | |
| 2.  identifying the location of the theater | | | | |
| 3.  dressing appropriately for the event and weather | | | | |
| 4.  considering budget limitations for tickets, transportation, food, etc. | | | | |
| 5.  allocating adequate time | | | | |
| 6.  calling to confirm accessibility | | | | |
| **B. Transportation** | | | | |
| Upon learning the address and location of the theater, the patient demonstrated the ability to arrange transportation by: | | | | |
| 1.  considering all transportation alternatives and choosing one | | | | |
| 2.  obtaining fare and schedule information, if needed | | | | |
| 3.  making a reservation, if needed | | | | |
| 4.  considering parking arrangements, if needed | | | | |
| 5.  knowing emergency transportation options | | | | |
| **C. Accessibility** | | | | |
| The patient compensated for barriers to accessibility by: | | | | |
| 1.  managing street barriers (curbs, crosswalks, rough sidewalks, and crowds) | | | | |
| 2.  managing architectural barriers (doors, stairs, turnstiles, escalators, elevators) | | | | |
| 3.  managing the public restrooms and food services | | | | |
| 4.  directing others to assist as appropriate and needed | | | | |
| **D. Emergency/Safety** | | | | |
| When presented with a hypothetical emergency situation, the patient demonstrated the ability to respond appropriately by: | | | | |
| 1.  showing awareness of and consideration for the options available | | | | |
| 2.  choosing the safest and most reasonable option with regard to the situation at hand | | | | |
| **E. Equipment** | | | | |
| The patient demonstrated the ability to anticipate the types of equipment and supplies that s/he needed by: | | | | |
| 1.  having the necessary equipment throughout the trip | | | | |
| 2.  having the necessary medical supplies throughout the trip | | | | |

**Summary:**




Score: _____ out of _____ appropriate questions.

Patient: _____ Therapist: _____ Date: _____

# Module 2B  Restaurant

You have been invited out to dinner. You should consider the following to assure the success of your evening.

## A. Pre-arrangements
1. Will you need to make reservations?
2. Do you need to tell the restaurant of your special needs?
3. Do you know the restaurant location?
4. Will you be drinking alcoholic beverages? Will you need identification?
5. How much money will you needs?

## B. Transportation
1. How will you get to and from the restaurant?
2. Where will you park?
3. If you travel with friends, is their vehicle eligible to park in the disabled parking?

## C. Accessibility
1. Is the restaurant accessible?
2. How can you find out?
3. Does space in the restaurant require that you be able to transfer?
4. Where will you sit? Are there booths?
5. If you transfer, where will you put your wheelchair?
6. Are the tables high enough for you to get your chair close enough to eat? If not, do you have a lap tray, or could you use one of the restaurant trays?
7. Are the bathrooms in the restaurant accessible?

## D. Ordering
1. How will you take care of special dietary requests?
2. If you must serve yourself, how will you carry your food?
3. Will you drink alcohol with your meal?
4. If so, what is a safe consumption level for you?
5. If you are dining alone, would the kitchen cut your meal for you?

## E. Emergency/Safety
1. What will you do if the fire alarm suddenly rings?
2. Are the bathrooms accessible?
3. Do you know how to signal if you are choking?
4. Would you be able to assist someone else if they are choking? How?
5. How would you explain to someone the type of help that you need?
6. Do you have a medical identification card on you in case you are not able to give the information to someone?
7. Will you need to bring any medications so that you don't miss your next dose?
8. Do you recognize the symptoms of concern for your diagnosis, i.e., dysreflexia, disabetes, seizures?
9. Are the bathrooms accessible?

## F. Equipment
1. What equipment will you take with you?
2. What special equipment do you need for eating?

Flesch Grade Level: 7.1

Score: _____ out of _____ applicable questions

Patient: _____   Therapist: _____   Date: _____

# Community Integration - Restaurant
## Field Trial Score Sheet

| A. Pre arrangements | score | cues | unable | N/A |
|---|---|---|---|---|
| Upon being asked to plan a trip to a restaurant, the patient demonstrated the ability to plan ahead for the trip by: | | | | |
| 1.  choosing and locating a restaurant | | | | |
| 2.  deciding if special arrangements are needed | | | | |
| 3.  identifying what identification, if any, is required | | | | |
| 4.  considering budget limitations | | | | |
| 5.  calling to confirm accessibility | | | | |
| 6.  allocating enough time | | | | |
| **B. Transportation** | | | | |
| Upon learning the address and location of the restaurant, the patient demonstrated the ability to arrange transportation by: | | | | |
| 1.  considering all transportation alternatives and choosing one | | | | |
| 2.  obtaining fare and schedule information, if needed | | | | |
| 3.  making a reservation, if needed | | | | |
| 4.  considering parking arrangements, if needed | | | | |
| 5.  knowing emergency transportation options | | | | |
| **C. Accessibility** | | | | |
| The patient compensated for barriers to accessibility by: | | | | |
| 1.  managing street barriers (curbs, crosswalks, and rough sidewalks) | | | | |
| 2.  managing architectural barriers (doors, stairs, tables, benches, escalators, elevators) | | | | |
| 3.  transferring self to chair/booth and supervising placement/storage of wheelchair | | | | |
| 4.  determining the best way to access the bathroom | | | | |
| 5.  interacting appropriately with others to solve problems | | | | |
| **D. Ordering** | | | | |
| The patient demonstrated the ability to order his/her meal as shown by: | | | | |
| 1.  determining any special dietary consideration - esp. with fluids and/or alcohol | | | | |
| 2.  reading menu and placing order | | | | |
| 3.  being able to serve self and feed self | | | | |
| **E. Emergency/Safety** | | | | |
| When presented with a hypothetical emergency situation, the patient demonstrated the ability to respond appropriately by: | | | | |
| 1.  showing awareness of and consideration for the options available | | | | |
| 2.  choosing the safest and most reasonable option with regard to the situation at hand | | | | |
| **F. Equipment** | | | | |
| The patient demonstrated the ability to anticipate the types of equipment and supplies that s/he needed by: | | | | |
| 1.  having the necessary equipment throughout the trip | | | | |
| 2.  having the necessary medical supplies throughout the trip | | | | |

**Summary:**


Score: _____ out of _____ applicable questions.

Patient: _____  Therapist: _____  Date: _____

# Module 2C  Library

You want to go to the library to look at magazines or to check out some books. You need to consider the following before visiting the library.

## A. Pre-arrangements
1. Do you have a library card?
2. Will you have access to the city library? The county library?
3. Do you need a different card for each library?
4. What identification do you need to apply for a card?
5. What is the telephone number of the library you plan to visit?
6. What hours and days is the library open?
7. What special information services does the library provide?
8. How will you return the items on time?

## B. Transportation
1. How far is the library from your home?
2. Could you walk?
3. What would be the safest route to walk?
4. What other transportation is available?
5. Is there special parking for individuals with disabilities?
6. Do you have a permit to park?
7. What do you need to do to obtain a permit?

## C. Accessibility
1. Is the building accessible?
2. Is there a special entrance for wheelchairs?
3. How will you enter and exit if there are turnstiles?
4. Where could you ask for assistance or information?
5. How can you reach books on upper and lower shelves?
6. Can you access the computers, audio and video equipment?
7. How will you get from one floor to the next?
8. How will you check out books if the check out aisle is too narrow for your wheelchair?
9. Does the library offer a map locating the books, magazines, bathrooms, and elevators?
10.  Does the library have a mobile unit that serves your area?

## D. Emergency/Safety
1. How will you gather information from non-accessible parts of the library?
2. What will you do if the fire alarm suddenly sounds?
3. What will you do if you have to go to the bathroom or cath yourself?
4. Do you recognize all symptoms related to your disability i.e. diabetes, dysreflexia?
5. Do you carry all supplies necessary for your symptoms?
6. Will you need to bring any medications so that you don't miss your next dose?
7. Are the bathrooms accessible?

## E. Equipment
1. What equipment will you need for your library visit?
2. How will you carry your supplies and books?

Flesch Grade Level 7.9


Score: _____ out of _____ applicable questions

Patient: _____    Therapist: _____    Date: _____

# Community Integration - Library
## Field Trial Score Sheet

| A. Pre arrangements | score | cues | unable | N/A |
|---|---|---|---|---|
| Upon being asked to plan a trip to the library, the patient demonstrated the ability to plan ahead for the trip by: | | | | |
| 1.  choosing a convenient branch and identifying its location | | | | |
| 2.  determining the hours of operation | | | | |
| 3.  knowing how to apply for a library card | | | | |
| 4.  determining services available | | | | |
| 5.  allocating adequate time | | | | |
| 6.  calling to confirm accessibility | | | | |
| **B. Transportation** | | | | |
| Upon learning the address and location of the library, the patient demonstrated the ability to arrange transportation by: | | | | |
| 1.  considering all transportation alternatives and choosing one | | | | |
| 2.  obtaining fare and schedule information, if needed | | | | |
| 3.  making a reservation, if needed | | | | |
| 4.  considering parking arrangements, if needed | | | | |
| 5.  knowing emergency transportation | | | | |
| **C. Accessibility** | | | | |
| The patient compensated for barriers to accessibility by: | | | | |
| 1.  choosing the best entrance and entering the library | | | | |
| 2.  managing aisles, turnstiles, and architectural barriers | | | | |
| 3.  determining the best way to reach items on the upper and lower shelves | | | | |
| 4.  choosing an appropriate method to carry books and other items | | | | |
| 5.  managing the check out procedure | | | | |
| 6.  being able to direct others to assist as needed | | | | |
| **D. Emergency/Safety** | | | | |
| When presented with a hypothetical emergency situation, the patient demonstrated the ability to respond appropriately by: | | | | |
| 1.  showing awareness of and consideration for the options available | | | | |
| 2.  choosing the safest and most reasonable option with regard to the situation at hand | | | | |
| **E. Equipment** | | | | |
| The patient demonstrated the ability to anticipate the types of equipment and supplies that s/he needed by: | | | | |
| 1.  having the necessary equipment throughout the trip | | | | |
| 2.  having the necessary medical supplies throughout the trip | | | | |

**Summary:**

Score: _____ out of _____ applicable questions.

Patient: _____ Therapist: _____ Date: _____

# Module 2D  Sporting Event

Your favorite team is playing tomorrow and you have tickets to attend the game. Prior to leaving there are many alternatives to consider to assure yourself a safe and enjoyable trip.

## A. Pre-arrangements
1. Will you need to buy tickets in advance?
2. How will you manage this?
3. Will you be protected if it rains or snows?
4. Will you need to arrange for special seating?
5. Who will you need to contact for special seating?
6. Will your attendant have to purchase a ticket?
7. Does the company managing the tickets know the layout of the stadium or field? If not, can they provide a number for someone who does?

## B. Transportation
1. How will you travel to and from the event?
2. Will you need to consider parking?
3. How will you find out about accessible parking?
4. Is there parking near the entrance and elevators?
5. Do you have a permit to park in the disabled parking section?
6. (If your friends drive) Can you use your parking permit in your friend's car?

## C. Accessibility
1. Is there an entrance convenient to the elevators?
2. Will you sit in your wheelchair or in an arena seat?
3. How will you manage turnstile entrances?
4. Are the bathrooms accessible?
5. How will you move up to your seat if it is in the grandstands?
6. (If the seats are tiered) What special precautions must you take in finding a place to sit?
7. What precautions do you need to take to do pressure releases?

## D. Equipment/Supplies
1. What equipment will you plan to take?
2. Can you access the concession stands or will you need to take your own food?

## E. Emergency
1. If the bathrooms are not accessible, is there a bathroom at the First Aid station that can accommodate you?
2. Do you know where the first aid station is in the stadium?
3. Do you recognize the symptoms of concern for your diagnosis i.e. dysreflexia, diabetes?
4. Will you need to bring any medications so that you don't miss your next dose?

Flesch Grade Level 8.9

Score: _____ out of _____ applicable questions

Patient: _____  Therapist: _____  Date: _____

# Community Integration - Sporting Event
## Field Trial Score Sheet

| A. Pre arrangements | score | cues | unable | N/A |
|---|---|---|---|---|
| Upon being asked to plan a trip to a sporting event, the patient demonstrated the ability to plan ahead for the trip by: | | | | |
| 1.   arranging to purchase tickets | | | | |
| 2.   determining if attendant also needed a ticket | | | | |
| 3.   ensuring that appropriate seating was available | | | | |
| 4.   explaining the layout of field/stadium | | | | |
| 5.   allocating adequate time | | | | |
| 6.   calling to confirm accessibility | | | | |
| **B. Transportation** | | | | |
| Upon learning the address and location of the sporting event, the patient demonstrated the ability to arrange transportation by: | | | | |
| 1.   considering all transportation alternatives and choosing one | | | | |
| 2.   obtaining fare and schedule information, if needed | | | | |
| 3.   making a reservation, if needed | | | | |
| 4.   considering parking arrangements, if needed | | | | |
| 5.   knowing emergency transportation options | | | | |
| **C. Accessibility** | | | | |
| The patient compensated for architectural barriers by: | | | | |
| 1.   managing street barriers (curbs, crosswalks, rough sidewalks, and crowds) | | | | |
| 2.   managing architectural barriers (doors, stairs, turnstiles) | | | | |
| 3.   managing geographical barriers (hills, dips, water) | | | | |
| 4.   choosing the best alternatives for carrying supplies | | | | |
| 5.   managing the public restrooms and food services | | | | |
| 6.   being able to appropriately direct others to help | | | | |
| **D. Emergency/Safety** | | | | |
| When presented with a hypothetical emergency situation, the patient demonstrated the ability to respond appropriately by: | | | | |
| 1.   showing awareness of and consideration for the options available | | | | |
| 2.   choosing the safest and most reasonable option with regard to the situation at hand | | | | |
| **E. Equipment** | | | | |
| The patient demonstrated the ability to anticipate the types of equipment and supplies that s/he needed by: | | | | |
| 1.   having the necessary equipment throughout the trip | | | | |
| 2.   having the necessary medical supplies throughout the trip | | | | |

**Summary:**

Score: _____ out of _____ applicable questions.

Patient: _____  Therapist: _____  Date: _____

# 10. Community Activities

While many people would name a baseball game, a party, or hiking as a normal leisure activity, most of our leisure time is actually spent using the businesses and parks in our community. This chapter contains five modules related to the normal, day to day activities which take up so much of our leisure time.

These evaluations are often considered the domain of other disciplines. At Harborview, the treatment team decided that these modules would be done by the discipline that is always out in the community – the therapeutic recreation specialists. Make sure that you are aware of interdisciplinary concerns when you discuss using these modules in team meetings.

We use an informal group approach, including families whenever possible, for all of these modules. Harborview is conveniently close to an area with a bank, a small shopping mall, and a grocery store. The businesses are close enough together that we often go through all of the modules in this chapter in one trip downtown. They are far enough apart that the patients have to negotiate streets, organize their time, carry packages, maneuver through crowds, and deal with architectural barriers.

This practical experience promotes patient and family education through the support of the group problem solving and the supervision of the trained CTRS. Often it promotes the concept of anticipating needs or issues for the next community outing.

This kind of group, requires additional staffing, family support or volunteers. It is conducive to pairing patients with staff supervision. (Once it was considered acceptable to pair a patient using a wheelchair with an ambulatory patient who has a head injury, but check the example below for reasons why the therapist may want to think twice before doing this.) It is important to emphasize to your untrained helpers that things can go wrong. Pairs of people need to stay together. Patients with TBI's do not have the same level of judgment that they had before their injury. Having enough trained staff and/or volunteers on the outing is mandatory

Just as an example of how rough it can get ...

> The staff at Harborview took a group of four individuals and some of their family members to a local mall. The two individuals with traumatic brain injuries were paired with patients who had spinal cord injuries. The parents of one patient became hysterical at one point when they realized the actual limitations of their son. This patient was in a wheelchair and required volunteer and staff assistance. The other patient with a spinal cord injury became so distracted watching the scene that he lost his partner who had a traumatic brain injury. Security was notified, and while they were getting the description from the therapist, security received notice that a downstairs bathroom was overflowing. The therapist, aware that the lost patient had a toilet paper fetish, asked for directions to the downstairs bathroom and located the patient. During this same

*outing, a family member of one of the patients with a traumatic brain injury allowed him to go on his own because they didn't feel that he had any problems. The patient was picked up by security for shoplifting, not because he didn't have any money, but because he forgot to pay.*

Escorting patients into the community for cultural events are not without learning opportunities for the therapist.

*One outing involved a young male with a bilateral lower extremity traumatic amputation secondary to a train vs. pedestrian accident. The patient was very reluctant to go on community integration outings, nervous about being seen, concerned about negotiating in a wheelchair, etc. The therapist opted for more social vs. physical experience with peer support. The group was taken to the Old Spaghetti Factory and seated in the wheelchair accessible portion of the restaurant, an area decorated as a working train station. The patient relaxed, appeared to enjoy himself and participated in conversation. However, the therapist realized half way through the meal that the patient was sitting directly in front of a train that appeared to be coming into the restaurant, giving the illusion that he "could" get hit again — fortunately he never noticed and the therapist was able to control herself.*

At times both the therapist and the patient will need to do some serious problem solving together (as well as to develop some effective assertiveness skills).

*The staff at Harborview had a young male with a C4 quadriplegia and a permanent stoma trach secondary to a gun shot wound through the neck and cord. Several months into the recuperative phase with only one previous ground pass outing the patient decided that he was ready for his first outing into the community. His choice for his first outing was the horse race track. During the pre-test phase the therapist and the patient determined that the area was wheelchair accessible and they were assured that a Medical Aid Unit was available at the track for their use. Emergency procedures were cleared during medical rounds, training was given to the therapist in charge in case the young man required suctioning. (The increased need for and frequency of suctioning is common to this type of injury during new, high anxiety producing activities.) While at the track, the wind picked up spreading dust everywhere. The patient then maneuvered his chair to the smoking section and persuaded a young woman to give him a drag through his stoma. Shortly thereafter the patient indicated distress, requesting suctioning. The medical unit turned out not to be wheelchair accessible and no phone was available (a protection established by the track, to prevent illegal betting). A temper tantrum by the therapist got assistance to access the medical unit, suctioning was completed, the hospital was called through security's two way radio, and approval was given by medical staff at the hospital to stay for the last few races.*

# Module 3A  Shopping Mall

You have decided that you need to have some new clothes and household goods after discharge. Most of the stores that you want to go to are in the local mall.

### A. Pre-arrangements
1. How will you plan your shopping trip?
2. Which stores will you visit first and last? Why?

### B. Transportation
1. How will you get to the shopping mall?
2. Do you know the route to the mall?
3. Is there special parking available for the disabled? Is it conveniently located?
4. How will you carry your purchases between stores?
5. What is the safest and most efficient way to carry your items?
6. How will you carry your purchases home?
7. Will you need assistance?

### C. Accessibility
1. Are the stores you plan to shop in accessible?
2. How are you going to get from one floor to another?
3. How will you enter and exit if there are turnstiles?
4. Will you be able to move around the clothes racks and through the aisles?
5. Are the dressing rooms accessible?
6. If not, can you try the clothes on at home and return them later?
7. Will you need a receipt?

### D. Money Management
1. Where will you usually be able to pay for your purchases?
2. How do you check to see that the salesperson has included all your purchases at the correct price?
3. How will you pay for your purchases?
4. Should you save you receipt? Why?

### E. Emergency/Safety
1. What will you do if you have to cath yourself or go to the bathroom in the middle of your shopping trip?
2. What would you do if the building fire alarm sounded?
3. Will you need to bring any medications so that you don't miss your next dose?
4. Do you recognize the symptoms of concern for your diagnosis, i.e., dysreflexia, diabetes, seizures?
5. Are the bathrooms accessible?

### F. Equipment
1. What medical equipment will you require for the trip?
2. What special equipment will you require to help you with your shopping?

Flesch Grade Level 6.9

Score: _____ out of _____ applicable questions

Patient: _____ Therapist: _____ Date: _____

113

# Community Integration - Shopping Mall
## Field Trial Score Sheet

| A. Pre arrangements | score | cues | unable | N/A |
|---|---|---|---|---|
| Upon being asked to plan a trip to the shopping mall, the patient demonstrated the ability to plan ahead for the trip by: | | | | |
| 1.   choosing a convenient mall | | | | |
| 2.   making a shopping list | | | | |
| 3.   identifying its location and selecting order of stops | | | | |
| 4.   allocating adequate time | | | | |
| 5.   calling to confirm accessibility | | | | |
| **B. Transportation** | | | | |
| Upon learning the address and location of the shopping mall, the patient demonstrated the ability to arrange transportation by: | | | | |
| 1.   considering all transportation alternatives and choosing one | | | | |
| 2.   obtaining fare and schedule information, if needed | | | | |
| 3.   making a reservation, if needed | | | | |
| 4.   considering parking arrangements, if needed | | | | |
| 5.   knowing emergency transportation options | | | | |
| **C. Accessibility** | | | | |
| The patient compensated for architectural barriers by: | | | | |
| 1.   determining the best way to reach each store | | | | |
| 2.   managing entrance, exits, and movement through the mall | | | | |
| 3.   determining the best way to reach items on selves and on racks | | | | |
| 4.   choosing the best alternatives for carrying items and supplies | | | | |
| 5.   being able to appropriately direct others to assist | | | | |
| **D. Money Management** | | | | |
| The patient demonstrated the ability to manage money by: | | | | |
| 1.   ensuring that all purchases are rung up and correctly placed in a bag | | | | |
| 2.   considering budget limitations | | | | |
| 3.   managing the check out procedure | | | | |
| **E. Emergency/Safety** | | | | |
| When presented with a hypothetical emergency situation, the patient demonstrated the ability to respond appropriately by: | | | | |
| 1.   showing awareness of and consideration for the options available | | | | |
| 2.   choosing the safest and most reasonable option with regard to the situation at hand | | | | |
| **F. Equipment** | | | | |
| The patient demonstrated the ability to anticipate the types of equipment and supplies that s/he needed by: | | | | |
| 1.   having the necessary equipment throughout the trip | | | | |
| 2.   having the necessary medical supplies throughout the trip | | | | |

Summary:




Score: _____ out of _____ applicable questions.

Patient: _____  Therapist: _____  Date: _____

# Module 3B  Grocery Store

You have decided to have a few of your best friends over for dinner. You look in your refrigerator and realize that you need to go shopping for food.

### A. Pre-arrangements
1.  Which grocery store will you choose? Why?
2.  Will you plan to take a grocery list with you?
3.  How will you pay for your groceries?

### B. Transportation
1.  How will you get to and from the store?
2.  How will you transfer in and out of the vehicle?
3.  Where is the store located?
4.  Where will you park?

### C. Accessibility
1.  Where will you enter the store?
2.  Is the store accessible?
3.  How will you get in and out through turnstile entrances?
4.  How will you reach items on the top shelves?
5.  How will you reach items from the cold storage section?
6.  How will you carry your groceries while shopping?
7.  How will you check out, if the cashier's aisle is too narrow for your wheelchair?
8.  How will you carry the grocery bags to your car, bus or taxi?

### D. Emergency/Safety
1.  As you are checking out, you learn that you do not have enough money for all that you've chosen. What will you do?
2.  What while you do if you have to cath yourself or go to the bathroom while you are shopping?
3.  Will you need to bring any medications so that you don't miss your next dose?
4.  Do you recognize the symptoms of concern for your diagnosis, i.e., dysreflexia, diabetes, seizures?
5.  Are the bathrooms accessible?

### E. Equipment
1.  What medical equipment will you require for your trip?
2.  What special equipment or supplies will you take to make your shopping more convenient?

Flesch Grade Level 6.4

Score: _____ out of _____ applicable questions

Patient: _____ Therapist: _____ Date: _____

# Community Integration - Grocery Store
## Field Trial Score Sheet

| A. Pre arrangements | score | cues | unable | N/A |
|---|---|---|---|---|
| Upon being asked to plan a trip to the grocery store, the patient demonstrated the ability to plan ahead for the trip by: | | | | |
| 1. choosing a convenient store | | | | |
| 2. identifying its location | | | | |
| 3. making a grocery list | | | | |
| 4. considering budget limitations | | | | |
| 5. allocating adequate time | | | | |
| 6. calling to confirm accessibility | | | | |
| **B. Transportation** | | | | |
| Upon learning the address and location of the grocery store, the patient demonstrated the ability to arrange transportation by: | | | | |
| 1. considering all transportation alternatives and choosing one | | | | |
| 2. obtaining fare and schedule information, if needed | | | | |
| 3. making a reservation, if needed | | | | |
| 4. considering parking arrangements, if needed | | | | |
| 5. knowing emergency transportation options | | | | |
| **C. Accessibility** | | | | |
| The patient compensated for barriers to accessibility by: | | | | |
| 1. choosing the best entrance and entering the store | | | | |
| 2. managing entrance and exit through turnstiles | | | | |
| 3. determining the best way to reach food in the cold storage section and on the upper shelves | | | | |
| 4. choosing the best alternatives for carrying groceries | | | | |
| 5. managing the check out procedure | | | | |
| 6. being able to direct others to assist in an appropriate manner | | | | |
| **D. Emergency/Safety** | | | | |
| When presented with a hypothetical emergency situation, the patient demonstrated the ability to respond appropriately by: | | | | |
| 1. showing awareness of and consideration for the options available | | | | |
| 2. choosing the safest and most reasonable option with regard to the situation at hand | | | | |
| **E. Equipment** | | | | |
| The patient demonstrated the ability to anticipate the types of equipment and supplies that s/he needed by: | | | | |
| 1. having the necessary equipment throughout the trip | | | | |
| 2. having the necessary medical supplies throughout the trip | | | | |

**Summary:**

Score: _____ out of _____ applicable questions.

Patient: _____ Therapist: _____ Date: _____

The following four pages show chart notes that have been developed at Harborview Medical Center. The first note is the one used by the Rehabilitation group. The second note is used by the Psychiatric team. They should help you develop chart notes that you can use for your facility for this module and also the other modules in this chapter.

# Therapeutic Recreation: Community Integration Evaluation

## Assessment of Skills in a Grocery Store - Rehabilitation

Key:     (+) = independent function, affirmative response, or demonstrates appropriate knowledge
          (-) = patient needs assistance, negative response, or the lack of appropriate knowledge
          (N/A) = not applicable
          (N/T) = not tested

Patient is a _____ with a diagnosis of _____
seen on _____ to assess the following skills:

## 1. Pre-plan phase
### A. Demonstrates orientation, knowledge, or memory of:
_____ date and time of evaluation
_____ appropriate dress and grooming needed for weather
_____ purpose of evaluation
_____ items necessary (list, cart, etc.)
_____ money needed
_____ medical necessities (i.e., pressure releases, meds., splints/braces)

**Comments:**

## II. Future Leisure phase
### A. Demonstrates orientation to:
_____ shopping available at d/c site
_____ transportation available to shopping at d/c site
_____ leisure options with food/cooking (i.e., entertaining, gourmet or holiday
         cooking)

**Comments:**

## III. Management phase
### A. Functional behaviors: Demonstrates ability to:
_____ negotiate architectural barriers
_____ grasp, hold, and carry items
_____ reach and lift
_____ scan and locate items
_____ tolerate activity related to shopping

**Comments:**

**B. Cognitive behaviors: Demonstrates ability to:**

_____ locate all areas requested in store
_____ sequence/categorize items
_____ count back correct change
_____ follow directions
_____ identify/discriminate (items on list)
_____ remain task oriented
_____ complete task in an appropriate time

**Comments:**

**C. Social behaviors: Demonstrates:**

_____ consistently positive social interactions
_____ appropriate and realistic comfort level in community setting
_____ appropriate response to authority or conflict

**Comments:**

**Assessment:**

**Recommendations:**

**Therapist** _____ **Date** _____ **Time Spent** _____

# Therapeutic Recreation: Community Integration Evaluation

**Assessment of Skills in a Grocery Store - Psychiatric**

Key:     (+) = independent function, affirmative response, or demonstrates appropriate knowledge
          (-) = patient needs assistance, negative response, or the lack of appropriate knowledge
          (N/A) = not applicable
          (N/T) = not tested

Patient is a _____ with a diagnosis of _____
seen on _____ to assess the following skills:

## I. Pre-plan Phase

### A. Demonstrates orientation/knowledge or memory of:
_____ date and time of evaluation
_____ appropriate dress and grooming needed for weather
_____ purpose of evaluation
**Comments:**

## II. Management Phase

### A. Functional behaviors: Demonstrates ability to:
_____ scan items in the store
_____ ask for assistance from appropriate store personnel
**Comments:**

### B. Cognitive behaviors: Demonstrates ability to:
_____ pathfind to/from grocery store
_____ monitor traffic, use of signals for safe crossing
_____ identify items on list
_____ sequence/categorize items
_____ locate all areas requested in store
_____ compare values of like items
_____ remain task oriented
_____ complete task in appropriate time frame
_____ stay within given budget
_____ count back change correctly
**Comments:**

**C. Social Behaviors: Demonstrates:**
\_\_\_\_\_ consistently appropriate social interactions
\_\_\_\_\_ appropriate and realistic comfort level in community
\_\_\_\_\_ appropriate response to authority or conflict
**Comments:**

## III. Future Leisure Phase
### A. Demonstrates orientation to:
\_\_\_\_\_ location of store nearest discharge site
\_\_\_\_\_ transportation needs to store
\_\_\_\_\_ leisure options involving food/cooking
**Comments:**

**Assessment:**

**Recommendations:**

**Therapist** _____ **Date** _____ **Time Spent** _____

# Module 3C  Downtown

There are things that you need to do, and this means that you will be spending part of your day downtown. To make the trip worth your time, you've decided to combine business with pleasure. You will go shopping after your business is taken care of, meeting friends for lunch later. You must decide how to plan and organize your day.

## A. Pre-arrangements
1. Do you know the addresses and locations of the buildings?
2. Where will you park?
3. What should you take into consideration in planning the order of your errands?
4. How will you organize and order your errands?
5. Will you park in one spot and travel by wheelchair, or will you need to use the car or public transit to get from place to place?
6. How will you carry your packages?
7. How much will you have to carry?
8. How will you safely carry your money?

## B. Transportation
1. How will you travel to and from the downtown area?
2. Where does your disabled parking sticker enable you to park?
3. If traveling by public transit, how close to your destination will it take you?
4. How will you travel the remaining distance?
5. Will your electric wheelchair hold enough charge for your trip?
6. If using a manual wheelchair, are you strong enough to wheel the distance alone?
7. Will you need assistance?

## C. Accessibility
1. Is the downtown area accessible?
2. Where are curb cuts located?
3. Are there crosswalks?
4. How will you get up steep hills or ramps?
5. How will you pass through the turnstile entrances?
6. How will you get from one floor to another?

## D. Emergency/Safety
1. What emergency conditions might you encounter?
2. How will you be prepared to meet an emergency?
3. Will you need to bring any medications so that you don't miss your next dose?
4. Do you recognize the symptoms of concern for your diagnosis, i.e., dysreflexia, diabetes, seizures?
5. Are the bathrooms accessible?

## E. Equipment
1. What equipment will you require to help you plan a safe and comfortable day?
2. What resources are available to you that will identify accessibility, short routes?

Flesch Grade Level 6.8

Score: _____ out of _____ applicable questions

Patient: _____   Therapist: _____   Date: _____

# Community Integration - Downtown
## Field Trial Score Sheet

| A. Pre arrangements | score | cues | unable | N/A |
|---|---|---|---|---|
| Upon being asked to plan a trip downtown, the patient demonstrated the ability to plan ahead for the trip by: | | | | |
| 1.  identifying the locations of the sites to be visited | | | | |
| 2.  making a list and indicating a reasonable order for stops | | | | |
| 3.  knowing how to get from one location to another | | | | |
| 4.  considering budget limitations and package carrying limitations | | | | |
| 5.  allocating adequate time | | | | |
| 6.  calling to confirm accessibility | | | | |
| **B. Transportation** | | | | |
| Upon learning the address and location of the various stops, the patient demonstrated the ability to arrange transportation by: | | | | |
| 1.  considering all transportation alternatives and choosing one | | | | |
| 2.  obtaining fare and schedule information, if needed | | | | |
| 3.  making a reservation, if needed | | | | |
| 4.  considering parking arrangements, if needed | | | | |
| 5.  knowing emergency transportation options | | | | |
| **C. Accessibility** | | | | |
| The patient compensated for architectural barriers by: | | | | |
| 1.  managing street barriers (curbs, crosswalks, and rough sidewalks) | | | | |
| 2.  managing architectural barriers (doors, stairs, turnstiles) | | | | |
| 3.  managing geographical barriers (hills, dips, water) | | | | |
| 4.  choosing the best alternatives for carrying supplies and purchases | | | | |
| 5.  managing the public bathrooms and food services | | | | |
| 6.  being able to direct others to assist in an appropriate manner | | | | |
| **D. Emergency/Safety** | | | | |
| When presented with a hypothetical emergency situation, the patient demonstrated the ability to respond appropriately by: | | | | |
| 1.  showing awareness of and consideration for the options available | | | | |
| 2.  choosing the safest and most reasonable option with regard to the situation at hand | | | | |
| **E. Equipment** | | | | |
| The patient demonstrated the ability to anticipate the types of equipment and supplies that s/he needed by: | | | | |
| 1.  having the necessary equipment throughout the trip | | | | |
| 2.  having the necessary medical supplies throughout the trip | | | | |

**Summary:**

Score: _____ out of _____ applicable questions.

Patient: _____   Therapist: _____   Date: _____

# Module 3D  Bank

In order to organize your income and plan ahead for future savings and expenditures, you have decided that you need to open a checking and savings account at a local bank. There are many choices for you to consider in making these arrangements.

## A. Pre-arrangements
1. What do you need to consider when choosing a bank? (Accessibility, location, convenience, and services provided)
2. What information do you need to give the bank to open an account?

## B. Transportation
1. How will you get to the bank?
2. Will you park and enter the bank?

## C. Accessibility
1. Is the bank you've chosen accessible? How can you find out?
2. Can you reach to the back of the desks provided for your use?
3. Many banks make waiting lines using cords strung from posts. Can you get through this type of line?

## D. Bank Business
1. What identification must you have to prove who you are?
2. Is a social security card appropriate identification? If not, what is?
3. What type of identification do you need to cash a check at a different branch?
4. What kind of checks will the bank accept?
5. Will you plan to use your home or hospital address? How will you make these arrangements?
6. Who at the bank can help you open an account?
7. Are there special services or accounts available for individuals with disabilities?
8. Who will you see about getting a safety deposit box?
9. What other special services does the bank offer its customers?
10. Do you know your ATM number?
11. Can you access the machine? The card?

## E. Emergency/Safety
1. What will you do if your account is overdrawn?
2. What would you do if your medications were lost?
3. Do you recognize the symptoms of conditions related to your disability i.e. dysreflexia, seizure, diabetes.
4. Do you carry information about these conditions (a medical ID card)?
5. Will you need to bring any medications so that you don't miss your next dose?
6. Are the bathrooms accessible?

## F. Equipment
1. What medical equipment will you require for your outing?
2. How will you carry your money and documents safely?
3. Will you use the drive-up window?

Flesch Grade Level 8.2

Score: _____ out of _____ applicable questions

Patient: _____ Therapist: _____ Date: _____

# Community Integration - Bank
## Field Trial Score Sheet

| A. Pre arrangements | score | cues | unable | N/A |
|---|---|---|---|---|
| Upon being asked to plan a trip to the bank, the patient demonstrated the ability to plan ahead for the trip by: | | | | |
| 1.   choosing a convenient bank which provides the required services | | | | |
| 2.   identifying and obtaining necessary papers to bring along | | | | |
| 3.   allocating adequate time | | | | |
| 4.   calling to confirm accessibility | | | | |
| **B. Transportation** | | | | |
| Upon learning the address and location of the bank, the patient demonstrated the ability to arrange transportation by: | | | | |
| 1.   considering all transportation alternatives and choosing one | | | | |
| 2.   obtaining fare and schedule information, if needed | | | | |
| 3.   making a reservation, if needed | | | | |
| 4.   considering parking arrangements, if needed | | | | |
| 5.   knowing emergency transportation options | | | | |
| **C. Accessibility** | | | | |
| The patient compensated for barriers to accessibility by: | | | | |
| 1.   managing street barriers (curbs, crosswalks, crowds, and rough sidewalks) | | | | |
| 2.   managing architectural barriers (doors, stairs, turnstiles) | | | | |
| 3.   managing geographical barriers (hills, dips, water) | | | | |
| 4.   being able to direct others to help in an appropriate manner | | | | |
| **D. Bank Business** | | | | |
| While at the bank the patient demonstrated the ability to carry out his/her banking business by: | | | | |
| 1.   presenting appropriate identification and other papers | | | | |
| 2.   giving address and other information upon request | | | | |
| 3.   make reasonable decisions as to the services needed/desired | | | | |
| 4.   demonstrating an ability to use the various machines and services | | | | |
| **E. Emergency/Safety** | | | | |
| When presented with a hypothetical emergency situation, the patient demonstrated the ability to respond appropriately by: | | | | |
| 1.   showing awareness of and consideration for the options available | | | | |
| 2.   choosing the safest and most reasonable option with regard to the situation at hand | | | | |
| **F. Equipment** | | | | |
| The patient demonstrated the ability to anticipate the types of equipment and supplies that s/he needed by: | | | | |
| 1.   having the necessary equipment throughout the trip | | | | |
| 2.   having the necessary medical supplies throughout the trip | | | | |

**Summary**

Score: _____ out of _____ applicable questions.

Patient: _____   Therapist: _____   Date: _____

# Module 3E  Laundromat

You have just moved into your new apartment, and luckily you have discovered a laundromat is located nearby. Before you set out, you must decide exactly how best to plan your trip to the laundromat.

## A. Pre-arrangements
1.  What will you need to take with you?
2.  Will you have clothes that require hanging or ironing?
3.  How will you manage this?
4.  Do you have the correct amount of change to run the machines?

## B. Transportation
1.  How will you get to and from the laundromat?
2.  How will you carry your dirty clothes and extra supplies?
3.  Where will you park?
4.  If taking public transportation, how close is the stop to the laundromat?

## C. Accessibility
1.  Is the laundromat accessible?
2.  Are the restrooms accessible?
3.  Will you be able to reach the counters? Will you be able to reach the machine control dials?
4.  If not, how will you fold your clothes? Turn on the machine?
5.  How will you get your clothes in and out of the washer and dryer?
6.  If you need assistance, who will you ask?

## D. Emergency
1.  Will you need to bring any medications so that you don't miss your next dose?
2.  Do you recognize the symptoms of concern for your diagnosis, i.e., dysreflexia, diabetes, seizures?
3.  Are the bathrooms accessible?

## E. Equipment
1.  What equipment will you need to take?
2.  What laundry supplies will you need to remember? (money, clothes basket or bag, laundry soap, bleach, hangers, etc.)

Flesch Grade Level 7.6

Score: _____ out of _____ applicable questions

Patient: _____ Therapist: _____ Date: _____

# Community Integration - Laundromat
## Field Trial Score Sheet

| A. Pre arrangements | score | cues | unable | N/A |
|---|---|---|---|---|
| Upon being asked to plan a trip to the laundromat, the patient demonstrated the ability to plan ahead for the trip by: | | | | |
| 1. choosing a convenient laundromat | | | | |
| 2. identifying its location | | | | |
| 3. explaining how to wash clothing and use machines | | | | |
| 4. making a list, collecting supplies, and getting change (coins) | | | | |
| 5. allocating adequate time | | | | |
| 6. calling to confirm accessibility | | | | |
| **B. Transportation** | | | | |
| Upon learning the address and location of the laundromat, the patient demonstrated the ability to arrange transportation by: | | | | |
| 1. considering all transportation alternatives and choosing one | | | | |
| 2. obtaining fare and schedule information, if needed | | | | |
| 3. making a reservation, if needed | | | | |
| 4. considering parking arrangements, if needed | | | | |
| 5. knowing emergency transportation options | | | | |
| **C. Accessibility** | | | | |
| The patient compensated for barriers to accessibility by: | | | | |
| 1. choosing the best entrance and entering the laundromat | | | | |
| 2. managing moving around and running the machines | | | | |
| 3. managing architectural barriers (doors, stairs, turnstiles) | | | | |
| 4. choosing the best alternatives for carrying clothing and supplies | | | | |
| 5. managing or finding alternatives to the hand function required | | | | |
| 6. interacting appropriately with others to solve problems | | | | |
| **D. Emergency/Safety** | | | | |
| When presented with a hypothetical emergency situation, the patient demonstrated the ability to respond appropriately by: | | | | |
| 1. showing awareness of and consideration for the options available | | | | |
| 2. choosing the safest and most reasonable option with regard to the situation at hand | | | | |
| **E. Equipment** | | | | |
| The patient demonstrated the ability to anticipate the types of equipment and supplies that s/he needed by: | | | | |
| 1. having the necessary equipment throughout the trip | | | | |
| 2. having the necessary medical supplies throughout the trip | | | | |

**Summary**

Score: _____ out of _____ applicable questions.

Patient: _____ Therapist: _____ Date: _____

# 11. Transportation

Transportation is the most significant barrier to successful integration. Repeatedly patients tell us that they would become involved if they could only find efficient and independent transportation. These modules represent all the ground and air transportation presently available and covered by ADA legislation. Many commercial and passenger boats have floors that are barrier free. However, multiple exemptions make accessibility review difficult. No module has been written to represent this area yet. Formal ADA guidelines for accessibility are not anticipated before 1998 with implementation sometime around the year 2000.

The formal evaluation we use most is the community bus. Through an agreement with the county, we can furnish Reduced Fare Bus Permits from our office. In order to not affect the bus schedule, most evaluations occur during non-high peak ridership periods: the middle of the day and weekend mornings. We suggested that you wait on transportation evaluations until an environmental awareness module in a high stimulus area has been successfully completed. It is unsafe to assume that a patient with both physical and cognitive disabilities who can move on and off a bus lift using adaptive aides is also able to locate a specific place. Their path finding, particularly in an unfamiliar neighborhood, may be impaired. The perfect example of this was the evaluation completed with a patient who had a brain injury.

> *The patient's ambulation status was independent. The discharge plan included having him return for continued cognitive re-training, but only if we could determine he had the functional ability to use the bus and could structure his leisure time appropriately. Rather than extend his stay in the hospital, a multiple part evaluation was planned. The path finding part was from the hospital to his apartment to the community center where he would get one meal a day after discharge. All appeared to be going well, until the therapist requested a change in route to review banks and post offices. She got off, the patient did not. He got caught in the crowd on the bus. The therapist ran up a steep three block hill to the hospital where she noted to her delight that the patient was disembarking from the bus. Her appreciation of his skills was short-lived, however. Just outside of shouting distance, the patient got onto another bus and rode away. After the emergency plan was put into effect, the patient returned to the hospital. When he was asked what happened, he said that he just forgot. That by the time he remembered that he was still in the hospital he was already on the other bus, and that then he was to embarrassed to ask how to get off.*

As in all patient plans, an individual's personal needs will indicate what transportation modules should be reviewed. It is very common for us to evaluate a patient's functionality using the bus system and suggest it as an alternative or emergency backup if other transportation is not available. Often you will find that teaching the patient the skills to ride the bus is enough to make it an acceptable mode of transportation. In any case you will note that every module asks what alternative form of transportation the patient plans to use during an emergency.

Patients who are insensate need to identify specific needs for their seating if they are required to transfer. One solution may be as simple as using their own cushion, for example, on top of the car seat or airline seat. However, any adjustment to the standard seat may require additional support to the trunk for stability.

A complete field trial for air travel is probably beyond the financial abilities of most hospitals. This module is given to the patient when they are taking a trip by plane. We also give them the most recent list of travel resources and reviews of architectural barriers. However, the airport by itself is a powerful learning environment for solving problems with architectural barriers including escalators, small elevators, and ramps. Support systems can be designed for airport transport through pre-arrangements made with the airlines and/or travelers aide. In any case, an individual with a disability will want to read the handbook called New Horizons for the Air Traveler with a Disability by the United States Department of Transportation (1991). A complete copy of that handbook can be found in Section 3 of this book.

> *We discovered all the barriers in our local airport during the 1981 National Wheelchair games. Two hundred and fifty athletes arrived within a period of 8 hours. Advanced training with all airlines and a host of boy scouts made meeting the planes and the transfer of luggage easy. However, there were only four elevators from the level where the passengers disembark to the baggage claim area and they hold just two wheelchairs each. Seeing the long lines waiting to ride the elevators down to baggage claim, seven of the athletes headed for the escalators. One woman at the bottom feared that they were going to injure themselves and screamed for support. Then she fainted. The athletes simply avoided her at the bottom of the escalators. (The Seattle-Tacoma airport has made some gains since then. However, the elevators are still the same and parking for oversize vans with roof top extensions is not accessible from the terminal.)*

# Module 4A  Personal Travel

You and a friend have decided to go out in his car. It may be for a short drive to the store or a long vacation drive. Privately owned vehicles differ in their structure and adaptability. Consider the advantages and disadvantages of traveling in different vehicles.

## A. Pre-arrangements
1. How would you schedule or organize a full day of travel? Consider meals, cath times, rest, and driving intervals.
2. How will you do your pressure releases? Will you be able to do them on a bench car seat? Are space and leverage available?
3. How will you plan your route of travel?
4. Do you carry proper identification? Does your identification include special medical precautions?
5. What will you take on the trip?
6. How will you pack?
7. What type of luggage will you choose to use? Why?
8. Have you labeled your luggage?
9. How will you carry your luggage?
10. Where will your luggage, equipment and wheelchair be stored for the ride?
11. How will you store these items so they are easy to get to?

## B. Transportation
1. What type of vehicle will you be traveling in?
2. Does it meet your comfort and safety needs?
3. Is one type of vehicle more accessible to you than another?
4. Which do you prefer? Why?
5. Is there special equipment that can be installed to aid your entrance and exit from the vehicle?
6. Will you be driving yourself or riding with someone?
7. What type of seat belt and wheelchair tie down system will you need?

## C. Accessibility
1. Is it accessible? How would you know?
2. Where will you park your vehicle to ensure easier transfers and access to buildings?
3. How will you plan to transfer in and out of the vehicle? Will you need assistance?

## E. Emergency/Safety
1. If a special medical problem flares up during your trip, what will you do?
2. Will you need to bring any medications so that you don't miss any doses?
3. Do you recognize the symptoms of concern for your diagnosis, i.e., dysreflexia, disabetes, seizures?
4. Are the bathrooms accessible?
5. Is it safe for you to sit in the car seat?
6. Will you need to do pressure releases?
7. Should you wear a seat belt? Shoulder harness? Both?

Flesch Grade Level 8.1

Score: _____ out of _____ applicable questions

Patient: _____ Therapist: _____ Date: _____

# Community Integration - Personal Travel
## Field Trial Score Sheet

| A. Pre arrangements | score | cues | unable | N/A |
|---|---|---|---|---|
| Upon being asked to plan a trip using a privately owned vehicle, the patient demonstrated the ability to plan ahead for the trip by: | | | | |
| 1. outlining a reasonable travel schedule, including time for pressure releases, cathing, etc. | | | | |
| 2. determining routes and needed items (maps, identification, etc.) | | | | |
| 3. determining supplies, clothing, and packing strategies | | | | |
| 4. considering budget limitations | | | | |
| 5. allowing adequate time | | | | |
| **B. Transportation** | | | | |
| The patient demonstrated the ability to arrange transportation by: | | | | |
| 1. considering comfort and safety needs in selecting a vehicle | | | | |
| 2. determining the accessibility of the vehicle | | | | |
| 3. determining the types of adapted equipment needed to be able to use the vehicle | | | | |
| 4. considering parking arrangements, if needed | | | | |
| 5. knowing emergency transportation options | | | | |
| **C. Accessibility** | | | | |
| The patient compensated for accessibility barriers by: | | | | |
| 1. choosing a reasonable method of entering and exiting the vehicle | | | | |
| 2. demonstrating the ability to use appropriate restraining devices | | | | |
| 3. determining the ability to ensure easy access when using the vehicle | | | | |
| 4. demonstrating the ability to utilize the controls, knobs, etc. inside the vehicle | | | | |
| 5. interacting appropriately with others to solve problems | | | | |
| **D. Emergency/Safety** | | | | |
| When presented with a hypothetical emergency situation, the patient demonstrated the ability to respond appropriately by: | | | | |
| 1. showing awareness of and consideration for the options available | | | | |
| 2. choosing the safest and most reasonable option with regard to the situation at hand | | | | |
| **E. Equipment** | | | | |
| The patient demonstrated the ability to anticipate the types of equipment and supplies that s/he needed by: | | | | |
| 1. having the necessary equipment throughout the trip | | | | |
| 2. having the necessary medical supplies throughout the trip | | | | |

**Summary:**

Score: _____ out of _____ applicable questions.

Patient: _____ Therapist: _____ Date: _____

# Module 4B  Taxi/Taxi Vans

☐ pre-test   ☐ post-test

Your travel plans require your arrangement of transportation from the airport to the train station. The city does not have an accessible bus system so you will be required to use the taxi system.

## A. Pre-arrangements
1. Where will you find information regarding taxi schedules and reservation procedures?
2. What resources are available to you to find out this information?
3. Can you call and reserve a taxi? How far in advance will you need to reserve the taxi?
4. What information should you call and give the taxi service about your needs?
5. How can you find out how much your ride will cost?
6. Do you know how much to tip the driver?
7. Does the cab company have special regulations for disabled individuals traveling with their company?
8. How close to your destination will the cab take you?
9. How will you travel the remaining distance?
10. Do you know the address and directions?

## B. Packing and Luggage
1. Will you have packages or baggage to carry?
2. How will you carry the load?
3. Will you require assistance?

## C. Accessibility
1. How will you get to the cab?
2. Will you know where to tell the driver to drop you off?
3. Is there a special entrance for wheelchairs or is there a more convenient entrance into the building?
4. How will you ride in the taxi?
5. Where will you put your wheelchair?
6. Can you describe how to break down your chair, if that is necessary?
7. Can you describe how to assist with transfers?
8. Should you use your own cushion or will the car seat be safe?

## D. Emergency/Safety
1. Will you need to bring any medications so that you don't miss any doses?
2. Do you recognize the symptoms of concern for your diagnosis, i.e., dysreflexia, diabetes, seizures?
3. How would you get to a bathroom if you needed one?

## E. Equipment
1. What equipment will you need for the taxi ride?
2. What equipment will you need upon arrival at your destination?

Flesch Grade Level 7.7

Score: _____ out of _____ applicable questions

Patient: _____  Therapist: _____  Date: _____

# Community Integration - Taxi
## Field Trial Score Sheet

| A. Pre arrangements | score | cues | unable | N/A |
|---|---|---|---|---|
| Upon being asked to plan a trip using a taxi, the patient demonstrated the ability to plan ahead for the trip by: | | | | |
| 1. obtaining scheduling and reservation information | | | | |
| 2. identifying location of drop off site | | | | |
| 3. calling taxi service and giving appropriate information | | | | |
| 4. considering budget limitations (cost of fare, tip, etc.) | | | | |
| 5. allowing adequate time | | | | |
| 6. calling to confirm accessibility | | | | |
| **B. Transportation** | | | | |
| Upon learning the address and location where the patient needs to go, the patient demonstrated the ability to arrange transportation by: | | | | |
| 1. obtaining fare and schedule information, if needed | | | | |
| 2. making a reservation | | | | |
| 3. knowing emergency transportation options | | | | |
| **C. Accessibility** | | | | |
| The patient compensated for accessibility barriers by: | | | | |
| 1. choosing an appropriate site to meet the taxi | | | | |
| 2. managing to enter and exit the taxi and to use appropriate restraints | | | | |
| 3. determining the best way to reach, carry, and stow luggage and equipment. | | | | |
| 4. interacting appropriately with others to solve problems | | | | |
| **D. Emergency/Safety** | | | | |
| When presented with a hypothetical emergency situation, the patient demonstrated the ability to respond appropriately by: | | | | |
| 1. showing awareness of and consideration for the options available | | | | |
| 2. choosing the safest and most reasonable option with regard to the situation at hand | | | | |
| **E. Equipment** | | | | |
| The patient demonstrated the ability to anticipate the types of equipment and supplies that s/he needed by: | | | | |
| 1. having the necessary equipment throughout the trip | | | | |
| 2. having the necessary medical supplies throughout the trip | | | | |

**Summary:**

Score: _____ out of _____ applicable questions.

Patient: _____ Therapist: _____ Date: _____

# Module 4C  Train

You have decided to visit your relatives who live two states away. Since you have always wanted to travel by train, you decide to take the opportunity. In planning your trip, there are several decisions to make in order to assure a safe and comfortable journey.

## A. Pre-arrangements
1. Where will you find information about train schedules and routes?
2. What resources are available to you?
3. How much in advance should you make reservations?
4. How will you pay for your ticket?
5. Where will you pay for and pick up your ticket?
6. Will they provide you with written information about accessibility?
7. How close to your destination will the train take you?
8. How will you travel the remaining distance?
9. Are there special dietary arrangements you need to make?
10. How should you arrange this?

## B. Packing and Luggage
1. What will you need to take on the trip?
2. How will you pack?
3. What type of luggage will you choose to use? Why?
4. Have you labeled your luggage?
5. How will you transport your luggage?
6. Where will your extra equipment be stored?
7. How and where will your wheelchair be stored?

## C. Transportation
1. How will you travel to and from the train station?
2. Do you know the route to the station? Might traffic be a problem for you?
3. Is special parking available for individuals with disabilities?
4. How will you get into the station from the parking lot?
5. How will you get to your departure gate?

## D. Accessibility
1. Is the train accessible?
2. Will you need assistance boarding the train?
3. Where will you sit?
4. Will you transfer to a seat or sit in your wheelchair?
5. Will the seat cushion on the train offer adequate support for you?
6. When will you board the train?
7. Will you be able to move from car to car?
8. How can you find out about accessibility and special services at the other stations?

## E. Emergency
1. What will you do if your train is late, and you have to cath yourself or go to the bathroom?
2. What could you do to be prepared for cathing?
3. Are the bathrooms accessible?
4. What would you do if your medications were lost?
5. Will you need to bring any medications so that you don't miss any doses?

6. Do you recognize the symptoms of concern related to your disability i.e. dysreflexia, seizure, diabetes.
7. Do you carry information about these conditions to be used in emergencies?

**F. Equipment**
1. What equipment will you need for the train ride?
2. What equipment will you need once you arrive at your destination?

Flesch Grade Level 7.5

Score: _____ out of _____ applicable questions

Patient: _____ Therapist: _____ Date: _____

# Community Integration - Train
## Field Trial Score Sheet

| A. Pre arrangements | score | cues | unable | N/A |
|---|---|---|---|---|
| Upon being asked to plan a trip on the train, the patient demonstrated the ability to plan ahead by: | | | | |
| 1.  obtaining information on schedules and location(s) of stations | | | | |
| 2.  paying for and picking up tickets | | | | |
| 3.  understanding basic rights granted to travelers who are disabled | | | | |
| 4.  arranging food and beverage service as needed | | | | |
| 5.  determining the clothing supplies, and equipment needed for the trip | | | | |
| 6.  allowing adequate time | | | | |
| 7.  calling to confirm accessibility | | | | |
| **B. Transportation** | | | | |
| Upon learning the address and location of the departure and destination train stations, the patient demonstrated the ability to arrange further transportation to and from the train by: | | | | |
| 1.  considering all transportation alternatives and choosing one | | | | |
| 2.  obtaining fare and schedule information, if needed | | | | |
| 3.  making a reservation, if needed | | | | |
| 4.  considering parking arrangements, if needed | | | | |
| 5.  knowing emergency transportation options | | | | |
| **C. Accessibility** | | | | |
| The patient compensated for accessibility barriers by: | | | | |
| 1.  choosing the best entrance and entering the station and the train | | | | |
| 2.  managing entrance and exit through turnstiles | | | | |
| 3.  determining the best way to reach, carry, and stow luggage and equipment | | | | |
| 4.  managing the check in procedure | | | | |
| 5.  interacting appropriately with others to solve problems | | | | |
| **D. Emergency/Safety** | | | | |
| When presented with a hypothetical emergency situation, the patient demonstrated the ability to respond appropriately by: | | | | |
| 1.  showing awareness of and consideration for the options available | | | | |
| 2.  choosing the safest and most reasonable option with regard to the situation at hand | | | | |
| **E. Equipment** | | | | |
| The patient demonstrated the ability to anticipate the types of equipment and supplies that s/he needed by: | | | | |
| 1.  having the necessary equipment throughout the trip | | | | |
| 2.  having the necessary medical supplies throughout the trip | | | | |

**Summary:**



Score: _____ out of _____ applicable questions.

Patient: _____ Therapist: _____ Date: _____

# Module 4D  Air Travel

Because of the low fares, you are planning a trip by air and there are many questions that you need to answer prior getting on to the plane.

You will be expected to visit with airport personnel or other air travelers so that they can assist you in learning answers to the following questions.

## A. Pre-arrangements

1. How far in advance should you make reservations?
2. How will you pay for your ticket?
3. Where will you pay for and pick up your ticket?
4. Will the airline require that you travel with an attendant? Must you pay for your attendant's ticket?
5. Can you get your boarding pass in advance?
6. Will you require an aisle seat? Does that aisle have removable aisle armrests?
7. What are the dimensions of your wheelchair?
8. Will the aisle of the airplane accommodate your chair?
9. Does the carrier have an on-board wheelchair?
10. Are the bathrooms accessible?
11. If you use an electric wheelchair will your battery need to be packaged to meet hazardous material concerns?
12. Do you want to purchase insurance?
13. Where do you do that?
14. Does the airline have a printed statement describing the rules or regulations for disabled individuals flying on their airline?
15. Where could you write for this information?
16. Do you have special dietary restrictions?
17. Are there special dietary arrangements you need to make?
18. How should you do this?
19. How much in advance would the airlines like you to be at the airport departure gate?

## B. Packing and Luggage

1. What will you need to take on the trip?
2. How will you pack?
3. What type of luggage will you choose to use? Why?
4. Have you labeled your luggage?
5. How will you transport your luggage?
6. Where will your extra equipment be stored?
7. How and where will your wheelchair be stored?
8. Have you considered the your medical needs during the trip? Are those items including any medications and adapted equipment packed separately?
9. How many bags are you allowed to take with you?
10. Is there a charge per bag if you exceed this number?

## C. Transportation

1. How will you travel to and from the airport?
2. Is there special parking available for the disabled?
3. How will you get into the airport from the parking lot?
4. How will you get to your departure gate?
5. If you plan to drive a van, does it have an oversize roof? Does this need special parking? How convenient is the parking to the airport?

6. If you plan to leave your car, which long term parking lot is accessible, and are the vans that transport you to the airport accessible?
7. What transportation will you need once you reach your destination?
8. How much time do you assume you will need to get to the airport?
9. Do you know the route to the airport and have you considered traffic conditions?

### D. Accessibility
1. Is there a special entrance for wheelchairs?
2. How will you get from one floor to another?
3. How will you enter or exit if there are turnstiles?
4. How will you get to your departure gate?
5. How will you go through the airport security system?
6. Do you need any special letters for metal implants?
7. Are the airplane aisles accessible?
8. Must you transfer to a passenger seat, or is there space for your chair?
9. How will you board the plane?
10. When?
11. How will you learn about accessibility and special assistance available at other airports?

### E. Emergency/Safety
1. Are the bathrooms accessible?
2. If not, what alternative do you have?
3. How should you brace yourself in the event of an emergency landing?
4. Will you need to bring any medications so that you don't miss any doses?
5. Do you recognize the symptoms of concern for your diagnosis, i.e., dysreflexia, disabetes, seizures?
6. Are the bathrooms accessible?

### F. Equipment
1. What equipment will you need to take on the plane?
2. What equipment will you need with you?
3. What equipment will you need once you've reached your destination?

Flesch Grade Level 7.9

Score: _____ out of _____ applicable questions

Patient: _____ Therapist: _____ Date: _____

# Community Integration - Air Travel
## Field Trial Score Sheet

| A. Pre arrangements | score | cues | unable | N/A |
|---|---|---|---|---|
| Upon being asked to plan a trip using an airplane, the patient demonstrated the ability to plan ahead for the trip by: | | | | |
| 1.   determining how and when to get tickets | | | | |
| 2.   determining if an attendant will be needed, and who will be paying for the attendant's ticket | | | | |
| 3.   determining when and where to use the mobility equipment provided by the airlines | | | | |
| 4.   planning adequate time to carry out needed functions | | | | |
| 5.   determining dietary needs and how to satisfy them | | | | |
| 6.   calling to confirm accessibility | | | | |
| **B. Packing and Luggage** | | | | |
| Once deciding to take the trip, the patient demonstrated the ability to select appropriate luggage and to pack by: | | | | |
| 1.   determining the correct amount of each item required for the trip | | | | |
| 2.   selecting the appropriate containers in which to pack the items | | | | |
| 3.   determining which items must be carried on the plane and which items may be stowed in the luggage compartment | | | | |
| **C. Transportation** | | | | |
| The patient will be able to demonstrate the ability to get to and from the airport by: | | | | |
| 1.   considering all transportation alternatives and choosing one | | | | |
| 2.   obtaining fare and schedule information, if needed | | | | |
| 3.   making a reservation, if needed | | | | |
| 4.   considering parking arrangements, if needed | | | | |
| 5.   knowing emergency transportation options | | | | |
| **D. Accessibility** | | | | |
| The patient compensated for accessibility barriers by: | | | | |
| 1.   choosing the best entrance and entering the airport | | | | |
| 2.   determining accessibility of the jetway, armrests, and bathrooms. | | | | |
| 3.   determining the best way to reach, carry, and stow luggage and equipment | | | | |
| 4.   managing the check in procedure | | | | |
| 5.   interacting appropriately with others to solve problems | | | | |
| **E. Emergency/Safety** | | | | |
| When presented with a hypothetical emergency situation, the patient demonstrated the ability to respond appropriately by: | | | | |
| 1.   showing awareness of and consideration for the options available | | | | |
| 2.   choosing the safest and most reasonable option with regard to the situation at hand | | | | |
| **F. Equipment** | | | | |
| The patient demonstrated the ability to anticipate the types of equipment and supplies that s/he needed by: | | | | |
| 1.   having the necessary equipment throughout the trip | | | | |
| 2.   having the necessary medical supplies throughout the trip | | | | |

**Summary:**




Score: _____ out of _____ applicable questions.


Patient: _____ Therapist: _____ Date: _____

# Module 4E  City Bus

You have decided to spend the day visiting friends. The city bus offers the easiest transportation to your destination. You have several choices and things to consider before making this outing.

*Note: This evaluation should be completed after an environmental awareness evaluation determining your pathfinding and understanding of safety in the community.*

### A. Pre-arrangements
1. Where will you find information for the city bus schedules and routes? What resources are available to you? Is there a phone number for you to call?
2. How much time will you allow yourself to catch the bus?
3. How much does a one-way or a round trip bus fare cost? When will you pay the driver?
4. Will you need exact change?
5. If you plan to ride the bus often, have you considered purchasing a bus pass? How much do they cost?
6. Where can you buy them?
7. How close to where you want to go will the bus take you?
8. Is the area in which you will be dropped off accessible?
9. How will you travel the remaining distance?

### B. Transportation
1. What reasonable changes in the route or the service will the bus be able to make for you?
2. Is there a van service in your area?
3. What are the requirements for this service?

### C. Accessibility
1. How will you tell which buses are accessible?
2. Will you need help boarding the bus?
3. Do you know if the bus drivers are allowed to physically help you?
4. Where will you sit on the bus?
5. Once on the bus, will you transfer to a seat?
6. If not, how will you secure your wheelchair for the bus ride?
7. What help will you need on the ride? Who will you ask for help?
8. How will you let the driver know you want to get off the bus?
9. What safety features do you need to know about the bus?

### D. Emergency/Safety
1. How will you brace yourself in the event of an accident?
2. What will you do if the bus is full or has a broken lift and can't pick you up?
3. Will you need to bring any medications so that you don't miss any doses?
4. Do you recognize the symptoms of concern for your diagnosis?
5. What will you do if you need a bathroom?
6. What will you do if you get on the wrong bus?

### E. Equipment
1. What special equipment will you need for the bus trip?
2. What equipment will you need for your planned outing?

Flesch Grade Level 8.3

Score: _____ out of _____ applicable questions

Patient: _____ Therapist: _____ Date: _____

# Community Integration - City Bus
## Field Trial Score Sheet

| A. Pre arrangements | score | cues | unable | N/A |
|---|---|---|---|---|
| Upon being asked to plan a trip using the city bus, the patient demonstrated the ability to plan ahead for the trip by: | | | | |
| 1.   obtaining scheduling and route information | | | | |
| 2.   identifying the locations of the bus stops s/he needed | | | | |
| 3.   ensuring that s/he knew what the bus fare was and had appropriate change (or a pass) | | | | |
| 4.   considering time limitations | | | | |
| 5.   calling to confirm accessibility | | | | |
| **B. Transportation** | | | | |
| Upon learning the bus route(s) and time schedule, the patient demonstrated the ability to use the city bus as demonstrated by: | | | | |
| 1.   considering all route and schedule alternatives and choosing one | | | | |
| 2.   obtaining fare information, if needed | | | | |
| 3.   determining when and if s/he qualified for special services, and how to ask for those services | | | | |
| 4.   determining how to travel from the bus stop to his/her destination | | | | |
| 5.   knowing emergency transportation options | | | | |
| **C. Accessibility** | | | | |
| The patient compensated for accessibility barriers by: | | | | |
| 1.   choosing routes, scheduled buses, and stops that were accessible | | | | |
| 2.   managing getting in and of the vehicle and using appropriate restraint systems | | | | |
| 3.   choosing the best alternatives for carrying packages and equipment | | | | |
| 4.   managing the fare paying procedure | | | | |
| 5.   interacting appropriately with others to solve problems | | | | |
| **D. Emergency/Safety** | | | | |
| When presented with a hypothetical emergency situation, the patient demonstrated the ability to respond appropriately by: | | | | |
| 1.   showing awareness of and consideration for the options available | | | | |
| 2.   choosing the safest and most reasonable option with regard to the situation at hand | | | | |
| **E. Equipment** | | | | |
| The patient demonstrated the ability to anticipate the types of equipment and supplies that s/he needed by: | | | | |
| 1.   having the necessary equipment throughout the trip | | | | |
| 2.   having the necessary medical supplies throughout the trip | | | | |

**Summary:**




Score: _____ out of _____ applicable questions.


Patient: _____ Therapist: _____ Date: _____

# Therapeutic Recreation: Community Integration Evaluation

**Assessment of City Bus Skills**

Key:    (+) = independent function, affirmative response, or demonstrates appropriate knowledge
(-) = patient needs assistance, negative response, or the lack of appropriate knowledge
(N/A) = not applicable
(N/T) = not tested

Patient is a _____ with a diagnosis of _____
evaluated on _____ to assess the following skills:

## I. Pre-phase

**A. Demonstrates orientation, knowledge, or memory of:**
_____ date and time of evaluation
_____ appropriate dress and grooming needed for weather
_____ purpose of the evaluation
_____ information regarding bus system (i.e., schedule, information
       phone numbers, bus station/stops)
**Comments:**

**B. Demonstrates memory of:**
_____ destination and correct bus number
_____ money needed
_____ medical necessities (i.e., pressure release, meds., splints/braces)
**Comments:**

## II. Future Leisure Phase

**A. Demonstrates orientation, knowledge, and memory of:**
_____ destination and correct bus number(s)
_____ alternative means of transportation
_____ bus schedule
_____ recreation/leisure sites or facilities accessible by bus system
       (i.e., parks, malls, health clubs)
**Comments:**

### III. Management phase

**A. Functional Behaviors: Demonstrates ability to:**
_____ negotiate curbs, ramps, doorways, board and depart bus
_____ tolerate activity
_____ scan/locate all necessary information: signs, bus number, bus schedule
**Comments:**

**B. Cognitive Behaviors: Demonstrates ability to:**
_____ locate all areas requested
_____ manage money during outing
_____ stay on task
_____ make safe judgments about traffic
_____ communicate needs to others
**Comments:**

**C. Social Behaviors: Demonstrates:**
_____ consistently positive social interactions
_____ appropriate and realistic comfort level in community setting
_____ appropriate response to authority or conflict
**Comments:**

**Assessment:**

**Recommendations:**

**Bus pass received:**
    **Permanent** _____
    **Temporary** _____

**Therapist** _____ **Date** _____ **Time Spent** _____

# Module 4F  Bus Station

With extra time on your hands, you have decided to travel cross country for a month. You have plenty of time set aside for a leisurely trip, so you've chosen to travel by bus to see more of the country.

There are several decisions you need to make to assure a safe and comfortable trip.

## A. Pre-arrangements
1. Where will you find information regarding different bus company schedules, routes, and fares?
2. What information resources are available to you?
3. How much in advance should you make reservations?
4. How will you pay for your ticket?
5. Where will you pay for and pick up your ticket?
6. Does the bus company have special regulations regarding travel by the disabled on their bus line?
7. How can you find out?
8. How close to your final destination will the bus take you?
9. How will you travel the remaining distance?

## B. Packing and Luggage
1. What will you need to take on the trip?
2. How will you pack?
3. What type of luggage will you choose to use? Why?
4. Have you labeled your luggage?
5. How will you transport your luggage between the bus and other transportation?
6. Where will your extra equipment be stored?
7. How and where will your wheelchair be stored?
8. Do you want to take your own food?

## C. Transportation
1. How will you travel to and from the bus station?
2. Do you know the route to the bus depot, and have you considered traffic conditions?
3. Is there special parking for the disabled?
4. How will you get into the station from the parking lot?
5. How will you get to your departure gate?

## D. Accessibility
1. Is the bus accessible?
2. Will you require assistance boarding the bus?
3. Are the aisles of the bus accessible?
4. Where will you sit on the bus?
5. Will you transfer to a seat or use your wheelchair?
6. When will you board the bus?
7. How will you learn about accessibility and special assistance available at other bus terminals?

## E. Emergency/Safety
1. How will you brace yourself in the event of an accident?
2. What will you do if you have to cath yourself or go to the bathroom?
3. What could you do to prepare for this?
4. Will you need to bring any medications so that you don't miss any doses?

5. Do you recognize the symptoms of concern for your diagnosis, i.e., dysreflexia, disabetes, seizures?
6. Are the bathrooms accessible?

**F. Equipment**
1. What special equipment will you need for the bus trip?
2. What equipment will you need once you've reached your destination?

Flesch Grade Level 7.2

Score: _____ out of _____ applicable questions

Patient: _____ Therapist: _____ Date: _____

# Community Integration - Bus Station
## Field Trial Score Sheet

| A. Pre arrangements | score | cues | unable | N/A |
|---|---|---|---|---|
| Upon being asked to plan a trip to the bus station, the patient demonstrated the ability to plan ahead for the trip by: | | | | |
| 1. being able to find information on bus companies, schedules, routes, and fares | | | | |
| 2. determining how to obtain a ticket | | | | |
| 3. determining if any regulations concerning disabled travelers apply to him/her | | | | |
| 4. determining how to get from the bus station to final destination | | | | |
| 5. considering budget limitations | | | | |
| 6. considering time limitations | | | | |
| 7. calling to confirm accessibility | | | | |
| **B. Transportation** | | | | |
| Upon learning the address and location of the bus station, the patient demonstrated the ability to arrange transportation by: | | | | |
| 1. considering all transportation alternatives and choosing one | | | | |
| 2. obtaining fare and schedule information, if needed | | | | |
| 3. making a reservation, if needed | | | | |
| 4. considering parking arrangements, if needed | | | | |
| 5. knowing emergency transportation options | | | | |
| **C. Accessibility** | | | | |
| The patient compensated for barriers to accessibility by: | | | | |
| 1. managing street barriers (curbs, crosswalks, and rough sidewalks) | | | | |
| 2. managing architectural barriers (doors, stairs, turnstiles) | | | | |
| 3. choosing the best alternatives for carrying luggage and equipment | | | | |
| 4. managing the public bathrooms and food services | | | | |
| 5. managing the check in procedure | | | | |
| 6. knowing emergency transportation options | | | | |
| **D. Emergency/Safety** | | | | |
| When presented with a hypothetical emergency situation, the patient demonstrated the ability to respond appropriately by: | | | | |
| 1. showing awareness of and consideration for the options available | | | | |
| 2. choosing the safest and most reasonable option with regard to the situation at hand | | | | |
| **E. Equipment** | | | | |
| The patient demonstrated the ability to anticipate the types of equipment and supplies that s/he needed by: | | | | |
| 1. having the necessary equipment throughout the trip | | | | |
| 2. having the necessary medical supplies throughout the trip | | | | |

**Summary:**


Score: _____ out of _____ applicable questions.


Patient: _____ Therapist: _____ Date: _____

# 12. Physical Activity

One of the main focuses of our program is to introduce leisure activities that encourage physical fitness. We do this for each patient by determining his/her interest and potential, reviewing adaptations and community resources available in the discharge area, and considering significant medical concerns. One observation that is worth passing along is that activities with peers are often better received than reintegration into mainstream activities.

We run a once a week aquatics program, off site. Our goal is to promote not only the physical activity of swimming, but also to encourage the activity for positive social and emotional benefits.

Wheel chair sports are promoted as a potential leisure based physical activity in our area. However, as hospital stays are shortened, the medical condition of the patient is usually still compromised at discharge. Instead of expecting active participation during the short stays, we make sure that the patient has all of the information s/he will need to participate when his/her condition allows it. This may include community outings to local wheelchair sports training or events. The information includes:

- resources for participation in wheelchair sports
- adaptations for activity
- newsletter resource for updates
- outpatient referrals for training

# Module 5A  Aquatics

It is a hot sunny day and your friends have asked you to go swimming with them. Please consider the following before you leave your home.

## A. Pre-arrangements/Transportation
1. How are you going to the swimming area?
2. What resources are available to determine whether the swimming area is accessible?
3. How are you going to get home?
4. Will you need money for admission and locker fees?

## B. Dressing Skills
1. Are you going to change clothes once you get to the swimming area?
2. Would it be more convenient to change clothes at home?
3. Will you need assistance dressing? If so, will there be someone you may ask for help?
4. Are there dressing facilities available at the swimming area? Do they include accessible mats, benches and lower lockers?
5. Can you direct someone to assist you?
6. How will you carry your wet clothes and equipment?

## C. Transfers
1. How do you plan to get into the water?
2. How will you get out?
3. Will you need assistance? If so, will you know whom to ask for help? Can you direct them?

## D. Swimming Skills and Safety Precautions
1. Have you been swimming since your hospitalization?
2. Do you know how to swim? Can you float?
3. Which strokes do you know?
4. Which stroke is your strongest?
5. What floatation devices do you plan to use?
6. Will these devices be available?
7. Will you swim alone?
8. Will you swim in an area with a lifeguard?
9. Will you need assistance while you are in the water? If so, whom will you ask for help?
10. Will you jump into the water without testing the depth first?
11. Where will be your best place to enter the water? Why? (lifts, stairs, ramps)
12. How are you going to protect your legs and feet from dragging on the bottom?

## E. Emergency
1. What will you do in an emergency?
2. Do you carry identification on your person?
3. Does your identification include phone numbers of family or friends to contact? Medical doctor? Special precautions?
4. Should you inform the lifeguards of special needs you might have?
5. Will you need to bring any medications so that you don't miss your next dose?
6. Do you recognize the symptoms of concern for your diagnosis, i.e., dysreflexia, disabetes, seizures?
7. Are the bathrooms accessible?

**F. Equipment**

1. What clothes and supplies are you going to need for swimming? (bathing suit, cap, towel, goggles, soap, shampoo, brush and comb, flotation equipment, clean clothes)
2. Do you need special medical equipment? (cath kit, cath clip, gizmo)
3. What other equipment needs can you think of?
4. Do you have sunscreen? Are you taking any photo sensitive drugs?

Flesch Grade Level 7.0

Score: _____ out of _____ applicable questions

Patient: _____ Therapist: _____ Date: _____

# Community Integration - Aquatics
## Field Trial Score Sheet

| A. Pre arrangements/Transportation | score | cues | unable | N/A |
|---|---|---|---|---|
| Upon being asked to plan a trip to go swimming, the patient demonstrated the ability to plan ahead by: | | | | |
| 1.   determining an appropriate means to get to/from the swimming area | | | | |
| 2.   determining if, and how much of, the swimming area was accessible (including the bathrooms) | | | | |
| 3.   considering budget limitations (admission, locker fees, etc.) | | | | |
| 4.   considering time limitations | | | | |
| **B. Dressing Skills** | | | | |
| Upon deciding to go swimming, the patient demonstrated the ability to manage dressing and clothing issues by: | | | | |
| 1.   determining an appropriate place to change clothes | | | | |
| 2.   determining needed assistance with dressing and helpers | | | | |
| 3.   determining if the dressing areas were accessible and had mats, benches, and lower lockers | | | | |
| 4.   being able to describe and direct the assistance that was needed | | | | |
| 5.   determining how to carry wet clothing and other equipment | | | | |
| **C. Transfers** | | | | |
| When asked to discuss/problem solve issues related to transfers, the patient was able to: | | | | |
| 1.   determine how to get into and out of the water | | | | |
| 2.   describe/direct the type(s) of assistance that s/he needed | | | | |
| **D. Swimming Skills and Safety Precautions** | | | | |
| Once the patient decided to go swimming, s/he was able to identify personal swimming skills and safety precautions by: | | | | |
| 1.   being able to identify the special skills that s/he was able to do | | | | |
| 2.   being able to identify the types of flotation devices that s/he required and where to get these devices | | | | |
| 3.   explaining the pros and cons of swimming without a lifeguard and/or a partner | | | | |
| 4.   demonstrating an adequate knowledge of safety rules related to entering the water | | | | |
| 5.   demonstrating an adequate knowledge of the mechanical steps to getting it and out of the water | | | | |
| 6.    demonstrating the ability to maintain skin integrity while swimming | | | | |
| **D. Emergency/Safety** | | | | |
| When presented with a hypothetical emergency situation, the patient demonstrated the ability to respond appropriately by: | | | | |
| 1.   showing awareness of and consideration for the options available | | | | |
| 2.   choosing the safest and most reasonable option with regard to the situation at hand | | | | |
| **E. Equipment** | | | | |
| The patient demonstrated the ability to anticipate the types of equipment and supplies that s/he needed by: | | | | |
| 1.   having the necessary equipment throughout the trip | | | | |
| 2.   having the necessary medical supplies throughout the trip | | | | |

**Summary:**


Score: _____ out of _____ applicable questions.

Patient: _____ Therapist: _____ Date: _____

# Therapeutic Recreation: Community Integration Evaluation

**Aquatics Program**

Key:    (+) = independent function, affirmative response, or demonstrates appropriate knowledge
          (-) = patient needs assistance, negative response, or the lack of appropriate knowledge
          (N/A) = not applicable
          (N/T) = not tested

Patient is a _____ with a diagnosis of _____
seen on _____ to assess the following skills:

## I. Pre-planning

### A. Demonstrates orientation, knowledge, and/or memory of:
_____ commitment
_____ timeliness
_____ appropriate dress/equipment/medical needs

**Comments:**

## II. Clinical ADL Carryover

### A. Demonstrates ability to carry over:
_____ dressing
_____ lower extremity
_____ upper extremity
_____ safety/judgment

**Comments:**

## III. Community Skills

### A. Demonstrates knowledge and ability regarding:
_____ wheelchair mobility
_____ architectural barriers: door, rough ground, level surfaces
_____ entering and exiting pool
_____ following directions
_____ general pathfinding
_____ safety/judgment

**Comments:**

**IV. Adaptive Aquatics/Techniques**
    **A. Demonstrates ability of:**
    \_\_\_\_\_ flotation
    \_\_\_\_\_ ROM
    \_\_\_\_\_ balance/ambulation
    \_\_\_\_\_ adaptive technique
    \_\_\_\_\_ back float
    \_\_\_\_\_ safety/judgment
**Comments:**

**V. Family Education**
    **A. Investment/knowledge**
    \_\_\_\_\_ family involvement
    \_\_\_\_\_ continued involvement
**Comments:**

**Previous Swimming Ability: \_\_\_\_\_ participated \_\_\_\_\_ did not participate**
**Assessment:**

**Recommendations:**

**Therapist _____ Date _____ Time Spent: _____**

# Module 5B  Wheelchair Sports

This module is organized differently from the other modules. It is designed more for orientation and observation than as a treatment protocol. Wheelchair athletes, equipment displays and demonstrations, slide presentations, and patient observation of various sports in action will serve as the main teaching tools. Patients will be expected to attend the orientation sessions, and participation will be optional.

Suggested areas of concentration for this module may include:

1. Resources describing community sports activities
2. Transportation and accessibility
3. Special skills required for individual sports
4. Adapted rules and regulations
5. Skin care
6. Equipment

Suggested orientation sessions might include:

1. Community speakers representing various sports interests for the disabled
2. Slide shows depicting equipment
3. Athletes demonstrating equipment
4. Athletes demonstrating the sport as well as rule adaptations
5. Equipment displays that include required and optional equipment for each individual sport

# Module 5C  Leisure Activities

You are going to (scuba dive, camp, hike, hunt, sail, ride horses, etc.) this weekend. Consider the following questions to be sure that you will have a successful leisure experience.

## A. Pre-arrangements
1. Will you need to apply for a license?
2. Will you require re-certification?
3. Have you been medically cleared for the activity?
4. Do you know where you are going?
5. Do you need to let the place know you have special needs?
6. Are there special newspapers or magazines that tell you about new leisure opportunities?
7. How much money will you need to spend?
8. Will you need special training or tests?
9. Can the facility provide lessons?
10. Have they worked with people with disabilities? Should you check for special resources?

## B. Transportation
1. How will you get to the leisure site?
2. How close will you able to get to the site by car if there is rough ground?
3. If you need transportation (i.e., back to the launch site for white water rafting), is it accessible?
4. Is accessible parking available? Will your disabled parking permit be valid, even if you cross state lines?

## C. Accessibility
1. Is the area accessible? Will you need to provide equipment such as ramps to take full advantage of the area? Will you need an attendant?
2. Are the bathrooms accessible? What about showering facilities, water fountains, barbecue or cook areas? Are the campsites accessible?
3. How will you access, for example, the boat for fishing or water-skiing?
4. How should you secure yourself or your wheelchair in a boat?
5. Will you need supported seating?
6. Should you wear seat belts or shoulder harnesses?
7. Should you wear a helmet for safety?

## D. Emergency/Safety
1. Will you need to take special precautions to ensure skin integrity?
2. What special precautions should you take to ensure your safety and health?
3. Will you need to bring any medications so that you don't miss any doses?
4. Do you recognize the symptoms of concern for your diagnosis, i.e., dysreflexia, disabetes, seizures?
5. Are the bathrooms accessible?
6. How will you get out of, for example, a boat should there be an emergency?
7. Are you sensitive to heat or cold? Do you need to take special equipment because of the temperature?

## E. Equipment
1. What equipment will you need to meet your medical needs?
2. Do you need to regulate your fluids? Would dehydration be a concern in hot weather? What equipment or clothes should you take?

Flesch Grade Level 8.9

Score: _____ out of _____ applicable questions

Patient: _____ Therapist: _____ Date: _____

# Community Integration - Leisure Activities
## Field Trial Score Sheet

| A. Pre arrangements | score | cues | unable | N/A |
|---|---|---|---|---|
| Upon being asked to plan a leisure activity, the patient demonstrated the ability to plan ahead for the activity by: | | | | |
| 1.  obtaining the appropriate licenses, re-certifications, and clearances | | | | |
| 2.  identifying its location and the types of services available | | | | |
| 3.  identifying the amount of training and supervision needed | | | | |
| 4.  considering budget and equipment limitations | | | | |
| 5.  allocating adequate time | | | | |
| 6.  calling to confirm accessibility | | | | |
| **B. Transportation** | | | | |
| Upon learning the address and location of the activity, the patient demonstrated the ability to arrange transportation to the activity by: | | | | |
| 1.  considering all transportation alternatives and choosing one | | | | |
| 2.  obtaining fare and schedule information, if needed | | | | |
| 3.  making a reservation, if needed | | | | |
| 4.  considering parking arrangements, if needed | | | | |
| 5.  knowing emergency transportation options | | | | |
| **C. Accessibility** | | | | |
| The patient compensated for accessibility barriers by: | | | | |
| 1.  choosing the best method of entering and moving through the site (pathfinding) | | | | |
| 2.  determining the best way to access the bathrooms, etc. | | | | |
| 3.  choosing the best way to access the activity | | | | |
| 4.  choosing appropriate seating, harnessing, and other safety equipment | | | | |
| 5.  interacting appropriately with others to solve problems | | | | |
| **D. Emergency/Safety** | | | | |
| When presented with a hypothetical emergency situation, the patient demonstrated the ability to respond appropriately by: | | | | |
| 1.  showing awareness of and consideration for the options available | | | | |
| 2.  choosing the safest and most reasonable option with regard to the situation at hand | | | | |
| **E. Equipment** | | | | |
| The patient demonstrated the ability to anticipate the types of equipment and supplies that s/he needed by: | | | | |
| 1.  having the necessary equipment throughout the duration of the activity | | | | |
| 2.  having the necessary medical supplies throughout the duration of the activity | | | | |

**Summary**


Score: _____ out of _____ applicable questions.

Patient: _____ Therapist: _____ Date: _____

# 13. Independent Plan

The purpose of this module is to provide a final chapter to the community integration program by giving the patient a chance to use all of his skills to successfully integrate into the community. In this module the individual patient takes the leadership role by doing all of the planning for an activity. Whether the activity is for a group of patients or a family outing, the patient will need to:

- determine the interests and preferences of the rest of the group,
- consider everyone's physical and cognitive limitations,
- recognize how much support is needed to complete the activity safely,
- identify medical needs for all of the participants,
- identify architectural barriers, transportation and financial concerns,
- combine a leisure activity with a learning experience.

We do not use a pre-test, field trial, and post-test for this module. Usually the plan is developed informally with the therapist and other patients during leisure education sessions.

After the environmental and transportation modules this is the module that gets the most attention from the patients. Some are appalled at being asked to do the "therapist's job". Some comment how unaware they were of all the things that the therapist considered.

Taking a patient into the community whose etiology is suicide requires extra thought from the CTRS and the rest of the treatment team. The following story shows a situation that the therapeutic recreation staff was presented with ...

*A middle aged male, clinically depressed, attempted suicide by jumping from a bridge This resulted in a bilateral amputation of the lower extremity. Toward the end of his rehabilitation stay this patient was ready for an outing using the Independent Patient Plan. The patient selected the 605 foot high Seattle Space Needle for a group community outing and fulfilled all obligations of pre-planning and organization. The therapist was faced with several questions regarding the advisability of this outing such as: Why does he want to go to the Space Needle? Is he considering another suicide attempt or does he just like high places? Should I cancel the outing for the safety of the patient? (The therapist called the Space Needle to confirm that the new "jump proof" fence had been installed around the entire observatory platform prior to agreeing to the outing.)*

Giving the patient the opportunity to plan his/her own leisure activity outside of the hospital, gives the patient valuable insight into the real impact of his/her disability and the real difficulties of participating independently in leisure activities. By being able to solve the problems, even one time, with the support of a knowledgeable and supportive therapist, the patient greatly increases his/her chances of taking charge of his/her leisure lifestyle after discharge.

We recommend, if possible, that each patient plan two independent activities. This allows the therapist and the patient time to work out the various barriers to leisure involvement prior to being discharged from the therapeutic recreation service.

# Module 6A  Independent Patient Plan

☐ pre-test   ☐ post-test

You have decided to plan an outing of your choice. Below you will find some general questions for you to consider before leaving for your outing.

**Type of Activity:** _____

## A. Pre-arrangements

1. Have you decided where you and the group would like to go?
2. What resources are available to help you make your plans?
3. How much time will you allow for the activity? Have you allowed enough time to meet your commitments?
4. Will you need reservations?
5. How will you handle this?
6. Will you be taking other people?
7. Have you considered their leisure interests?
8. Have you thought about how to support the patients who are coming with you? Will you need additional volunteers?
9. Have you told the staff and participating patients when you will need to leave?
10. Will you need money?

## B. Transportation

1. How do you plan to travel to your destination? (If traveling by bus, train, taxi, airplane or personal vehicle, see appropriate module and related questions.)
2. What alternative transportation might you need?

## C. Accessibility

1. Is the site accessible?
2. How can you learn more about the accessibility to the area?
3. Are the bathrooms accessible?
4. Do you know about the standards established by the Americans with Disabilities Act?

## D. Emergency/Safety

1. What emergency conditions might you encounter?
2. How will you be prepared to handle an emergency?
3. Will you need to bring any medications so that you don't miss any doses?
4. Do you recognize the symptoms of concern for your diagnosis, i.e., dysreflexia, disabetes, seizures?

## E. Equipment

1. What equipment will you require for your outing?

Flesch Grade Level 8.4

Score: _____ out of _____ applicable questions

Patient: _____   Therapist: _____   Date: _____

# Community Integration - Independent Plan
## Field Trial Score Sheet

| | score | cues | unable | N/A |
|---|---|---|---|---|
| **A. Pre arrangements** | | | | |
| Upon being asked to plan a leisure activity, the patient demonstrated the ability to plan ahead for the activity by: | | | | |
| 1.  choosing an appropriate activity | | | | |
| 2.  identifying the types of resources and equipment needed to participate in the activity | | | | |
| 3.  determining if (and how) to make reservations/obtain a ticket | | | | |
| 4.  considering budget limitations | | | | |
| 5.  determining how much time should be scheduled for the activity | | | | |
| 6.  calling to confirm accessibility | | | | |
| **B. Transportation** | | | | |
| Upon determining the address and location of the activity, the patient demonstrated the ability to arrange transportation by: | | | | |
| 1.  considering all transportation alternatives and choosing one | | | | |
| 2.  obtaining fare and schedule information, if needed | | | | |
| 3.  making a reservation, if needed | | | | |
| 4.  considering parking arrangements, if needed | | | | |
| 5.  knowing emergency transportation options | | | | |
| **C. Accessibility** | | | | |
| The patient compensated for accessibility barriers by: | | | | |
| 1.  managing street/path barriers (curbs, crosswalks, and rough sidewalks/terrain) | | | | |
| 2.  managing architectural barriers (doors, stairs, turnstiles) | | | | |
| 3.  managing geographical barriers (hills, dips, water) | | | | |
| 4.  choosing the best alternatives for carrying supplies and purchases | | | | |
| 5.  managing the public bathrooms and food services | | | | |
| 6.  interacting appropriately with others to solve problems | | | | |
| **D. Emergency/Safety** | | | | |
| When presented with a hypothetical emergency situation, the patient demonstrated the ability to respond appropriately by: | | | | |
| 1.  showing awareness of and consideration for the options available | | | | |
| 2.  choosing the safest and most reasonable option with regard to the situation at hand | | | | |
| **E. Equipment** | | | | |
| The patient demonstrated the ability to anticipate the types of equipment and supplies that s/he needed by: | | | | |
| 1.  having the necessary equipment throughout the trip | | | | |
| 2.  having the necessary medical supplies throughout the trip | | | | |

**Summary:**




Score: _____ out of _____ applicable questions.

Patient: _____  Therapist: _____  Date: _____

# 14. Summary

The Community Integration Program has been in existence since 1980. It was originally designed to meet the needs of patients with new spinal cord injuries. Since that time it has been expanded at Harborview Medical Center to meet the needs of patients with traumatic brain injuries and psychiatric problems. In other facilities it has been used successfully in long term care, congregate care, hospice care, community transition programs, community special recreation programs, and community support programs. Modified versions have been successfully used with all age groups.

The program has been successful in educating individuals with physical, cognitive, and emotional disabilities how to successfully integrate into the community. In addition we had the added benefit that the rehabilitation team accepted therapeutic recreation as the community integration expert.

The patient response to the program has been a positive one. Initially, some patients expressed reluctance to participate in the program, indicating they felt the tasks were silly and the experiences all too familiar. It wasn't until these patients had completed the program that they expressed a positive attitude about it. Patients realized that, "Talking and thinking about an experience is one thing, but doing it is another."

Some patients realized that their ability to talk about doing something may be much better than their actual performance level. The modules provided a way to help the patients realize what their actual skill levels were and to help increase those skill levels so that they could participate in community activities successfully. Rehabilitation patient re-admitted to the hospital remarked that though they wouldn't have tackled the activity alone before, doing it once made it easier, and they felt that they would be more confident in future attempts.

Families have also responded with interest and support. They accompanied the patient on the evaluations, and modules were often distributed to family members to be used once the patient arrived home. This was particularly helpful for parents who were over-protective and reluctant to let the patient adventure into the community on his/her own. By following the module format and the therapist's role model, parents have the opportunity to learn to allow the patient greater independence. This eventually rewarded both the patient and the family by demonstrating to both exactly how many skills they both had. It was as much a learning process for the family as it was for the patient.

For example, one young wife, whose husband was on the rehabilitation unit, told us that she was convinced that they were still together 10 years later because she had gotten so much community experience before they left, and they had so much fun doing it that early on they recognized that there was life after rehabilitation.

We hope that you will be as successful using the Community Integration Program as we have been at Harborview Medical Center. Remember, if you have any suggestions, problems, or concerns, feel free to write us care of Idyll Arbor. We are always looking for ways to make the program better.

# Section 3

# *Related Information*

*"I'm going to turn these guys in. This damn building is not accessible."*

*"How do you know?"*

*"What do you mean, 'How do I know?' I can't get my wheelchair into the half the tables in this room. That's how I know!"*

*"Yeah, but look here. The ADA standards say that the building needs to handle 48" wheel chairs. Your wheelchair is just too big."*

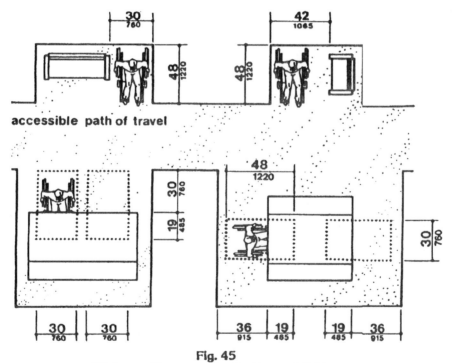

**Fig. 45**
**Minimum Clearances for Seating and Tables**

*"Oh."*

# 15. Glossary

By joan burlingame © 1994 Idyll Arbor, Inc.

*Note: The definitions contained in this glossary which have "(ADA)" before the definition indicate that the definition is the official definition found in the Americans with Disabilities Act regulations.*

**Abduction** Abduction refers to the process of moving a body part away from midline. In the case of the digits (the fingers or toes), abduction refers to the process of moving the digit away from the axis of the limb. Most leisure activities require some degree of abduction. These include walking (abduction of lower limbs, arms), cooking (abduction of arms in mixing), etc.

**Acceleration Factors in Head Injuries** If the patient has received an injury to his/her brain as a result of an accident involving movement, the therapist should expect significant neurological deficits. The movement of the brain against the skull (an acceleration injury) causes far more neurological damage to the brain then the action of crushing the stationary skull. An acceleration injury to the head causes significantly more damage to the brain then a crushing blow twenty times as intense to the skull. (Ylvisaker, 1985 p. 5)

**Access Aisle** (ADA) An accessible pedestrian space between elements, such as parking spaces, seating, and desks, that provides clearances appropriate for use of the elements.

**Accessible** (ADA) Legally defined, a site, building, or facility, (or a portion of one of these) is accessible if it complies with the ADA Accessibility Guidelines. Practically defined, a site, building, or facility (or a portion of one of these) is accessible to a patient if the patient can engage in normal uses.

**Accessible Element** (ADA) An element specified by the ADA regulations (for example, telephone, controls, and the like).

**Accessible Route** (ADA) A continuous unobstructed path connecting all accessible elements and spaces of a building or facility. Interior accessible routes may include corridors, floors, ramps, elevators, lifts, and clear floor space at fixtures. Exterior accessible routes may include parking access aisles, curb ramps, crosswalks at vehicular ways, walks, ramps, and lifts.

**Accessible Space** (ADA) Space that complies with the ADA regulations.

**Activity Intolerance** When a patient has insufficient physiological or psychological energy to endure or complete a required task. Some of the measurable/observable characteristics would include the patient's verbal report of fatigue or weakness; an abnormal heart rate or blood pressure in response to activity; discomfort upon exertion; or an abnormal change in the patient's heart beat (e.g., arrhythmias).

**Acute Stage** The first of two or more phases of an illness or disease. This stage is usually somewhat severe and short in duration. The acute stage of tissue and bone damage usually involves a decrease in leisure options caused by pain without exertion, inflammation, immobilization (both voluntary and as treatment) and the sedating effects of pain medications. (See Subacute Stage and Chronic Stage.)

**Adaptability** (ADA) The ability of certain building spaces and elements, such as kitchen counters, sinks, and grab bars, to be added or altered so as to accommodate the needs of individuals with or without disabilities or to accommodate the needs of persons with different types or degrees of disability. In therapy (related to patient ability) it is the ability of the patient to modify his/her behavior and performance to accommodate to the situation and to adjust to the environment, allowing the successful completion of the desired activity.

**Addition** (ADA) An expansion, extension, or increase in the gross floor area of a building or facility.

**Adduction** The process of moving a body part toward midline. In the case of the digits (fingers and toes) adduction refers to the process of moving the digit toward the axis of the limb.

**Adhesions** Collagen fibers which adhere to surrounding structures and cause a reduction in the normal elasticity and movement of those structures. Adhesions are frequently a complication of surgery, trauma, or immobilization.

**Administrative Authority** (ADA) A governmental agency that adopts or enforces regulations and guidelines for the design, construction, or alteration of buildings and facilities.

**Aerobic** Activities which provide a paced activity which:
1. allows the heart and circulatory system to keep up with oxygen needs of the body
2. uses a continuous amount of energy for muscle contraction
3. maintains a heart beat faster than resting rate for a minimum of 10 minutes.
When leading exercise activities for patients with heart conditions, the recreational therapist should delay arm exercises until after both the warm up exercises and aerobic activities of the lower extremity (e.g., walking, leg raises). This delay will decrease the chance of having the patient experience angina episodes (chest pain), dysrhythmias (uneven heart beat), muscle soreness, and fatigue (Karam, page 8). The safest aerobic schedule for most patients is 20 minutes of exercise three or four times a week. Individuals who exercise over 30 minutes at a time and/or five or more days a week do not significantly increase their aerobic ability and significantly increase the risk of orthopedic injury (Karam, pages 16, 17). When using aerobic activities with patients with diabetes the biggest challenge is to balance the exercise with diet modifications, especially in Type I diabetes mellitus. This balance is the responsibility of the physician and the dietitian. The therapist should also limit the aerobic activity to under 40 minutes, even with a patient who has a balanced program (Karam page 63).

**Agitation** The appearance that a patient is anxious because s/he is demonstrating motor restlessness. Agitation is frequently due to neurological damage in individuals who have sustained a traumatic brain injury.

**Air Carrier Access Rules** In 1986 the United States Government passed the Air Carrier Access Act of 1986, which was further updated in the Americans With Disabilities Act of 1990. This Act required the Department of Transportation (DOT) to develop regulations which ensure that individuals with disabilities are treated without discrimination in a way consistent with the safe carriage of all passengers.

**Alteration** (ADA) An alteration is a change to a building or facility made by, on behalf of, or for the use of a public accommodation or commercial facility, that affects or could affect the usability of the building or facility or part thereof. Alterations include, but are not limited to, remodeling, renovation, rehabilitation, reconstruction, historic restoration, changes or rearrangement of the structural parts or elements, and changes or rearrangement in the plan configuration of walls and full-height partitions. Normal maintenance, reroofing, painting or wallpapering, or changes to mechanical and electrical systems are not alterations unless they affect the usability of the building or facility.

**Altered Body Image**  A change in the way that a patient perceives his/her own body image. The patient may actually have a change in his/her body function or structure, or it may be a perceived change in his/her body function or structure.

**Ambulatory Status**  The current functional level of the patient when walking or moving about.

**Americans with Disabilities Act 1990**  The Americans with Disabilities Act (ADA) is a federal civil rights law. This law has five sections, called "Titles". Title I covers equal employment opportunities for individuals with disabilities. Title II covers nondiscrimination on the basis of disability in the receipt and use of state and local government services. Title III covers nondiscrimination on the basis of disability by public accommodations and in commercial facilities. Title IV covers telecommunications relay services for individuals who have a hearing impairment or a speech impairment. Title V covers miscellaneous provisions including construction, (lack of) state immunity, prohibition against retaliation and coercion, regulations by the Architectural and Transportation Barriers Compliance Board, attorney's fees, technical assistance, federal wilderness areas, coverage of Congress and the agencies of the legislative branch, illegal use of drugs, definitions, amendments to the Rehabilitation Act, and alternative means of dispute resolution. The ADA opens up many opportunities in recreation and leisure to individuals with disabilities as it helps break down architectural and attitudinal barriers.

**Amnesia**  An inability to recall past events. Some types of amnesia include post-traumatic amnesia (due to trauma to the brain), anterograde amnesia (an inability to recall events after the onset of amnesia), and retrograde (an inability to recall events which happened prior to the onset of amnesia).

**Amputation**  Amputation refers to the removal of a part of the body through the bone. An amputation is usually the last choice of a medical team. However, injury caused by trauma or burns, infection, malignancy, or a loss of the circulatory system may dictate the need for an amputation. Occasionally a nonviable limb is amputated to allow the fitting and use of a prosthetic limb to increase function.

**Anaerobic Activities**  Activities of short duration which deplete energy stores in the body by using oxygen faster than the heart and lungs can replace it.

**Aneurysm**  The dilation or bulging out of the wall of an artery or vein. It may rupture and cause a spontaneous hemorrhage.

**Ankle and Foot**  The ankle and foot have three primary functions:
1.  To provide a means of mobility including being able to provide a rigid structure to push the body forward and a flexible structure to absorb the shock of foot contact with hard surfaces.
2.  To provide a means of stability on even and uneven surfaces.
3.  To provide a means to bear weight using a limited amount of energy.

**Antalgic Gait**  Caused by pain the patient modifies his/her gait by:
1.  avoiding weight bearing on the painful side and/or
2.  shortening of the gait and stance and/or
3.  supporting of the injured area with one hand while the other hand is outstretched or otherwise held to assist with balance.

**Anterior**  Referring to the front of the body or organ, or indicating a location toward the head.

**Aphasia**  The loss or decrease in the ability to speak, understand, read, or write.

**Apraxia** The inability to carry out purposeful, voluntary movements without presence of muscle weakness, paralysis, or impaired sensations. This can be found in physical activities and speech.

**Architectural Barriers Act of 1968** This federal law requires that buildings and facilities be designed and constructed to be accessible to and usable by individuals with disabilities. It also requires that when major changes are made in a building, the issue of architectural barriers in that building must be addressed and corrected. The significant limitation to this law, which the ADA has corrected, is that this law only applied to buildings that received federal funds.

**Area of Rescue Assistance** (ADA) An area, which has direct access to an exit, where people who are unable to use stairs may remain temporarily in safety to await further instructions or assistance during emergency evacuation.

**Arthogenic Gait** A gait noted by the elevation of one hip and the swinging out of the leg (instead of a straight through swing). This gait is often caused by a deformity or stiffness of either the hip or the knee.

**Arthrodesis** At times the limitations on a patient's activity level caused by chronic joint pain or chronic joint instability require the fusing of bony surfaces. These limitations are so severe that the loss of range of motion caused by the fusion (called arthrodesis) is secondary to the pain or instability. The internal fusion is usually done using plates, pins, or by bone grafts. A patient who has undergone arthrodesis may need significant re education in movement and balance during leisure activities. Not only is it likely that the pre morbid movement pattern was abnormal because of pain and/or instability, but the post morbid movement pattern will also be different because of a loss of normal range of motion. Re education of movement patterns as well as balance may be required, as well as the potential need for adapted equipment.

**Artificial Airway** A surgically placed alternative passage for air to reach the lungs. The two most common types of artificial airways are the endotracheal tube and the tracheostomy. Between 20% and 40% of patients with burns treated at burn centers have a secondary complication of an associated respiratory insult requiring an artificial airway (DiGregorio).

**Assembly Area** (ADA) A room or space accommodating a group of individuals for recreational, educational, political, social, or amusement purposes, or for the consumption of food and drink.

**Assessment** The process of placing a value on something through measurement and qualification. Assessment is not the same thing as an evaluation. See evaluation.

**Ataxic Gait** This gait is characterized by an unsteady, wide gate and has two different forms:
1. Spinal Ataxia is caused by a disruption of sensory pathways in the central nervous system. This gait is frequently seen in patients with either tabes dorsalis or multiple sclerosis or other disease processes which affect the central nervous system. The ataxic gait tends to become worse when the patient closes his/her eyes. In addition to the broad based gait, spinal ataxia is also identified by "double tapping" (the heel comes down first followed by the toes making a double slapping sound).(Rothstein, et al., 1990 page 727).
2. Cerebellar Ataxia is caused by lesions in the cerebellum. Cerebellar ataxia is characterized by an inability to walk in a straight line but does not worsen went the patient's eyes are closed.

This type of gait limits the patient's ability to participate in mainstream activities like basketball, soccer, and football. While activities like hiking and swimming may need some modification, these should be a realistic option to all but the most involved patients.

**Attending Physician** The physician who is ultimately responsible for the type and quality of care received by the patient.

**Attention Deficits**  The inability to attend to a task or a thought due to a lack of 1. duration of attention, 2. appropriate selectivity of attention, 3. appropriate filtering of attention, or 4. ability to maintain attention.

**Augmentative Communication**  The use of tools or techniques to allow communication with another person when the individual's ability to communicate is impaired.

**Automated Guideway Transit (AGT)** (ADA) An AGT system is a fixed guideway transportation system which operates with automated (driverless) individual vehicles or multi car trains. Service may be on a fixed schedule or in response to passenger activated call buttons. Such systems using small, slow moving vehicles, often operated in airports and amusement parks, are sometimes called "people movers". These vehicles must comply with the ADA accessibility standards. The ADA accessibility guidelines for Automated Guideway Transit may be found in the **Automated Guideway Transit Vehicles and Systems Technical Assistance Manual** (US Architectural and Transportation Barriers Compliance Board).

**Automatic Door**  (ADA) A door equipped with a power-operated mechanism and controls that open and close the door automatically upon receipt of a momentary actuating signal. The switch that begins the automatic cycle may be a photoelectric device, floor mat, or manual switch (see power-assisted door).

**Autonomic Dysreflexia**  A serious medical problem that can occur in individuals with a spinal cord injury above the 7th thoracic level. Autonomic dysreflexia can be caused by many type of noxious stimuli below the level of the spinal cord injury, and its symptoms may be mild or severe. Severe autonomic dysreflexia is a medical emergency which, if not properly treated, can result in a cerebral vascular hemorrhage (stroke) and possibly death. Severe autonomic dysreflexia, if not addressed immediately on a community integration outing, can lead to the death of a patient prior to the therapist being able to return to the hospital with the patient. Common stimuli which cause autonomic dysreflexia include full or spastic bladders, a full rectum, tight or irritating clothing, a fracture or another undiscovered, painful stimulus.

**Auxiliary Aides and Services**  (ADA) At times a facility is required to provide auxiliary aides or services for individuals who are disabled because of a hearing or vision impairments. Legally this is defined as qualified interpreters, note takers, transcription services, written materials, telephone headset amplifiers, assistive listening devices, assistive listening systems, telephones compatible with hearing aides, closed caption decoders, open and closed captioning, telecommunications devices for individuals who are deaf (TDDs), video text displays, or other effective methods of making aurally delivered materials available to individuals with hearing impairments. Qualified readers, taped tests, audio recorders, Braille materials, large print materials, or other effective methods of making visually delivered materials available must be provided to individuals with visual impairments.

**Baclofen**  A medication which inhibits monosynaptic and polysynaptic reflexes at the spinal cord level. It is used primarily as a means to reduce spasticity. Baclofen may cause drowsiness, dizziness, and fatigue. While on community integration outing the patient should avoid substances that depress the central nervous system (like alcohol). Not known to cause sun sensitivity.

**Baroreceptor Sensitivity**  The baroreceptor nerve detects pressure applied to body parts. As a person ages s/he may experience a natural loss of baroreceptor sensitivity. An individual with a baroreceptor sensitivity has hypersensitivity to touch and pressure.

**Behavioral Lability**  A patient's inability to regulate his/her moods and behaviors due to cognitive deficits. The patient may fluctuate between being confused/oriented, overly emotional/flat affect, emotional and behavioral outburst/calm, sexually inappropriate behavior/socially and sexually appropriate, failure to recognize behavior as inappropriate/able to recognize inappropriateness of behavior.

**Brain Plasticity** The brain's ability to adjust to a physiological insult (e.g., traumatic brain injury) by developing the ability to manage a specific function in a part of the brain which usually is responsible for other functions. It is thought that the younger the patient is at the time of the insult, the greater potential for relearning due to a greater brain plasticity.

**Brain-Skull Differential** During an acceleration or deceleration of the body, the skull tends to accelerate or decelerate with a faster reaction time then the brain. It is because of this differential that a person sustains coup and contrecoup lesions during a traumatic brain injury.

**Brainstem** The part of the brain that controls breathing, heart beat and involuntary functions. Also known as the Medulla.

**Building** (ADA) Any structure used and intended for supporting or sheltering any use or occupancy.

**Burn** Skin damage caused by open flame, scalding, chemicals, and/or contact with electrical currents.

**Bus** (ADA) Bus means any of several types of self propelled vehicles, other than an over the road bus, generally rubber tired, intended for use on city streets, highways, and busways, including but not limited to minibuses, forty and thirty foot transit buses, articulated buses, double decked buses, and electric powered trolley buses, used to provide designated or specific public transportation services. Self propelled, rubber tire vehicles designed to look like antique or vintage trolleys or street cars are considered buses. The ADA accessibility guidelines for buses may be found in the **Buses, Vans, and Systems Technical Assistance Manual** (US Architectural and Transportation Barriers Compliance Board).

**Cardiorespiratory Endurance** The ability of both the heart and lungs to move oxygen efficiently enough to muscle groups to allow normal activity with reasonable endurance over a period of time. May be increased with the systematic use of leisure activities which stress the heart and other muscle tissues usually at least 3 times a week and without causing undue fatigue. Cardiorespiratory endurance can be significantly hindered when the patient has second and third degree burns to the anterior trunk area. After consultation with the physician, the recreational therapist may want to encourage the patient's daily involvement in leisure activities which involve diaphragmatic breathing. Fun activities involving the blowing around balloons suspended from overhead or a game of air hockey using a ping pong ball on a table are good places to begin.

**CAT Scan** See Computerized Axial Tomography.

**Cath.** See Catheterization

**Catheterization** Insertion of a tube into a cavity (in this context, into the bladder) to allow drainage. The Certified Therapeutic Recreation Specialist may need to catheterize a patient while out in the community to help reduce the symptoms of autonomic dysreflexia.

**Caudal** (caudad) The end, tail, inferior to or the bottom of a point; away from the head.

**Cerebellum** Second largest part of the brain. It is responsible for the coordination of voluntary muscular movements.

**Cerebral Embolism** An occlusion of a cerebral artery, a type of stroke.

**Cerebral Hemorrhage** The rupturing of a cerebral vessel with bleeding into the brain tissues, a type of stroke.

**Cerebral Thrombosis** The formation of a blood clot within a cerebral artery, leading to an occlusion of the vessel, a type of stroke.

**Cerebrovascular Accident** (CVA) Stroke, restricted blood supply to some part of the brain.

**Cerebrum** The main and largest portion of the brain consisting of two hemispheres. This is the area responsible for memory, speech, sensation, intellect, and for directing our conscious movements.

**Chronic Arteriosclerotic Vascular Disease** The blood flow to the extremities decreases over time because of a narrowing and fibrosis of the medium to large arteries. This disease is most commonly seen in patients who are elderly or have a long history of diabetes mellitus. (Abbreviated ASVD, this disease is sometimes also called arteriosclerosis.) Some of the clinical signs include:
1. decreased skin temperature in extremities
2. chalky white coloring of skin and/or with blanching of the skin in the affected limbs
3. decreased hair growth over affected area
4. increased susceptibility to skin ulceration
5. pain

The patient may experience a decreased tolerance to temperature extremes leading to discomfort during certain leisure activities. The pain experienced by the patient may fall into two separate categories:
- pain upon exertion (intermittent claudication)
- pain during periods of inactivity

Intermittent claudication (which feels like cramping muscles) is caused by a lack of oxygen to the muscles which are being used. Because of the nature of ASVD, a progressive conditioning program may do little more than increase the patient's tolerance of activity and to decrease the occurrence of claudication. Patients may be encouraged to exercise through the use of leisure activities multiple times a day to the point of discomfort (and not beyond). Pain subsides slowly with rest. Pain upon rest (which usually has a burning, tingling feeling) is the result of a decreased oxygen flow to the affected limb. This decreased flow may be, in part, caused by positioning (the limb placed above the level of the heart and/or pressure over the arteries leading to the muscles) and/or caused by long periods of rest. (The heart tends to be less productive during sleep and/or during events which lead to Deconditioning.) Encouraging the patient to engage in leisure activities which allow the affected limb(s) to be positioned below the heart will help decrease the pain caused by rest.

**Chronic Inflammation** When a patient has long term inflammation caused by a disease like arthritis, the recreational therapist must guard against promoting activities which cause the inflamed area excessive stress or cause irritation. When the affected scar tissues are in the healing and remodeling process, such stress will significantly increase the occurrence of fibroblasts, which in turn increase the production of collagen. The outcome may be an actual weakening of the affected area and a decrease in ROM. The therapist will be able to tell if too much movement, stress, or irritation has occurred by noting increased pain and inflammation which lasts more than two hours after the activity. The patient may restrict movement (muscle guarding) because of pain. After a rest period the patient will experience increased stiffness, and after 24 hours the patient will experience a slight loss of ROM.

**Chronic Stage** The third and last stage of healing, maturation, and remodeling after an injury or illness is called the chronic stage. There are two subclassifications within the chronic stage. The first involves an injury after the 21st day, when inflammation is no longer present but when the patient's functional ability has not returned to normal. The second involves a continuous state of pain or recurring episodes of pain with a suboptimal return to the patient's normal functional ability. The collagen fibers which are thickening as a result of the injury will not mature for up to 14 weeks. Up to that time the fibers and scar tissue are able to be remodeled through therapeutic activity to lessen the severity of the disability. After around 14 weeks the scar tissue resists remodeling and stretching may only be achieved through surgery or the adaptive (over) lengthening of the tissues surrounding the scar. The over lengthening of tissue around the scar should be done only under the direction of a physician or a physical therapist.

**Circle of Willis**  The union of the anterior and posterior cerebral arteries, forming a loop near the base of the brain.

**Circulation Path**  (ADA) An exterior or interior way of passage from one place to another for pedestrians, including, but not limited to, walks, hallways, courtyards, stairways, and stair landings.

**Circumlocution**  Using many words to say what could be said in a few words.

**Classification**  Classification is the process of placing a single unit of something in the same group as similar objects/subjects following a pre established set of rules and guidelines.

**Clear**  (ADA) Unobstructed

**Clear Floor Space**  (ADA) The minimum unobstructed floor or ground space required to accommodate a single, stationary wheelchair and occupant.

**Clinical Decision Making**  Decisions about patient care and the types of services provided based on assessed patient needs, standards of practice, and institutional policies. Diagnoses and treatment protocols based on established scientific evidence, are two kinds of clinical decision making. When the therapist, using his or her knowledge base and experience, but without supporting evidence from research, makes a decision, it is called a clinical opinion.

**Clinical Opinion**  The belief or ideas that a professional holds regarding a patient. This opinion may be based on the use of tests and measurements but cannot be directly supported by evidence relating to those tests and measurements. Clinical opinions should be based on the therapist's evaluation of all available information; clinical decisions based on a therapist's synthesis of information are based on clinical opinions. (Rothstein, et al. 1990, page 925)

**Closed Circuit Telephone**  (ADA) A telephone with dedicated line(s) such as a house phone, courtesy phone or phone that must be used to gain entrance to a facility.

**Cognition**  The brain's ability to process information is what is usually considered "cognition". Obviously it takes quite a few different skills and processes to take in information; identify, classify, and organize the information; and to then be able to retrieve that information in a manner that it can be used. While there are many different philosophies about what cognition is, the therapist will find it useful to group cognition into three functional aspects: 1. information *processes* (which would include the patient's ability to attend to the information being received, understand the information received, remember the information, and organize the information to allow for reasoning and problem solving), 2. information *systems* (which would include a patient's ability to utilize his/her memory in a functional manner (both long and short term memory) and being able to utilize executive function skills based on learned information and reasoning), and 3. information *integration* (which would include the patient's being able to use his/her information processes and information systems to interact with the environment around him/her in a meaningful and functional manner).

**Cognitive Deficits**  An inability to perform normal cognitive functions (e.g., judgment, problem solving, communication, interpretation of environmental stimuli, insight, ability to follow commands, memory, abstract thought, attention span, etc.)

**Collagen**  The chief component of the fibrils of connective tissue and of the bones. Activities which promote mild to moderate stretching of muscles over a period of 15 minutes (with frequent short periods) allow the breaking down of the collagen crystals. A gentle, sustained stretch maintained for 15 to 20 minutes over 5 days will also allow measurable change in the muscles. With daily or every other day stretching during leisure activities the collagen crystals will actually rebind to other collagen crystals, allowing more plasticity. Not allowing the frequent rest periods or over stressing the muscles can cause tissue failure (rupture). A lighter stretch should be allowed when working with older patients. As a person gets older the collagen becomes less elastic. Combined with decreased capillary blood supply caused by age, the muscles are at greater risk for failure and require an increased length of time to recover.

**Commercial Facilities** (ADA) The ADA define commercial facilities as those facilities whose operations will affect commerce, that are intended for nonresidential use by a private entity; and that are not facilities that are covered or expressly exempted from coverage under the Fair Housing Act of 1968, as amended.

**Common Use** (ADA) Refers to the interior and exterior rooms, spaces, or elements that are made available for the use of a restricted group of people (for example, occupants of a homeless shelter, the occupants of an office building, or the guests of such occupants).

**Common Wheelchairs and Mobility Aids** (ADA) Common wheelchairs and mobility aids is a term used in the ADA and refers to equipment belonging to a class of three or four wheeled devices, usable indoors, designed for and used by individuals with mobility impairments which do not exceed 30 inches in width and 48 inches in length, measured 2 inches above the ground, and do not weigh more than 600 pounds when occupied. The ADA accessibility guidelines for these may be found in the **Buses, Vans, and Systems Technical Assistance Manual** (US Architectural and Transportation Barriers Compliance Board).

**Commuter Rail** (ADA) The United States Government defines a commuter rail system to be a short haul rail passenger service which operates in a metropolitan and/or suburban area, operated by a commuter authority whether within or across the geographical boundaries of a state, usually characterized by reduced fare, multiple ride, and commutation tickets and by morning and evening peak period operations. For ADA purposes, commuter rail does not include light or rapid rail transportation. The ADA accessibility guidelines for commuter rail may be found in the **Commuter Rail Cars and Systems Technical Assistance Manual** (US Architectural and Transportation Barriers Compliance Board).

**Commuter Rail Car** (ADA) A commuter rail car means a rail passenger car obtained by a commuter authority for use in commuter rail transport.

**Compression** Pressing together or on top of. A compression may cause an occlusion.

**Computerized Axial Tomography** (CAT Scan) The CAT scan uses x-rays and computers to visually examine the brain and other parts of the body in three dimensions. For stroke diagnosis, a CAT scan gives a clear view of the physical structure of the brain and its related arteries.

**Confabulation** Telling of false information without intending to deceive. Unintentional lying.

**Congenital** From birth, an illness or disability present at birth.

**Consulting Physician** Physicians who are not the patient's attending physician, but who have been asked to give their advice on certain aspects of the patient's care or problems.

**Contracture** The reduction of normal mobility and/or flexibility of a body part caused by a shortening or tightening of the skin, fascia, muscle, or joint capsule (Kisner and Colby, 1990 page 684). Contractures may be caused by immobility, injury, or scarring and, depending on the cause and degree of involvement, may require surgery to correct. The therapist's best approach to contractures (especially in long term care settings) is prevention. Assisting the patient in identifying enjoyable leisure activities which allow the daily range of motion of all body parts during various activities reduces the chance of contracture development.

**Contrecoup Lesions**  The lesions caused by the brain's hitting the skull wall after its initial impact (counter bounce) due to a significant acceleration or deceleration of the head. Because the brain is encased but free-moving inside the skull, it will impact the skull initially when the head impacts an object and then rebound in the opposite direction to impact the opposite side of the skull. The lesions are caused by the impact of hitting the skull. These lesions will translate to reduced neurological functioning in the months and years to come.

**Convenience Store**  A small to moderate sized store which offers a limited variety of food, drinks, and some general merchandise (e.g.; gas, over-the-counter medications, magazines). Smaller than a grocery store.

**Counter indicated**  Means that a treatment or action should not be taken because the situation does not call for it, in fact, the treatment or action may actually make the patient's condition worse.

**Coup Lesions**  The lesions caused by the impact of the brain against the skull during an impact. If the patient sustained a head injury by hitting his/her head on the dash board after hitting a telephone pole, the damage to the frontal lobes would be considered the coup lesions - or area of first impact.

**Covered Entity**  (ADA) When used in a federal law, covered entity refers to "an employer, employment agency, labor organization, or joint labor management committee" (ADA 1630.2(b)).

**Cross Slope**  (ADA) The slope that is perpendicular to the direction of travel (see running slope).

**Curb Ramp**  (ADA) A short ramp cutting through a curb or built up to it.

**Data**  The assignment of numerical values or symbols to help facilitate the evaluation of an event over a predetermined period of time. The information collected is based on a predetermined set of criteria which describes what is to be measured.

**Debridement**  Removing foreign material or contaminated cells through cleansing, usually once every shift. Debridement is frequently extremely painful, especially when associated with "tubbing" for patients with burns. The four primary goals of debridement are:
1.  to keep the injured area clean
2.  to remove dead tissue
3.  to remove bacteria
4.  to remove caked antimicrobials

**Deconditioning**  A decrease in the combined ability of the circulatory system, cognition, neuromuscular movement, and metabolic system to function as a direct result of prolonged immobility and/or bedrest. This decrease is a direct result of inactivity and not a result of an injury or illness. Typical loss of abilities may include:
1.  decreased brain wave activity caused by bedrest or chair rest (which produces the same EEG patterns as individuals placed in environments which promote sensory deprivation)
2.  noted decrease in cognitive ability including verbal fluency, color discrimination, reversible figures, distorted awareness of time
3.  potential decrease in thermoregulation
4.  noted increase in anxiety, irritability, depression, and possible hallucinatory experiences
5.  decrease in balance (after 2 to 3 weeks on bedrest)
6.  increase in resting heart rate (by the end of 3 weeks morning heart rate can increase by 21%, evening by 33%, or an average of 1 heart beat per 2 days of bedrest)

7. decrease in oxygen uptake (anticipated 15 to 30% decrease in uptake after just 3 weeks bedrest). (from burlingame and Blaschko, 1990, page 3)

**Demand Response Systems** (ADA) A demand response system is a system which transports individuals, including the provision of designated public transportation service by public entities and the provision of transportation service by private entities, including but not limited to specific public transportation service, which is not a fixed route system. The ADA accessibility guidelines for demand response systems may be found in the **Buses, Vans, and Systems Technical Assistance Manual** (US Architectural and Transportation Barriers Compliance Board).

**Dependent Position** Referring to the relaxed position of a limb which is hanging downward, held in place by gravity.

**Depression** A feeling of sadness or grief. In patients with strokes, this depression can be psychological or physiological. Studies have found that over 50% of patients with stroke have clinical depression. The closer the stroke to the left frontal pole of the brain, the greater risk for severe depression. Without intervention, this depression will normally last 9 to 12 months.

**Designated Public Transportation** (ADA) means a transportation system which is run by a public entity (other than public school transportation) by bus, rail, or other conveyance (other than transportation by aircraft or intercity or commuter rail transportation) that provides the general public with general or specific service, including charter service, on a regular and continuing basis. The ADA accessibility guidelines for designated public transportation may be found in the **Buses, Vans, and Systems Technical Assistance Manual** (US Architectural and Transportation Barriers Compliance Board).

**Detectable Warning** (ADA) A standardized surface feature built in or applied to walking surfaces or other elements to warn people who are visually impaired of hazards on a circulation path.

**Diagnostic Tool** An instrument or pen and paper assessment which is used to help the therapist to assign a diagnosis to a patient based on the results of the tool. At this point, the field of recreational therapy does not have any instruments or testing tools with enough scientific data and research to clearly assign diagnoses to patients.

**Disability** (ADA) Legally defined, disability means, with respect to an individual, a physical or mental impairment that substantially limits one or more of the major life activities of such individual; that there is a record of such an impairment; or being regarded as having such an impairment. The term disability does not include 1) transvestitism, transsexualism, pedophilia, exhibitionism, voyeurism, gender identity disorders not resulting from physical impairments, or other sexual behavior disorders, 2) compulsive gambling, kleptomania, or pyromania; or 3) psychoactive substance use disorders resulting from current illegal use of drugs.

**Distal** Opposite of close; away from the center or midline of the body. The fingers are more distal to the chest than the shoulder.

**Doppler-Ultrasound Test** The Doppler-Ultrasound listens for the turbulent blood flow caused by narrowing in the arteries which may be the cause of transient blockage of blood flow to the brain.

**Dorsiflexion** Moving a body part closer to the center plane of the body by flexing or bending. To dorsiflex the foot, the patient would flex the toes toward the body. To dorsiflex the hand, the patient would cock his/her hand back over the wrist, exposing the palm.

**Dressing** Putting on clothing. For a patient to be considered independent in dressing s/he would need to be able to complete the following tasks without cueing or other assistance:

1. ability to determine appropriate clothing for the situation, activity, and weather,
2. ability to identify where the clothing is kept, and then obtain the clothing,
3. ability to don (put on) and doff (take off) clothing, shoes, and appliances in a sequential fashion,
4. ability to manipulate buttons, zippers, ties, etc. as needed for clothing and appliances.

While the patient's initial training in these skills will most likely come from an occupational therapist, the CTRS will need to supervise, assist, and evaluate the patient in his/her skills related to dressing while on community integration outings.

**Dwelling Unit** (ADA) A single unit which provides a kitchen or food preparation area, in addition to rooms and spaces for living, bathing, sleeping, and the like. Dwelling units include a single family home or a townhouse used as a transient group home; an apartment building used as a shelter; guest rooms in a hotel that provide sleeping accommodations and food preparation area; and other similar facilities used on a transient basis. For purposes of these guidelines, use of the term "Dwelling Unit" does not imply the unit is used as a residence.

**Dysarthria** The loss of function in the muscles used for speech and voice production. The speech produced is difficult to understand. The individual may have all other language and comprehension centers intact, but be unable to physically to product speech.

**Dysesthesia** Alteration of any sense, but particularly to the sense of touch. This is usually experienced as pain and/or pinpricks.

**Dysphagia** Difficulty swallowing, due to loss of neurological function.

**Dystrophic Gait** Movement is achieved by rolling the hips from side to side producing a pronounced waddling or penguin gait. Because of the nature of this gait, the patient's ability to run or to climb up stairs or hike up inclines is greatly limited. The most common reason for this gait is muscular dystrophy but it is also seen in a variety of myopathies.

**Eccentric Lengthening Exercises** Prescriptive exercise programs which:
1. uses equipment to provide a pulling force on actively contracting muscles
2. lengthens and strengthens the muscles

**Edema** the excessive accumulation of fluid in the body's soft tissue causing swelling and discomfort. This swelling is controlled by:
1. positioning (using gravity to drain fluids)
2. pressure wraps (like ace bandages)
3. medications

The recreational therapist should be aware of the strategies used to reduce edema in the patient and ensure that the leisure activities that the patient engages in are not counter indicated. The use of ace bandages on extremities or pressure clothing (like jobst) may be required during leisure activities, even passive ones.

**Efficiency** The degree to which an individual is able to complete a task measured against the amount of energy and work required to complete the task. Usually a modification of movement to decrease unneeded movement combined with an increased endurance will result in increased efficiency. Increasing efficiency for individuals with neuromuscular disorders like cerebral palsy may require significant modifications to an activity or equipment that reduces tone or eliminates undesired movement.

**Egress, Means of** (ADA) A continuous and unobstructed way of exit travel from any point in a building or facility to a public way. A means of egress comprises vertical and horizontal travel and may include intervening room spaces, doorways, hallways, corridors, passageways, balconies, ramps, stairs, enclosures, lobbies, horizontal exits, courts and yards. An accessible means of egress is one that complies with the

ADA guidelines and does not include stairs, steps, or escalators. Areas of rescue assistance or evacuation elevators may be included as part of the accessible means of egress.

**Elasticity** The ability of soft tissue to return to its normal state after a period of gentle, passive stretching. Muscles are made up of bundles of fibers called myofibril. Each myofibril is made up of shorter, overlapping fibers called sarcomere made up of actin and myosin filaments. During contraction the actin and myosin filaments slide closer together (overlap more) causing the muscle fibers to contract. When the muscle is relaxed, the actin and myosin filaments pull apart a little, allowing the muscle to lengthen. When a patient remains immobile (or experiences a decrease in normal movement) over a period of time, the amount of connective tissue produced by the muscles will increase. At the same time the body increases its absorption of sarcomere fibers. This undesirable physiological event may be stopped and/or reduced through the prescriptive use of leisure activities. The recreational therapist should ensure that the leisure activities prescribed are enjoyable to the patient and at the same time adequately exercise all of the appropriate muscles. This exercise regimen may require combining numerous leisure activities to achieve the desired combination of muscle stretching.

**Element** (ADA) An architectural or mechanical component of a building, facility, space, or site, e.g., telephone, curb ramp, door, drinking fountain, seating, or water closet.

**Embolus** Sudden blocking of an artery by a blood clot or a foreign material that has been brought to that site by the blood. (See occlusion.)

**Employer** (ADA) The Americans with Disabilities Act defines an employer as: (1) In general, the term "employer" means a person engaged in an industry affecting commerce who has 15 or more employees for each working day in each of 20 or more calendar weeks in the current or preceding calendar year, and any agent of such person, except that from July 26, 1992 through July 25, 1994, an employer means a person engaged in an industry affecting commerce who has 25 or more employees for each working day in each of 20 or more calendar weeks in the current or preceding year and any agent of such person.
(2) Exceptions, the term employer does not include: (i) the United States, a corporation wholly owned by the government of the United States, or an Indian tribe; or (ii) a bona fide private membership club (other than a labor organization) that is exempt from taxation under Section 501(c) of the Internal Revenue Code of 1986. (ADA 1630.2 (e)

**Endarterectomy** A surgical process to remove the inner portion of an artery, particularly in the neck, to remove the build-up of plaque which may eventually result in stroke.

**Endotracheal Airway** When the patient requires assisted ventilation (usually for no more than 7 days), a tube is slipped down the trachea (windpipe) into the lungs. This tube may be placed into the trachea through the nose (nasotracheal), through the mouth (orotracheal), or through an existing hole (stoma) in the trachea (see tracheostomy).

**Endurance** The ability of:
1. the muscle to resist fatigue even with repeated contractions over a period of time
2. the cardiovascular system to resist fatigue through efficient delivery of oxygen over a period of time
3. the neuropsychological system to resist fatigue allowing the performance of cognitive functions over a period of time, and/or
4. the general ability to sustain low intensity activity over a period of time.

**Entrance** (ADA) Any access point to a building or portion of a building or facility used for the purpose of entering. An entrance includes the approach walk, the vertical access leading to the entrance platform, the entrance platform itself, vestibules if provided, the entry door(s) or gate(s), and the hardware of the entry door(s) or gate(s).

**Environmental Safety** A unit in the CIP which is intended to measure:
1. how well the patient anticipates and identifies threats to his/her own safety in the community and
2. how well the patient is able to problem solve to better ensure his/her own safety.

**Epicondyle** Referring to a bony prominence on the top of a condyle of a bone. An example would be the bump felt on the top of the femur on the outside of the hip. Skin tissue covering epicondyles are prone to skin breakdowns caused by pressure, sheer, inactivity, and poor circulation. The eight epicondyle locations on the body are
1.  external epicondyle of femur
2.  external epicondyle of humerus
3.  internal epicondyle of femur
4.  internal epicondyle of humerus
5.  lateral epicondyle of femur
6.  lateral epicondyle of humerus
7.  medial epicondyle of femur
8.  medial epicondyle of humerus

**Escharotomy** The surgical incision in scar tissue to allow elasticity in the skin. Especially in patients with burns encircling an entire body part (i.e.; arm, abdomen), the non elastic scar tissue is incised (cut) the length of the scar tissue, through the complete depth of the scar. This allows greater movement. Escharotomy is especially important for patients who have burns encircling the torso to allow the expansion of the thoracic cavity for breathing. The procedure leaves especially disfiguring scars, usually causing the patient concerns about cosmetic issues. The use of leisure activities to help increase feeling of self worth and control over one's environment are extremely important. The recreational therapist should be skilled in taking extremity pulses in patients with burns or know what to look for to call nursing staff. Extremities with circumferential burns will experience a tightening of the scar tissue throughout the hospitalization. The patient is at risk for a restricted blood flow below the circumferential scar. Peripheral pulses may be cut off, requiring immediate medical attention.

**Evaluation** A clinical opinion as a result of the therapist's review of data and assessment results. Evaluation is not the same as an assessment.

**Eversion** Turning outward of a body part.

**Extensibility** See flexibility.

**Extension** Straightening or unbending a flexed limb. Moving two ends of a jointed part away from each other. Opposite of flexion.

**Facility** (ADA) All or any portion of buildings, structures, site improvements, complexes, equipment, roads, walks, passageways, parking lots, or other real or personal property located on a site.

**Fatigue** The decreased ability of an individual to complete a task because of a lack of oxygen delivery, protective influences of the central nervous system, or a depletion of potassium in the elderly. The use of a muscle past the point of fatigue may lead to strain or to overuse syndrome. The idea of "No Pain, No Gain" is a phrase that the therapist may want to avoid. Too frequently it leads to over fatigue of a muscle. The intensity of exercise should cause a gentle "pulling" sensation in the tight tissue and not pain (Kisner and Colby, 1990, page 679). With patients who have experienced a recent prolonged reduction in normal leisure activity, the therapist may need to help the patient develop a schedule of modified activity until the appropriate level of endurance and strength can be achieved.

**Feeding/Eating** For a patient to be considered independent in eating s/he would need to be able to complete the following tasks without cueing or other assistance:

1.  ability to order and/or obtain and set up food and drink,
2.  ability to successfully and appropriately use regular or adapted tableware, utensils, and cups,
3.  ability to bring food and drink from the table or eating surface to mouth,
4.  ability to adequately chew food and swallow food/liquids so that threat of choking is not evident.

While the patient's initial training in these skills will most likely come from either the occupational therapist or the speech therapist, the CTRS will need to supervise, assist, and evaluate the patient in his/her skills related to feeding and eating while on community integration outings.

**Field Cut** Decrease or loss of a portion of a person's field of vision following a stroke.

**Fixed Route Systems** (ADA) Legally fixed route systems means a system of providing transportation of individuals (other than by aircraft) on which a vehicle is operated along a prescribed route according to a fixed schedule. The ADA accessibility guidelines for fixed route systems may be found in the **Buses, Vans, and Systems Technical Assistance Manual** (US Architectural and Transportation Barriers Compliance Board).

**Flaccid** A muscle or limb that is weak, lacks tone and voluntary control.

**Flaccid Bladder** A bladder that has a weakened capability to retain fluid without artificial help.

**Flaccid Gait** See Hemiplegic Gait

**Flesch Grade Level** To help determine the degree of difficulty (or ease) in reading text, an index was developed called the Flesch Grade Level Index. Through research, it was found that by determining the average number of words in a sentence and the average number of syllables per 100 words, a person could predict who could understand the material. After conducting norm studies, a grade level reading equivalent was determined. The number before the decimal indicates the grade level of the reading. The number after the decimal indicates the number of months the average reader in that grade would have been in that grade before being able to read the written text. (The CIP's Module 3B Grocery Store has a Flesch Grade Level of 6.4 which means a reader in the fourth month of sixth grade could understand the material.)

**Flexibility** The body's or mind's ability to yield (bend, move, change stance) when required. Muscle and other soft tissues responds when challenged with stretching force, the mind responds when challenged to format thoughts in a different manner. The maintenance of flexibility usually requires an individual's involvement in multiple leisure activities on a regular basis. For patients with a cardiac condition, flexibility is especially important. Being flexible allows the patient to maintain a better posture, decreases the change of injury, and relieves stress (Karam, page 1).

**Flexion** Bending at a joint moving two ends of a joint closer together. Opposite of extension.

**Fluent Aphasia** Speech is fluent with paraphasic errors. Auditory comprehension, reading comprehension, and writing comprehension are impaired.

**Foley Catheter** A tube inserted into the uretha to allow continuous emptying of the bladder. Patients with burns usually have both an intravenous line (IV) and a catheter placed because of the amount of intravenous fluid loss. The capillaries become more permeable, causing excess fluid loss and edema (as well as the loss of electrolytes). This permeability happens in both the involved (burned) and healthy parts of the body, especially in those patients with total body surface area burns of 30% or more (Livingstone, page 18). To help fight hypovolemic shock (too little fluid) an IV is placed and fluids which are electrolyte fortified, are pumped into the patient. Urine output is measured. The amount of fluid (and how it looks) is an important indicator of patient health. The recreational therapist will probably be expected to empty the Foley Catheter bag and accurately record the amount and appearance of the urine. Even when the patient has progressed to the point of being able to leave the hospital for short periods of time, s/he may still rely on a urine collection device. There are many different options for urine collection (especially for outings of three hours or less). Because Foley Catheter bags hang on the side of a wheelchair, the patient's urine is visible for all to see. The recreational therapist should work with the rest of the rehabilitation team and the patient to come up with a more normalizing alternative.

**Footdrop Gait** Frequently caused by weak or paralyzed dorsiflexor muscles, the patient is seen to slap the foot to the ground after lifting the knee high on the affected side only. This gait causes increased jarring to the body and limits to some degree the patient's ability to achieve a high skill level in physical activities which require grace.

**Four Point Gait** The four point gait refers to the use of two crutches in addition to the use of two weight bearing legs in ambulation. By alternating the movement of the crutches and the legs the patient is able to move while always having at least three points of support. This gait provides maximal support with stability but provides significant limitations to leisure activities. This type of gate is usually slower than other types of gaits and requires the use of the hands, providing limited or no use of the hands during leisure activities while ambulating. Backpacks are frequently used by patients who ambulate using the four point gait. The therapist may need to educate the patient on appropriate and safe ways of donning and doffing the pack, as well as how to determine a good pack weight and balance.

**Full Arc Extension** The movement of a joint from flexion to extension. Some leisure activities which may promote full arc extension are creative dance and swimming.

**Full Thickness Graft** A graft which contains the epidermis and the dermis of the skin, but does not contain the subcutaneous fat.

**Functional Independence Measure** The Functional Independence Measure, or the "FIM" is a standardized scoring method used when measuring a patient's functional ability. The FIM is a 7 point scale which is used to measure the patient's degree of independence in performing any observable skill.

**Gait Training** An initial element of rehabilitation intervention to treat ambulation/mobility deficits. The physical therapist may start the patient on the parallel bars, crutches, a walker, or a cane and provide the patient with specific exercises and instructions for the use of the equipment. This training may be supervised by appropriately in serviced professional staff, paraprofessional staff, or family members. After the patient has achieved a degree of success with his/her gait training, the patient is then ready to be cleared for gait training and practice in the community. It is frequently the recreational therapist who supervises this phase of the gait training.

**Gastrocnemius Soleus Gait** The affected side is dragged along because of the lack of heel lift on push off. Activities which involve going up inclines are most affected. Since this gait is usually caused by weakened gastrocnemius and/or soleus muscles, a strengthening program involving activities which mildly stress those muscles may lead to a decrease in the gait.

**Generalization** The ability to understand that one behavior or skill can be modified to work in a different situation or setting. This is a skill that is frequently impaired in patients who have experienced a traumatic brain injury or have other significant cognitive deficits. For integration to be successful, the patient needs to taught how to generalize the skills learned while in an institution or hospital to the functional abilities required in the community. The therapist will want to ensure that 1. the patient has the perception that the problem solving strategies taught during therapy were helpful, that 2. the patient has learned specific techniques to enhance generalization of the problem solving strategies, and 3. (the therapist had determined that) the problem solving strategy will work for that patient.

**Glasgow Coma Scale** The Glasgow Coma Scale (GCS) is routinely used to measure the severity of a coma and subsequent injury by grading eye, motor, and verbal responses. The numerical values of the scale run from 3 (low) to 15 (normal). The total score of a patient's GCS means: 3-8 = severe coma, 9-12 = moderate coma, and 13-15 = mild coma. A newer Glasgow type scale has been developed for children to be able to more accurately measure the early recovery in young children (under the age of three years). This assessment is called the Children's Coma Scale (CCS).

**Granulation** The normal, healthy reaction of the body to tissue damage. Small blood vessels increase significantly at the site of a wound to help promote healing. Granulation tissue will eventually be replaced by normal tissue but at first it appears red and raw. Granulation tissue is a desired tissue type to graft skin onto.

**Graphic Input** (Reading) Traumatic Brain Injuries often impact a patient's ability to read. Once the patient is able to recognize words and to consistently scan from left to right, s/he is ready to progress to reading safety and other information on community integration outings. Patients tend to progress from being able to find concrete information in reading passages (as found in menus) to being able to figure out implied abstract information (such as satire or subtle meanings found in parks program bulletins). In house therapy along with actual experience on community integration outings with the therapist helps the patient understand any visual/spatial deficits that s/he might have and to compensate for them. It is important that reading speed and accuracy increase together.

**Graphic Output** (Writing) Written communication is one of the key skills required of adults. Whether it is writing a check, filling out an insurance form, or just writing a letter to a friend, the use of the written word is vital to independence in the community. One of the primary uses of the written word prior to discharge is a memory book. The purpose of the memory book is to provide the patient with a visual reminder of his/her schedule as well as to provide a place to write down thoughts and questions which should not be forgotten. Patients who require the use of a memory book usually have difficulty with spelling, punctuation, sentence formation, paragraph organization. Unless these skills will be required soon (because of vocational or educational needs) it is best to focus on the content of the material and not the manner in which it is written.

**Grooming** For a patient to be considered independent in grooming s/he would need to be able to complete the following tasks without cueing or other assistance:
1. ability to identify and obtain the supplies needed for such activities as donning and doffing makeup, shaving, nail care, hair care, applying deodorant, etc.,
2. ability to identify the appropriate care and placement (storage) for grooming supplies.
While the patient's initial training in these skills may come from either the occupational therapist or the CTRS, the CTRS will need to supervise, assist, and evaluate the patient in his/her skills related to grooming while on community integration outings.

**Ground Floor** (ADA) Any occupiable floor less than one story above or below grade with direct access to grade. A building or facility always has at least one ground floor and may have more than one ground floor as where a split level has been provided or where a building is built into a hillside.

**Habilitation** The maintenance of an individual's current health status and functional ability.

**Halo** A splinting/traction device which has a metal ring placed around the head of the patient who has a spinal cord injury. The mental ring has supporting "arms" which extend down to the patient's torso to help stabilize the head. There are metal pins extending from the metal ring into the patient's skull to help further stabilize the vertebra and spinal cord. The use of a halo allows the patient to regain mobility faster then if s/he were placed in traction in bed.

**Hemianopsia**  Defective vision or blindness in half of the visual field. This is an anatomical problem. (Also called hemianopia.) *Note:* Do not confuse with neglect.

**Hemiparesis**  Weakness of one side of the body.

**Hemiplegia**  Paralysis of one side of the body.

**Hemiplegic Gait**  Also known as a flaccid gait, this gait has two primary elements:
1. a swinging (circumduction) or pushing of the affected leg forward
2. forefoot strike with a missing heel strike on the affected leg.
This gait is usually noted with patients who have a measurable difference in leg length or a deformity of one leg.

**Hemorrhage**  The escape of blood from a ruptured vessel—bleeding into the brain.

**Heterodermic Graft**  A temporary skin graft taken from a donor of a different species than the recipient.

**High Speed Rail**  (ADA) High speed rail refers to an intercity type rail service which operates primarily on a dedicated guideway or track not used, for the most part, by freight, including, but not limited to, trains on welded rail, magnetically levitated (meglev) vehicles on special guideway, or other advanced technology vehicles, designed to travel at speeds in excess of those possible on other types of railroads. The ADA accessibility guidelines for high speed rail may be found in the **High Speed Rail Cars, Monorails, and Systems Technical Assistance Manual** (US Architectural and Transportation Barriers Compliance Board).

**Hyperesthesia**  Abnormal increased sensitivity of the skin or an organ to sensory stimuli.

**Hyperflexia**  Excessive flexion of a joint or joints.

**Hypertension**  An elevation in blood pressure. Going above the normal range.

**Hypertonic**  An increased level of tension in a muscle or limb.

**Hypoflexia**  Less then normal flexion of a joint or joints.

**Hypotension**  Blood pressure well below what is considered normal. An individual with hypotension may experience dizziness if s/he stands up quickly.

**Impaired Adjustment**  A patient's inability to modify his/her style/behavior in a manner that is consistent with a change in his/her health status. The patient may either be purposeful (lack of acceptance) in his/her ability to recognize the change, or may be unaware of the change. Due to this impaired adjustment, the patient will probably demonstrate a lack of movement toward independence; experience an extended period of shock, disbelief, or anger toward his/her health change; or demonstrate an impaired ability to make plans for the future.

**Ineffective Individual Coping**  An impairment in the patient's adaptive behaviors and ability to solve problems related to his/her illness or disability. It is likely that a patient who demonstrates ineffective individual coping related to a newly acquired disability had poor coping skills premorbidly. The therapist may want to explore the patient's past coping strategies. This should help the therapist identify the specific skills lacking which need to be taught to the patient. A patient with a poor ability to cope with new, distressing situations is not likely to integrate successfully into community based leisure activities.

**Infarct**  An area of tissue that has died because of lack of blood supply.

**Inhibition**  Patients who lack inhibition will be unable to repress or terminate behavior appropriately.

**Instrument**  A tool used by the therapist to obtain a measurement during the assessment process. This instrument may be a questionnaire, a machine, or any other device which assists the therapist in obtaining the desired measurement.

**Intercity Rail Transportation**  (ADA) refers to transportation provided by Amtrak. The ADA accessibility guidelines for Intercity Rail Transportation may be found in the **Buses, Vans, and Systems Technical Assistance Manual** (US Architectural and Transportation Barriers Compliance Board).

**Intermittent Claudication**  The painful cramping of muscles following short periods of exercise. This usually indicates a suboptimal cardiovascular function frequently seen in patients with occlusive arterial disease. Resolution is usually fairly quick following a cessation of activity. (Also see Chronic Arteriosclerotic Vascular Disease.)

**Intern**  A student who has completed his/her training and is completing field placement. A medical intern is a physician who has completed all of his/her medical training and is completing his/her field placement. A medical intern is supervised by a medical resident or an attending physician.

**Internal Carotid Artery**  The artery originating in the common carotid artery that supplies blood to the frontal lobe (the front part of the brain).

**Internist**  A physician who has specialized in the study of internal medicine. They are experts in the areas of infectious diseases and diseases of the heart, gastrointestinal tract, and other internal organs.

**Inversion**  Turning inward of a body part toward midline.

**Ischemia**  A term which means a lack of blood flow and a lack of delivery of oxygen to the cells.

**Isokinetic Exercises**  Exercises which use of specialized equipment to provide:
1.  contraction of specific muscles through their full ROM
2.  measured resistance provided by the equipment which responds to the strength of the contracting muscles as it moves through the full ROM.

**Isometric**  A movement program consisting of either structured exercises or specified leisure activities which involve:
1.  contraction of muscles without joint movement
2.  increased circulation through muscles caused by activity
3.  resistance provided by a fixed object (wall, chair, etc.) or by the use of flexors versus extensors.

**Isotonic**  A movement program consisting of either structured exercise or specified leisure activities which involve:
1.  contraction of muscles with joint movement
2.  increased circulation through muscles caused by activity
3.  a predetermined amount of resistance provided through the use of exercise or leisure equipment and/or one's own body.

**Judgment**  The cognitive ability to decide to act based on a review of various aspects and factors related to the decision as well as being able to reasonably predict the results of the action under consideration.

**Knowledge Deficit**  An inability to call upon basic information required to survive in one's environment. A patient who has a knowledge deficit may demonstrate an inability to: accurately follow through on instructions given, accurately perform skills needed (although physically able to do so), perform within socially excepted norms for behavior and emotional expression, or otherwise function because of missing information.

**Lability**  Unable to control inappropriate laughing or crying.

**Lateral**  Referring to the side or portion of the body furthest away from the midline of the body.

**Leisure Planning Deficit**  An inability to experience self-initiated leisure activities as a result of a lack of knowledge about leisure opportunities, decreased stimulation from or a lack of interest in leisure activities, or an inability or unwillingness to use one's leisure time in a manner that is satisfying to the individual.

**Lethargy**  An abnormal and undesirable drowsiness or stupor frequently resulting in an increased indifference to one's environment. Lethargy, as a side effect of medication, can place the patient at greater risk of accidents and injury.

**Light Rail**  (ADA) refers to a streetcar type vehicle railway operated on city streets, semi private rights of way, or exclusive private rights of way. Service may be provided by step entry vehicles or by level boarding. The ADA accessibility guidelines for light rail may be found in the **Light Rail Vehicles and Systems Technical Assistance Manual** (US Architectural and Transportation Barriers Compliance Board).

**Magnetic Resonance Imaging**  (MRI)  The MRI uses a magnetic field instead of radiation to make a three-dimensional image similar to the CAT scan. The MRI produces the clearest and crispest picture available today.

**Major Life Activities**  (ADA) Major life activities means functions such as caring for oneself, performing manual tasks, walking, seeing, hearing, speaking, breathing, learning, and working.

**Marked Crosswalk**  (ADA) A crosswalk or other identified path intended for pedestrian use in crossing a vehicular way. For purposes of standardization for the CIP, a marked crosswalk is marked with obvious lines which define the path to be used to cross the street. Marked crosswalk does not mean that the crosswalk must have an electrical pedestrian cross walk light.

**Medial**  Referring to the middle portion or the midline of the body; closest to the midpoint.

**Medulla**  The part of the brain that controls breathing, heart beat, and involuntary functions. Also known as the Brainstem.

**Memory Deficit**  Inability to recall information stored in one's brain, either short (working) or long term. Depending on the cause of the memory deficit, the individual may exhibit a combination of the following symptoms: poor learning ability, reduced self-esteem, short term memory loss, long term memory loss, disorientation, confabulation, poor safety awareness. Short term memory refers to the storage of information that the individual is using or has just used. Thoughts are encoded and organized in short term memory. Because short term memory has limited ability to store large quantities of information, some of the information is selected, encoded and shifted to long term memory. Long term memory contains past learned information, including information related to concepts and words, rules and social/governmental expectations, organizational strategies, and other memories of past experiences.

**Mezzanine or Mezzanine Floor**  (ADA) That portion of a story which is an intermediate floor level placed within the story and having occupiable space above and below its floor.

**Mobility** Mobility refers to the patient's ability to move from one location to another. For a patient to be considered independent in mobility s/he would need to be able to complete the following tasks without cueing or other assistance:

1. ability to move from current position (point A) to desired position (point B). This would include ability to move in bed, with a wheelchair, to transfer, and/or to ambulate with prescribed mobility devices (if any),
2. ability to use prescribed mobility techniques and devices in a variety of settings found in the community.

While the patient's initial training in these skills most likely will come from a physical therapist, the CTRS will need to supervise, assist, and evaluate the patient in his/her skills related to mobility while on community integration outings.

**Movement** Referring to motion.

**MRI** See Magnetic Resonance Imaging

**Multifamily Dwelling** (ADA) Any building containing more than two dwelling units.

**Muscle Strength** The amount of power that a single muscle, or group of muscles, is able to demonstrate.

**Myopathy** Referring to a disease of a muscle.

**Nasogastric Tube (NG Tube)** A tube which is placed down the patient's nose into the patient's stomach. This tube is used to help provide nutritional supplement for those patient's who cannot eat because of a jaw injury, neurological damage, or coma.

**Neglect** Lack of awareness of one side of the body and space — usually seen in those individuals with a right CVA. Individuals with a right CVA show neglect to the left of mid-line. (Also known as visuospatial neglect, and unilateral neglect.)

**Neurologist** A physician who has specialized in the study of the brain, nerves, and muscles.

**Neuropathy** A measurable disability and/or undesirable change in the peripheral nervous system. Chronic alcoholism and diabetes are two common causes of neuropathy.

**Neuropsychologist** An individual with a Ph.D. in psychology who has additional training and experience in working with patients with traumatic brain injuries.

**Nonfluent Aphasia** Speech is effortful and halting. Auditory comprehension is relatively good but not perfect. Reading comprehension is better than written output.

**Occlusion** Closure of a blood vessel, closing off.

**Occupiable** (ADA) A room or enclosed space designed for human occupancy in which individuals congregate for amusement, educational, or similar purposes, or in which occupants are engaged at labor, and which is equipped with a means of egress, light, and ventilation.

**Operational Part** (ADA) A part of a piece of equipment or appliance used to insert or withdraw objects, or to activate, deactivate, or adjust the equipment or appliance (for example, coin slot, push button, handle).

**Organizational Deficit** The inability to mentally process information in an organized manner. This would include an inability to sequence, classify, prioritize, or identify relevant features of objects or events.

**Orientation** The ability to be cognitively aware of, and express time, place, personal data, relationship(s) of significant others to self, one's own condition, and purpose (identity/role).

**Overstretch** Overstretch refers to the excessive lengthening of soft muscle tissue which allows ROM beyond the normal limits. While this overstretching is beneficial in some leisure activities (i.e., gymnastics and yoga), for patients with mobility and/or balance problems, overstretch can be a hazard. Stability is compromised with overstretched tissue.

**Pain** A generally localized feeling of discomfort brought about by the stimulation of special nerve endings. It is thought that pain is an adapted state to help the individual protect the area that is uncomfortable. The degree of pain that a person "feels" is influenced by three factors (Cailliet, 1988):
1.  biologic factors
2.  psychological factors
3.  social factors
The recreational therapist can have a significant impact on the patient's tolerance (or lack there of) for pain, and change the degree to which the patient's leisure lifestyle is limited because of pain. Both the prevention of further movement which will actually cause biological damage as well as psychological training to increase tolerance are suitable areas for the recreational therapist to work. Also, increasing the patient's social skills to minimize the negative impact of pain is often addressed by the recreational therapist. The therapist can decrease the patient's need to talk about his/her pain by increasing awareness and interest in other things and by helping the patient redefine his/her role from "victim" to a healthier role. These changes will increase the patient's tolerance for pain.

**Paralysis** Complete loss of voluntary movement.

**Paraphasia** Condition characterized by fluent utterance of speech sounds in which unintended syllables, words, or phrases are prominent during speech.

**Paraxial Deficiencies** A weakness or other disabling condition which effects only one side of the limb along the axis, verse a transverse deficiency which may effect the entire width of the limb.

**Paresis** Weakness; partial or incomplete paralysis.

**Paresthesia** An abnormal, and frequently intense, feeling of burning and prickling ("biting ants") felt by the patient even though there is little or no pressure on the affected spot.

**Parkinsonian Gait** "This is a highly stereotypical gait in which the patient has impoverished movement of the lower limb. There is generalized lack of extension at the ankle, knee, hip, and trunk. Diminished step length and a loss of reciprocal arm swing are noted. Patients have trouble initiating movement, and this results in a slow and shuffling gait characterized by small steps. Because patients with Parkinsonism often exhibit flexed postures, their center of gravity project forward, causing a festinating gait. The patient, in an attempt to regain his balance, takes many small steps rapidly. The rapid stepping causes the patients to increase his walking speed. In some cases patients will break into a run and can only stop their forward progression when they run into an object. Less common than the forward propulsive gait pattern is a retropulsive pattern that occurs when patients lose their balance in a backward direction (retropulsion is more common in patients with cerebellar lesions)." (Rothstein et al., 1990 page 728)

**Perception Deficit** An inability to recognize objects or to misjudge one object's relationship to another object due to an inability to distinguish:

1. context (figure-ground),
2. significance of an object,
3. intensity of an object, or
4. the identity of a previously familiar object.

**Perseveration** The person gets "stuck" on the same response. This can be either a verbal or a motor response.

**Phantom Pain** Either a dull or sharp pain felt by a patient that seems to originate from a limb that is no longer present (has been amputated). This pain is very real and frequently limits the patient's ability to concentrate on leisure activities. The therapist may want to note the patient's description of the pain (burning, electrical, or throbbing) and the duration of the pain. Eventually the patient learns to localize the pain to the stump.

**Photosensitivity** The abnormal and undesirable response of the skin to sunlight. This response is a direct result of medications taken by the patient. The typical response is a heightened risk of sunburn.

**Physiatrist** A medical doctor who specializes in physical medicine.

**Physical Medicine and Rehabilitation (PM & R)** PM & R is an area of specialty in health care which is based on the bodies of knowledge in 1) cognition, 2) functional anatomy, 3) neuromuscular physiology, and 4) exercise physiology. The accrediting body for this specialty is Commission on Accreditation of Rehabilitation Facilities (CARF). For many of the treatment categories, CARF requires that the services of a Certified Therapeutic Recreation Specialist be available.

**Physical or Mental Impairment (ADA)** The phrase physical or mental impairment means: 1) any physiological disorder or condition, cosmetic disfigurement, or anatomical loss affecting one or more of the following body systems: neurological; musculoskeletal; special sense organs; respiratory, including speech organs; cardiovascular; reproductive; digestive; genitourinary; hemic and lymphatic; skin; and endocrine; 2) any mental or psychological disorder such as mental retardation, organic brain syndrome, emotional or mental illness, and specific learning disabilities; 3) the phrase physical or mental impairment includes, but is not limited to, such contagious and noncontagious diseases and conditions as orthopedic, visual, speech, and hearing impairments, cerebral palsy, epilepsy, muscular dystrophy, multiple sclerosis, cancer, heart disease, diabetes, mental retardation, emotional illness, specific learning disabilities, HIV disease (whether symptomatic or asymptomatic), tuberculosis, drug addiction, and alcoholism. The phrase physical or mental impairment does not include homosexuality or bisexuality.

**Plaque** A deposit of fatty material in the lining of a blood vessel. Build up of plaque in or near the brain can lead to the blockage of the blood vessel, resulting in a stroke.

**Plasticity** The tendency for soft tissue to resume a slightly longer length after a period of gentle passive stretching. Muscles are made up of bundles of fibers called myofibril. Each myofibril is made up of shorter, overlapping fibers called sarcomere which is made up of actin and myosin filaments. During contraction the actin and myosin filaments slide closer together (overlap more) causing the muscle fibers to contract. When the myofibrils experience repeated, prolonged periods of gentle stretching, the amount of sarcomeres are increased, allowing an actual lengthening of the muscle.

**Post Traumatic Stress Response** An individual's response to an unexpected extraordinary life event or events which produces a sustained painful response. The patient may experience an interruption in his/her normal sleep patterns, an inability to concentrate, a increased ability to be startled, and a decreased ability to initiate activity.

**Postural Drainage**  The use of gravity to help remove unwanted secretions from the airway. Patients frequently show a resistance to postural drainage because of boredom, agitation, pain, etc. The development of enjoyable leisure activities to be engaged in during drainage helps increase compliance.

**Postural Dysfunction**  The patient's decreased ability to engage in leisure activities caused by a shortening of soft tissue and muscle weakness. The patient experiences fatigue and a limiting range of motion which can frequently be overcome through the prescriptive use of leisure activities.

**Postural Fault**  An abnormal alignment of the body caused by pain, not caused by structural defects or postural dysfunction.

**Posterior**  Referring to the back part of a structure; the dorsal surface of the body.

**Power-Assisted Door**  (ADA) A door used for human passage with a mechanism that helps to open the door, or relieves the opening resistance of a door, upon the activation of a switch or a continued force applied to the door itself.

**Powerlessness**  A perception that one is unable to influence one's own life; that one is not able to significantly affect an outcome or a perceived lack of control over a current situation. A patient who feels powerless to control the events of his/her life will be less likely to initiate activity.

**Premorbid Leisure Lifestyle**  The combination of activities that the patient participated in prior to his/her injury or illness.

**Prescription**  A prescription is made up of four parts:
1.  the mode of treatment (i.e., type of activity (movement, cognition, etc.) required)
2.  duration of treatment program (i.e., 14 days)
3.  frequency of treatment (i.e., two times a day)
4.  intensity of treatment (i.e., maintenance of 120% resting heart rate for 15 minutes)

**Pressure Release**  The lifting or moving of the body to relieve pressure on areas compressed by gravity, constricting garments, or appliances.

**Problem Solving**  The process which takes place when an individual is not able to reach a desired goal directly. Some of the skills associated with problem solving include 1. the ability to identify the desired outcome, 2. the ability to gather and consider relevant information, 3. anticipating potential solutions, and 4. the selection of the action(s) which is most likely to get the desired outcome.

**Processing Deficits**  Processing deficits tend to fall into three categories: 1. the inability to *regulate the information being received* (e.g., not being able to handle: the rate of reception, the amount being received, the type of information being received, other noises and input, and manage (cope with) information overload in a productive manner); 2. the inability to *organize the information being received* (e.g., not being able to: maintain information in memory, group the information with similar information to allow analysis and problem solving, and use internal conversations to help retrieve information (Which way is it to the recreation center?); and 3. the inability to *regulate the manner in which information is expressed* (e.g., not being able to: monitor one's responses to ensure correctness and sequencing that make sense, plan the response to ensure that it is presented in an organized manner, and know when one needs more information before a response is appropriate (asking for clarification)).

**Proprioceptive Testing**  Any test which measures the patient's ability to sense the location and position of a body part while his/her eyes are closed.

**Proximal**  Referring to the nearest point to a person's midline.

**Public Accommodations** (ADA) As defined in the ADA, the following private entities are considered public accommodations for the purposes of this civil rights act, if the operations of such entities affect commerce: a) an inn, hotel, motel, or other place of lodging, except for an establishment located within a building that contains not more than five rooms for rent or hire and that is actually occupied by the proprietor of such establishment as the residence of such proprietor; b) a restaurant, bar, or other establishment serving food or drink; c) a motion picture house, theater, concert hall, stadium, or other place of exhibition or entertainment; d) an auditorium, convention center, lecture hall, or other place of public gathering; e) a bakery, grocery store, clothing store, hardware store, shopping center or other sales or retail establishment; f) a laundromat, dry cleaner, bank, barber shop, beauty shop, travel service, shoe repair service, funeral parlor, gas station, office of an accountant or lawyer, pharmacy, insurance office, professional office of a health care provider, hospital, or other service establishment; g) a terminal, depot, or other station used for specified public transportation; h) a museum, library, gallery, or other place of public display or collection; i) a park, zoo, amusement park, or other place of recreation; j) a nursery, elementary, secondary, undergraduate, or postgraduate private school, or other place of education; k) a day care center, senior citizen center, homeless shelter, food bank, adoption agency, or other social service center establishment; and l) a gymnasium, health spa, bowling alley, golf course, or other place of exercise or recreation.

**Public Use** (ADA) Describes interior or exterior rooms or spaces that are made available to the general public. Public use may be provided at a building or facility that is privately or publicly owned.

**Pulse** A pulse is the measurable surge of blood through the arteries and veins. The recreational therapist should be skilled in the techniques associated with taking a patient's pulse (Palpation of Pulses). The patient may already be experiencing a decreased pulse to various body parts for physiological reasons, or may experience ischemia (lack of blood flow and lack of delivery of oxygen) because of poorly fitted equipment and/or exposure to cold. Pulses are usually recorded as the number of beats per minute. In addition, the therapist will need to indicate whether the pulse was: 1. normal, 2. diminished, or 3. absent. An absent pulse is obviously an emergency situation. Pulses are "taken" at eight locations on the body: 1. carotid artery, 2. radial, 3. ulnar, 4. brachial, 5. femoral, 6. popliteal, 7. dorsalis pedis, and 8. posterior tibial.

**Qualified Interpreter** (ADA) an individual who is able to interpret effectively, accurately, and impartially both receptively and expressively, using any necessary specialized vocabulary.

**Ramp** (ADA) A walking surface which has a running slope greater than 1:20.

**Range of Motion (ROM)** Degree of motion (flexion and extension) of a joint. ROM exercises work to increase or maintain the maximum degree of movement. **PROM**—passive range of motion is when a joint is moved by some other person. In nursing homes PROM is usually done by aides and nursing staff. **AROM**—active range of motion is when the patient moves the joint by his/her own efforts. In some many states, occupational therapists, physical therapists, physicians, nurses, and aides are licensed to perform ROM exercises. However, most regulatory agencies expect all therapists to know enough about range of motion to be able to implement the appropriate type and use the appropriate precautions, while interacting with the patient. A recreational therapist may work with the physical therapist or occupational therapist to develop a set of leisure activities which promote the appropriate range of motion activity for a patient. The recreational therapist would then supervise the patient during these activities. There are five primary causes for a loss of ROM (Kisner and Colby 1990, page 109): 1. prolonged immobilization, 2. restricted mobility, 3. connective tissue or neuromuscular disease, 4. tissue pathology due to trauma, and 5. congenital or acquired deformities.

**Reasoning** The ability to consider information presented and then to create inferences and/or conclusions. The skill of reasoning requires that the individual is able to draw upon past experiences and is flexible in the possible interpretations of why an event occurred.

**Reflex Sympathetic Dystrophy** Seen frequently in individuals with hemiplegia caused by stroke, reflex sympathetic dystrophy is a painful condition caused by partial damage to the nerves in the shoulder area. Symptoms include severe pain, hypersensitivity, and paresthesias.

**Rehabilitation** The process of improving one's health and functional status through purposeful intervention.

**Rehabilitation Act of 1973** The Rehabilitation Act of 1973 (amended in 1992) is the principal federal legislation establishing programs aimed at promoting the employment and independent living of people with disabilities. The programs authorized under this Act are administered within the US Department of Education by the Rehabilitation Services Administration and the National Institute on Disability and Rehabilitation Research.

**Relaxation** The purposeful effort to release tension in one or more muscles. A patient's ability to decrease tension in muscles usually becomes more efficient with practice. While some patients may be able to increase this skill through self directed efforts, most will require some direct training from the therapist.

**Restraints** Restraints are objects or systems of limiting a patient's movement. Medications to control a patient's activity level and behavioral patterns are legally considered restraints. At times restraints may be medically indicated but too often they are overused and abused. It is the patient's right not to be restrained unless all other options have been tried and have failed.

**Rubor** Rubor refers to the normal coloring of the skin. A deep purple color in the extremities caused by poor venous return and dilated capillaries is called "dependent rubor". When treating patients with dependent rubor, the recreational therapist should try to encourage activities which allow raised positioning of the affected limb. Such simple solutions as having the patient sit in a Lazyboy type chair with the foot rest up allow a patient's legs to be raised, and yet a card table (or similar table) may be used over the foot rest to allow a game of cards or other leisure activities.

**Running Slope** (ADA) The slope that is parallel to the direction of travel (see cross slope).

**Scar** The tissue which replaces skin or other cells after the healing of a wound. Scar tissue lacks oil glands and lacks elastic tissue. As a scar ages, it usually contracts, causing a reduction in ROM to the affected area. A keloid scar is a scar with excess fibrous growth. Medical intervention is important during the healing process to reduce the development of keloid tissue. Keloid tissue, especially from untreated third degree burns, is at increased risk of malignancy.

**Secondary Brain Injury** Injury to the brain caused by subsequent physiological or pathophysiological response to the initial injury. Some secondary brain injury causes would include a re-bleed from a hemorrhage, increased pressure, cerebral edema; hydrocephalus; anoxia; or cerebral infections.

**Securement Devices (ADA)** A securement device is a mechanical object which ties the wheelchair or the mobility device to the vehicle. A securement device is not a seatbelt and should never be used to tie the passenger to his/her mobility device.

**Sensation** A message carried by the nerves as a result of some action or event.

**Sensorimotor** Those skills which require the coordination of one's senses with one's movement (motor behavior). Some of the functional skills which require a fair degree of sensorimotor skill are gross and fine motor coordination, muscle control, dexterity, strength and endurance, tactile awareness, and range of motion.

**Service Entrance**  (ADA) An entrance intended primarily for delivery of goods or services.

**Signage**  (ADA) Displayed verbal, symbolic, tactile, and pictorial information.

**Site**  (ADA) A parcel of land bounded by a property line or a designated portion of a public right-of-way.

**Site Improvement**  (ADA) Landscaping, paving for pedestrian and vehicular ways, outdoor lighting, recreational facilities, and the like, added to a site.

**Skill**  The ability to demonstrate a refined pattern of movements. Skill requires competence in five areas : 1. coordination, 2. agility, 3. balance, 4. timing, and 5. speed. (Kisner and Colby 1990, page 691)

**Sleeping Accommodations**  (ADA) Rooms in which people sleep; for example, dormitory and hotel or motel guest rooms or suites.

**Socket**  Refers to the cavity of a prosthetic device in which the stump is placed.

**Space**  (ADA) A definable area, e.g., room, toilet room, hall, assembly area, entrance, storage room, alcove, courtyard, or lobby.

**Space Boots**  Specially cushioned boots which help maintain the normal angle of the foot and ankle and to prevent pressure sores of the heal and foot.

**Spasm**  A sudden involuntary contraction of the muscles.

**Spastic**  Having a varying stiffness or tightness of a limb caused by spasms.

**Sprain**  Movement which result in severe stress, stretching, and/or tears of the soft tissues around a joint capsule, in a muscle, or the associated connecting ligaments or tendons is called a "sprain". Sprains are classified into three degrees of severity. Refer to Tissue Injury.

**Story**  (ADA) That portion of a building included between the upper surface of a floor and the upper surface of the floor or roof next above. If such portion of a building does not include occupiable space, it is not considered a story for purposes of these guidelines, There may be more than one floor level within a story as in the case of a mezzanine or mezzanines.

**Strain**  When a patient participates in activities which involve a range of motion in excess of the patient's normal range or involve repetitious movements in excess of the patient's accustomed level of activity, slight trauma occurs. This trauma usually occurs in the musculotendious unit. Good assessment of the patient's current level of activity combined with moderation and warm-up activities should decrease the chance of injury.

**Strength**  The measurable amount of force produced by a single muscle or a set of muscles. See muscle strength.

**Stretching**  A prescribed activity designed to lengthen soft tissue which has been pathologically shortened.
- *Passive Stretching*  The action of someone else (besides the patient) gently applying force to stretch tight tissue. Passive stretching is usually done by the PT, OT, or Certified Nursing Assistant using prescribed ROM exercises.

- *Active Stretching* Patient initiated movement designed to increase ROM in affected soft tissue and joints. This is usually carried out in physical therapy using a prescribed exercise program or in recreational therapy using a prescribed set of leisure activities designed to achieve the desired outcome.

The recreational therapist should encourage leisure activities which involve the slow static stretching of muscles lasting between 10 to 30 seconds. Activities which involve bouncing stretches or ballistic stretches increase the patient's change of injury, especially after a period of immobility (Karam page 1). Stretching Activities to Avoid with Patients (Karam page 2)

| | |
|---|---|
| Yoga Plow | places unusual pressure on the neck |
| Duck Walk | too much pressure on the knee |
| Deep Knee Bend | too much pressure on the knee |
| Standing Stiff Legged Toe Touch | too much strain placed on the back and the knee |
| Ballet Stretches | strain on ligaments, knees, lower back |
| Splits | strain on ligaments, knees, lower back |
| Stiff Double Leg Raise | places strain on the lower back |
| Sit-up with the Legs Extended | places strain on the lower back |

**Stretching Selective** Decreased ROM for selective muscle groups can greatly increase the level of independence for patients with thoracic and cervical spinal injuries. After a full examination the physician or the physical therapist will determine the amount of tightness for the extensor muscles of the lower back that will be needed to enhance the patient's balance. A slight tightness will allow greater balance while leaning forward in a wheelchair for patients with no active control of the back extensors. The recreational therapist should note the degree of tightness desired and ensure that the patient's leisure activities do not jeopardize that stability.

**Structural Frame** (ADA) The structural frame shall be considered to be the columns and the girders, beams, trusses, and spandrels having direct connections to the columns and all other members which are essential to the stability of the building as a whole.

**Subacute Stage** The second of three stages of the healing and maturation of an illness or injury. The subacute stage usually begins about the 4th day after an injury is marked by noted repair of the injured area. The subacute stage usually is over by the 21st day after the onset of an injury, but may last as long as 6 weeks (Kisner & Colby, 1990, page 216). During this time the remaining blood clots are absorbed and replaced by fibroblastic activity (which produces collagen). Immature connective tissue and granulation tissue form (to speed up the delivery of oxygen to the injured site). These tissues are very susceptible to damage by overstretching, overuse, or by being pulled/sheered in the wrong direction. Pain may be experienced by the patient as the immature tissue is stretched just past its normal limit. Some gentle stretching (in consultation with the physical therapist) is recommended to reduce the adherence to surrounding tissues during the healing process.

**Subclavian Artery** A branch of the innominate artery on the right and a branch of the aortic arch on the left that supplies blood to the neck, upper limbs, thoracic wall, spinal cord, brain, and meninges.

**Subcutaneous Tissue** The fatty and fibrous tissues which are situated just under the skin.

**Swing Through Gait** This gait involves the movement of the crutches in the direction that the patient is moving. The crutches are placed and then the patient swings his/her lower body beyond the point where the crutches are anchored before moving the crutches again. The swing through gait is most often used by those patients who have difficulty with alternate leg movements either because of balance difficulties or because of paralysis.

**Swing To Gait**  Once the patient places both crutches in front of him/her, the patient swings the legs to a position directly between the two crutches.

**Tactile**  (ADA) Describes an object that can be perceived using the sense of touch.

**Target Heart Rate**  The desired heart rate to be achieved during cardiovascular activity. The target heart rate is always determined before to the patient is involved in a prescribed program which increase a patient's cardiovascular endurance. The therapist may want to consult the patient's physician when determining the target heart rate. Some medications may modify the patient's responsive heart rate, making the use of standardized target heart rate scales undesirable.

**Tendon Reflex Examination**  A non standardized test which measures the degree of reactionary movement of a tendon when it is hit in a brisk manner. While tendon reflexes are generally graded from 1 (low) to 4 (high), there tends to be a large variation between one therapist and another. Treatment protocols and recreational therapy intervention/precautions should not rely heavily on a patient's tendon reflex grade unless the therapist is comfortable that s/he knows how the specific tester grades reflexes.

**Text Telephones (TTs)**  (ADA) Machinery or equipment that employs interactive graphic (i.e., typed) communications through the transmission of coded signals across a standard telephone network. Text telephones can include devices known as TDDs (telecommunication display devices or telecommunication devices for individuals who are deaf) or computers.

**Thalamic Pain**  A spontaneous pain or change so that a normal sensation feels painful .

**Three Point Gait**  When the patient is unable to ambulate because of intolerance of weight bearing on one of the legs, two crutches are used to bear the weight instead of the limb.

**Thromboangiitis Obliterans**  Inflammation of the small arteries caused by a decreased circulation in the extremities. This disease is a direct result of the patient's use of nicotine and/or smoking and will be resolved after the patient gives up the use of nicotine and/or smoking. The hands and the feet are the most affected, causing increased concern for frost bite when the patients are engaging in winter sporting events. This disease is sometimes referred to as Buerger's Disease.

**Thrombus**  A clot within the heart or a blood vessel that may lead to obstruction.

**Tightness**  A term describing a mild contracture of a group of muscles and tendons usually caused by inactivity and easily resolved through gentle, frequent enjoyable leisure activities which promote ROM of the involved area.

**Tissue Injury, Degree of**  Health care professionals usually divide injury to tissue into three levels or degrees. It is important for the therapist to be aware of the three degrees and to be able to make a reasonable determination of the degree of injury received during a leisure activity. Frequently an incident report will need to be written up for any tissue damage of a second or third degree and a continuing quality improvement program will be required to reduce the likelihood of a repeat incident.

**Toilet Hygiene**  For a patient to be able to be considered independent in toilet hygiene s/he would need to be able to complete the following tasks without cueing or other assistance:
1. ability to know the supplies needed, and where to obtain them
2. ability to use supplies and ability to perform toileting tasks to achieve cleanliness
3. ability to transfer to; maintain body position; and then transfer back from a bedpan, toilet, commode, or other similar equipment.

While the patient's initial training in these skills will most likely come from an occupational therapist, the CTRS will need to supervise, assist, and evaluate the patient in his/her skills related to toilet hygiene while on community integration outings.

**Tone**  The degree to which the muscles display strength and the ability to recover from normal stretching and contracting.

**Tracheostomy**  An opening through the skin and between the second and forth tracheal rings into the trachea (windpipe). A tracheostomy tube becomes flexible at body temperature to be able to move with the trachea. Depending on the patient's ability to breathe, a ventilator may or may not be hooked up to the cuff of the tube.

**Tram**  (ADA) Refers to several types of motor vehicles consisting of a tractor unit, with or without passenger accommodations, and one or more passenger trailer units, including but not limited to vehicles providing shuttle service to remote parking area, between hotels and other public accommodations, and between and within amusement parks and other recreation areas. The ADA accessibility guidelines for trams may be found in the **Trams, Similar Vehicles and Systems Technical Assistance Manual** (US Architectural and Transportation Barriers Compliance Board).

**Transient Ischemic Attack (TIA)**  Temporary symptoms of a stroke. Complete recovery usually results within 24 hours. A clot may have occluded the blood vessel and then released. People having TIAs are advised to seek medical attention immediately because they are signs of future strokes. People who have had a stroke may also have TIAs. Always alert a doctor to these "mini-strokes."

**Transient Lodging**  (ADA) A building, facility, or portion thereof, excluding inpatient medical care facilities, that contains one or more dwelling units or sleeping accommodations, Transient lodging may include, but is not limited to, resorts, group homes, hotels, motels, and dormitories.

**Transverse Deficiency**  A weakness or other disabling condition which effects the entire width of a limb.

**Two Point Discrimination Test**  This test measures the degree of sensation that a patient has on specific parts of his/her skin. The therapist or physician measures the patient's ability to perceive the difference between one or two points (measured in centimeters or millimeters). If a patient has been assessed to have poor two point discrimination, the therapist will need to ensure that appropriate safety measures are taken during leisure activities, as the patient will have a decreased ability to sense that his/her skin is being injured.

**Unilateral Neglect**  Lack of awareness of one side of the body. (See Neglect.)

**Vascular**  Pertaining to the blood vessels.

**Vasospasm**  Transient, abnormal constriction of a blood vessel.

**Vehicle Lift**  (ADA) The ADA outlines minimum size, function, and weight bearing ability of vehicle lifts used to help individuals access the vehicle.

**Vehicular Way**  (ADA) A route intended for vehicular traffic, such as a street, driveway, or parking lot.

**Vertebral Artery**  A branch of the subclavian artery which supplies blood to the brain.

**Visuospatial Neglect**  Lack of awareness of one side of the body. (See Neglect.)

**Walk**  (ADA) An exterior pathway with a prepared surface intended for pedestrian use, including general pedestrian areas such as plazas and courts.

**Weight Bearing**  Refers to the degree of one's own weight that can be supported by one or more body parts.
>Non weight bearing (NWB)
>Partial Weight bearing (PWB)
>Full Weight bearing (FWB)

**Wernicke's Aphasia**  (Fluent or Receptive Aphasia) Words that are easily spoken and grammatically correct, but have no meaning in the context spoken. Difficulty in understanding written or spoken words.

# 16. Americans with Disabilities Act Fact Sheet

The Americans with Disabilities Act (ADA) is a federal anti discrimination statute designed to remove barriers which prevent qualified individuals with disabilities from enjoying the same employment opportunities that are available to persons without disabilities.

Like the Civil Rights Act of 1964 that prohibits discrimination on the bases of race, color, religion, national origin, and sex, the ADA seeks to ensure access to equal employment opportunities based on merit. It does not guarantee equal results, establish quotas, or require preferences favoring individuals with disabilities over those without disabilities.

This chart was developed by the United States Architectural and Transportation Barriers Compliance Board in 1990.

**Abbreviations used in this chart:**

| | |
|---|---|
| **ADA** | Americans with Disabilities Act |
| **ATBCB** | Architectural and Transportation Barriers Compliance Board |
| **DOJ** | Department of Justice |
| **DOT** | Department of Transportation |
| **EEOC** | Equal Employment Opportunity Commission |
| **FCC** | Federal Communications Commission |
| **MGRAD** | Minimum Guidelines and Requirements for Accessible Design |
| **UFAS** | Uniform Federal Accessibility Standards |

| Accessibility Requirements | Effective Date | Regulations and Enforcement |
|---|---|---|
| **Title I - Employment**<br>Employers with 15 or more employees may not discriminate against qualified individuals with disabilities.<br><br><br><br>Employers must reasonably accommodate the disabilities of qualified applicants or employees, including modifying work stations and equipment, unless undue hardship would result. | July 26, 1992 - for employers with 25 or more employees.<br><br>July 26, 1994 - for employers with 15 to 24 employees. | EEOC to issue regulations by July 26, 1991.<br><br>Individuals may file complaints with EEOC. Individuals may also file a private lawsuit after exhausting administrative remedies.<br><br>Remedies are the same as available under Title VII of the Civil Rights Act of 1964. Court may order employer to hire or promote qualified individuals, reasonably accommodate their disabilities, and pay back wages and attorney's fees. |

| Accessibility Requirements | Effective Date | Regulations and Enforcement |
|---|---|---|
| **Title II - Public Services**<br>State and local governments may not discriminate against qualified individuals with disabilities.<br><br>Newly constructed state and local government buildings, including transit facilities, must be accessible.<br><br>Alterations to existing state and local government buildings must be done in an accessible manner.<br><br>When alterations could affect accessibility to "primary function" areas of a transit facility, an accessible path of travel must be provided to the altered areas and the restrooms, drinking fountains, and telephones serving the altered areas must also be accessible, to the extent that the additional accessibility cost are not disproportionate to the overall alterations costs.<br><br>New buses and rail vehicles for fixed route systems must be accessible.<br><br>New vehicles for demand responsive systems must be accessible unless the system provides individuals with disabilities a level of service equivalent to that provided to the general public.<br><br>One car per train must be accessible. | January 26, 1992 - unless otherwise noted below (Recipients of Federal financial assistance are presently required to comply with similar requirements under Section 504 of the Rehabilitation Act of 1973.)<br><br><br><br><br><br><br><br><br><br>Ordered after August 25, 1990.<br><br><br>Ordered after August 25, 1990.<br><br><br><br><br>By July 26, 1995 | DOJ to issue regulations except for public transportation by July 26, 1991.<br><br>DOT to issue regulations for public transportation by July 26, 1991.<br><br>ATBCB to supplement MGRAD by April 26, 1991. DOJ and DOT regulations must be consistent with supplemental MGRAD and may incorporate the supplemental MGRAD.<br><br>UFAS to be used as interim accessibility standard for transit facilities if final regulations have not been issued and if a building permit has been obtained prior to issuance of final regulations, work begins within one year of receipt of permit, and is completed under the terms of the permit. If final regulations have not been issued one year after MGRAD has been supplemented, MGRAD to be used as interim accessibility standard.<br><br>(Most facilities constructed or altered with Federal funds are presently required to comply with UFAS under the Architectural barriers Act of 1968. Facilities constructed or altered by recipients of Federal financial assistance are presently required to comply with UFAS under Section 504 of the Rehabilitation Act of 1973.) |

| Accessibility Requirements | Effective Date | Regulations and Enforcement |
|---|---|---|
| **Title II - Public Services** <u>**(cont.)**</u> <br> Existing "key stations" in rapid rail, commuter rail, and light rail systems must be accessible. | By July 26, 1993. Extensions may be granted up to July 2010 (commuter rail) and July 26, 2020 (rapid and light rail) for stations needing extraordinarily expensive structural changes. | Amtrak and commuter rail passenger cars must comply with MGRAD provisions for rail cars to the extent that they are in effect at the time the design of the cars is substantially completed, if final regulations have not been issued. |
| Comparable paratransit must be proved to individuals who cannot used fixed route bus service to the extent that an undue financial burden is not imposed. | By January 26, 1992 | Individuals may file complaints with DOT concerning public transportation and with other designated Federal agencies concerning matters other than public transportation. Individuals may also file a private lawsuit. |
| All existing Amtrak stations must be accessible. <br><br> Amtrak trains must have the same number of seating spaces for individuals who use wheelchairs as would be available if every car in the train were accessible to such individuals. | By July 26, 2010. <br><br> By July 26, 2000. Half of these seats must be available by July 26, 1995. | Remedies are the same as available under Section 505 of Rehabilitation Act of 1973. Court may order entity to make facilities accessible, provide auxiliary aids or services, modify policies, and pay attorney's fees. |

| Accessibility Requirements | Effective Date | Regulations and Enforcement |
|---|---|---|
| **Title III - Public Accommodations**<br><br>Restaurants, hotels, theaters, shopping centers and malls, retail stores, museums, libraries, parks, private schools, day care centers, and other similar places of public accommodation may not discriminate on the basis of disability.<br><br>Physical barriers in existing public accommodations must be removed if readily achievable (i.e., easily accomplishable and able to be carried out without much difficulty or expense). If not, alternative methods of providing services must be offered, if those methods are readily achievable.<br><br>New construction in public accommodations and commercial facilities (non-residential facilities affecting commerce) must be accessible.<br><br>Alterations to existing public accommodations and commercial facilities must be done in an accessible manner. When alterations could affect accessibility to "primary function" areas of a facility, an accessible path of travel must be provided to the altered areas and the rest rooms, telephones, and drinking fountains serving the altered areas must also be accessible, to the extent that the additional accessibility costs are not disproportionate to the overall alterations costs. | January 26, 1992 - unless otherwise noted below.<br><br><br><br><br><br><br><br><br><br><br><br><br><br><br><br><br>Facilities designed and constructed for first occupancy after January 26, 1993. | DOJ to issue regulations except for privately operated transportation by July 26, 1991.<br><br>DOT to issue regulations for privately operated transportation by July 26, 1991.<br><br>ATBCB to supplement MGRAD by April 26, 1991. DOJ and DOT regulations must be consistent with supplemental MGRAD and may incorporate the supplemental MGRAD.<br><br>UFAS to be used as interim accessibility standard if final regulations have not been issued and if a building permit has been obtained prior to issuance of final regulations, work beings within one year of receipt of permit, and is completed under the terms of the permit. If final regulations have not been issued one year after MGRAD has been supplemented, MGRAD to be used as interim accessibility standard.<br><br>On application by state or local government, Attorney General, in consultation with ATBCB, may certify that state or local building codes meet or exceed ADA accessibility requirements.<br><br>Individuals may file complaints with the Attorney General. Individuals may also file a private lawsuit. |

| Accessibility Requirements | Effective Date | Regulations and Enforcement |
|---|---|---|
| **Title III - Public Accommodations (cont.)** Elevators are not required in newly constructed or altered buildings under three stories or with less than 3,000 square feet per floor, unless the building is a shopping center, mall, or health provider's office. The Attorney General may determine that additional categories of such building require elevators. <br><br> New buses and other vehicles (except automobiles) operated by private entities must be accessible or system in which vehicles are used must provide individuals with disabilities a level of service equivalent to that provided to the general public depending on whether entity is primarily engaged in business of transporting people; whether system is fixed route or demand responsive; and vehicle seating capacity. <br><br> New over-the-road (buses with an elevated passenger deck located over a baggage compartment) must be accessible | Ordered after August 25, 1990 (February 25, 1992 for rail passenger cars and vans with a capacity of less than 8 persons when operated by an entity primarily engaged in the business of transporting people). <br><br><br> Ordered after July 26, 1996 (July 26, 1997, for small companies). Date may be extended by one year after completion of a study. | Remedies are the same as available under Title II of the Civil Rights Act of 1964. Court may order an entity to make facilities accessible, provide auxiliary aides or services, modify policies, and pay attorney's fees. <br><br> Court may award money damages and impose civil penalties in lawsuit filed by Attorney General but not in private lawsuit by individuals. <br><br> Small businesses with 25 or fewer employees and gross receipts of $1 million or less may not be sued for violations occurring before July 26, 1992; and small businesses with 10 or fewer employees and gross receipt of $.5 million or less may not be sued for violations occurring before January 26, 1993. However, such small businesses may be sued for violations relating to new construction and alterations to facilities occurring after the effective date. |
| **Title IV - Telecommunications** <br><br> Telephone Companies must provide telecommunications relay services for hearing-impaired and speech-impaired individuals 24 hours per day. | By July 26, 1993. | FCC to issue regulations by July 26, 1991. <br><br> Individuals may file complaints with the FCC. |

November 1990

**Access America Update**

The table above provides the reader with an overview of the American's with Disabilities Act. The United States Architectural and Transportation Barriers Compliance Board publishes the periodic newsletter called **Access America**. In the 1993, Number 2 issue of Access America the United States Architectural and Transportation Barriers Compliance Board announced some changes to the Americans with Disability Act Accessibility Guidelines. The following paragraphs are from this issue.

At its November 10, 1993, meeting in Washington, DC, the Access Board took four actions. Three were rulemaking actions; the fourth was adoption of a charter for an advisory committee.

Some of the rulemaking actions are carried out jointly with other agencies and require approval by those agencies. An individual action does not take effect until notice of the action has been published in the *Federal Register*. The Board expects publication in early 1994.

The three rulemaking actions taken by the Board in November are:

**Adoption of the final rule to amend the Americans with Disabilities Act (ADA) Accessibility Guidelines for Buildings and Facilities to include requirements for certain state and local government facilities.**

When it is published in the *Federal Register*, this new rule will add four sections to the ADA *Accessibility Guidelines (ADAAG) for Buildings and Facilities*, published by the Board in July 1991.

The guidelines will ensure that newly constructed and altered state and local government facilities covered by title II of the ADA, will be accessible to and usable by all people in terms of architecture, design, and communication.

The new sections of the ADAAG are:

- Section 11 — Judicial, Legislative, and Regulatory Facilities
- Section 12 — Detention and Correctional Facilities
- Section 13 — Accessible Residential Housing
- Section 14 — Public Rights-of-Way

**Adoption of a joint final rule to amend ADAAG by suspending temporarily, until July 26, 1996, requirements for detectable warnings at curb ramps, hazardous vehicular areas and reflecting pools.**

Detectable warnings are distinctively textured walking surfaces intended to be detectable by cane and under foot by people with visual impairments. The Board's action to suspend these provisions is based on a need for additional research on the necessity of detectable warnings at curb ramps, hazardous vehicular areas and reflecting pools, and on related safety factors. The actions does not affect the ADAAG requirement for detectable warnings at transit platforms.

The final rule will be published in the *Federal Register* jointly with the Department of Justice and Department of Transportation.

**Adoption of a joint notice of proposed rulemaking (NPRM) to amend ADAAG for Transportation Vehicles for over-the-road buses, to include additional requirements for people using mobility aids, including wheelchair users.**

Over-the-road buses are vehicles that have high passenger decks located over baggage compartments. They are frequently used for intercity fixed-route or charter tour bus service.

The NPRM will be published jointly with the Department of Transportation in early 1994. The Board and Department of Transportation are under statutory mandate to complete this rulemaking by May 16, 1994.

In addition to the rulemaking actions, the Board also approved:

**Adoption of a charter to establish an ADAAG Review Advisory Committee.**

The charter as adopted outlines three responsibilities for the committee: to recommend editorial revisions to the ADAAG; to review ADAAG, including a comparison with other model codes; and to recommend future coordination of the Board's ADAAG rulemaking and the processes used by the American National Standards Institute, Council of American National Standards Institute, Council of American Building Officials and other model code organizations.

**Other Actions:**

- A formal action to adopt ADAAG with special provisions for federally financed buildings will begin with the Board's publication of a notice of proposed rulemaking during 1995. A final rule is planned for 1996.

- Accessibility guidelines for recreation facilities and outdoor developed areas will be set forth in a proposed final rule targeted for 1996.

- Accessibility guidelines for such children's environments as day care centers, pre-school, kindergarten, elementary and other school programs, and children's museums, among others. The proposed rulemaking is expected in 1994, with a final rule in 1995.

- Accessibility guidelines for forms of water transportation, including passenger ships, ferries and docks is anticipated for final rule in 1997 or 1998.

Access America is a periodic newsletter published by the Architectural and Transportation Barriers Compliance Board, Suite 1000, 1331 F Street NW, Washington DC 20004-1111. There is no charge to receive a subscription to this publication.

# 17. Americans with Disabilities Act Accessibility Guidelines
## Checklist for Buildings and Facilities

*The material in this Chapter is included in the CIP manual because we felt that it was important to the therapist to know the actual standards required by the United States Government. The therapist may want to use the checklist on buildings and facilities where s/he will be taking patients prior to the community integration outing. By keeping the completed surveys on file in the therapeutic recreation office, other therapists, patients, and their families can use them to determine if they want to attempt an outing to that location.*

*The material contained in this Chapter was prepared by the United States Architectural and Transportation Barriers Compliance Board. The complete Checklist contains 29 forms. We have included 19 forms in this Chapter – the ones that we felt were most applicable to the modules in this book. For those therapists who plan to evaluate many types of buildings and facilities, we recommend that you obtain the entire book from the Compliance Board[11].*

This checklist has been prepared to assist individuals and entities with rights or duties under Title II, and Title III of the Americans with Disabilities Act (ADA) in applying the requirements of the ADA Accessibility Guidelines (ADAAG) to buildings and facilities subject to the law. The check list presents information in summary form on the Department of Transportation (DOT) and Department of Justice (DOJ) regulations implementing the ADA. The checklist must be used with the DOT and DOJ regulations and ADAAG to ensure accuracy.[12]

This checklist is intended for technical assistance purposes only. Individuals who use this checklist should be aware that the DOJ and the DOT, not the US Architectural and Transportation Barriers Compliance Board (Access Board), are responsible for the enforcement of Titles II and III of the ADA. Use of this

---

[11]US Architectural and Transpsortation Barriers Compliance Board, 1331 F Street N.W., Suite 1000, Washington D.C. 20004-111 1-800-USA-ABLE. The book may also be obtained through the U.S. Government Printing Office, Superintendent of Documents, Mailstop SSOP, Washington, DC 20402-9328. ISBN 0-16-041771-6.

[12]The Americans with Disabilities Act Handbook (ISBN 0-16-035847-7) is the United States Government's basic resource document on the ADA. This book contains ADA Regulations, the offical analysis and interpretation of those regulations, and the complete ADA Accessibility Guidelines. It is available from the U.S. Government Printing Office.

check list does not constitute a determination of your legal rights or responsibilities under the ADA, and it is not binding on the Department of Justice, Department of Transportation, or the Access Board.

Use of this checklist is voluntary. Individuals who use this checklist are not required to send the survey forms to DOJ, DOT, or the Access Board.

While ADAAG may be amended in the future, this checklist is based on ADAAG as published on July 26, 1991 (sections 1 through 4.35 and special application sections 5 through 9) and September 6, 1991 (section 10). See 56 FR 35408 (July 26, 1991) and 56 FR 45500 (September 6, 1991) as corrected at 57 FR 1393 (January 14, 1992).

# Introduction

The Americans with Disabilities Act (ADA), signed by President George Bush on July 26, 1990, is landmark legislation to extend civil rights protection with people with disabilities. The ADA prohibits discrimination on the basis of disability in employment, State and local government services, public transportation, public accommodations, commercial facilities, and telecommunications. The ADA requires the US Architectural and Transportation Barriers Compliance Board (Access Board) to supplement its Minimum Guidelines and Requirements for Accessible Design to serve as the basis for regulations to be issued by the Department of Justice and the Department of Transportation under Title II and Title II of the Act. On July 26, 1991, the Access Board published its ADA Accessibility Guidelines for Buildings and Facilities (ADAAG). These guidelines were amended and supplemented with provisions for transportation facilities on September 6, 1991. ADAAG is applicable to buildings and facilities covered by Title II and Title III of the ADA to the extent required by regulations issued by the Department of Justice and the Department of Transportation under the ADA.

The purpose of this checklist is to enable people to survey places of public accommodation, commercial facilities, and transportation facilities for compliance with the new construction and alterations requirements of Title II, Subtitle B (Public Transportation) and Title III of the ADA. It can also be used to identify barriers in existing buildings. No special training is needed to use this checklist. It can be used by businesses, building owners and managers, State and local governments, design professionals, or concerned citizens.

The checklist must be used in conjunction with the Department of Justice's regulations in 28 CFR Part 36, the Department of Transportation's Regulations in 49 CFR part 37, and the Americans with Disabilities Act Accessibility Guidelines which are reprinted in the appendices to those regulations. Appendix A of the Department of Transportation's regulations includes the section 10 of ADAAG, which specifies additional provisions for transportation facilities.

Buildings and facilities constructed or altered by, on behalf of, or for the use of State and local governments covered by Title II, Subtitle A of the ADA, (other than transportation facilities covered by the Department of Transportation's regulation), are allowed by 28 CFR 35.151 to follow either ADAAG without the elevator exception or the Uniform Federal Accessibility Standards (UFAS). A similar checklist, the UFAS Accessibility Checklist, is available from the Access Board.

### New Construction

Places of public Accommodation and commercial facilities covered by Title III of the ADA are required by 28 CFR 36.401 and 36.406 to comply with ADAAG if the facilities are designed and constructed for first occupancy after January 26, 1993. This requirement applies only if: 1. the last application for a building permit or permit extension for the facility is certified to be completed by a State, county, or local government after January 26, 1992 and 2. the first certificate of occupancy for the facility is issued after

January 26, 1993. Full compliance with the new construction requirements is not required where an entity can demonstrate that is structurally impracticable. The exception for structural impracticability, a very narrow one, is discussed in 28 CFR 36.401(c) and ADAAG 4.1.1(5)(a). Other exceptions for certain temporary structures, specific building areas and features (including elevators) are discussed in ADAAG 4.1.1.(4), 4.1.1(5)(b) and 4.1.3(5) and, where applicable, on the Minimum Requirements Summary Sheets or the Technical Requirement Survey Forms.

Transportation facilities covered by Title II, Subtitle B of the ADA are required by 49 CFR 37.9 and 37.41 to comply with ADAAG, including section 10, if a notice to proceed is issued _after_ January 25, 1992, for bus, light rail or rapid rail facilities; or _after_ October 7, 1991, for intercity or commuter rail stations.

## Employee Work Areas

Areas that are used only by employees as work areas must be designed and constructed so that individuals with disabilities can approach, enter, and exit the areas as required in ADAAG 4.1.1(3). The guidelines do not require that any areas used only by employees as work areas be constructed to permit maneuvering within the work area or be constructed or equipped (i.e., with racks or shelves) to be accessible.

## Equivalent Facilitation

Departures from the ADAAG technical and scoping provisions are permitted where the alternative designs and technologies used will provide substantially equivalent or greater access to and usability of the facility. See ADAAG 2.2 and other sections referenced in Appendix A2.2 of ADAAG for specific examples of equivalent facilitation.

For transportation facilities covered by Title II, Subtitle B of the ADA, a determination of equivalent facilitation must be made by the Administrator of the Federal Transit Administration or the Federal Railroad Administration, as applicable. The specific procedure for applying for such a determination is included in 49 CFR 37.9(d).

## Alterations

Alterations to a place of public accommodation or commercial facility covered by Title III of the ADA that are undertaken _after_ January 26, 1992 are required by 28 CFR 36.402 and 36.406 to be done in a manner so as to ensure that, to the maximum extent feasible, the altered portions of the facility comply with ADAAG. For transportation facilities covered by Title II, subtitle B of the ADA, 49 CFR 37.9 and 37.4 require that alterations must follow ADAAG if a notice to proceed or work order is issued _after_ January 25, 1992, for bus, light or rapid rail facilities; or _after_ October 7, 1991, for intercity or commuter rail stations.

In general, alterations of specific elements or portions of a facility must be completed in compliance with the requirements for new construction. However, full compliance with the alterations requirements is not required where it is technically infeasible, The exception for technical infeasibility is discussed in ADAAG 4.1.6(1)(j). This and other special provisions and exceptions for alterations contained in ADAAG 4.1.6 are discussed on the Minimum Requirements Summary Sheet I: Accessible Buildings – Additions and Alterations. Additional special provisions and exceptions for alterations for special facility types are found in ADAAG 5, 6, 7, 9, and 10 and on the Technical Requirements Survey Forms of the special facility types.

If an alteration affects or could affect the usability of or access to an area of a facility that contains a "primary function," an accessible path of travel must be provided to the altered area. In addition, restrooms, telephones, and drinking fountains serving the altered area must also be made accessible to the extent that the cost is not "disproportionate" to the cost of the overall alteration. Disproportionality is defined in 28 CFR 36.403 (f) and 49 CFR 37.43(e) as a sum not to exceed 20% of the cost of the alteration to the primary function area.

## Historic Preservation

Alterations to a qualified historic building or facility must comply with ADAAG unless it is determined in accordance with procedures described in ADAAG 4.1.7(2) that compliance with certain requirements would threaten or destroy the historic significance of the building or facility. In such a case, alternative requirements may be used. The alternative requirements are discussed in 28 CFR 36.405 and ADAAG 4.1.7(3) and on the Minimum Requirements Summary Sheet J: Accessible Buildings – Historic Preservation.

## Barrier Removal in Existing Facilities

Public accommodations covered by Title III of the ADA must remove architectural barriers in existing facilities, including communication barriers that are structural in nature, where such removal is readily achievable, The ADA generally defines readily achievable as "easily accomplishable and able to be carried out without much difficulty or expense." The requirement to remove architectural barriers where readily achievable is discussed in 28 CFR 36.304. Measures taken to comply with readily achievable barrier removal must comply with ADAAG unless it would not be readily achievable. Then, other readily achievable measures that do not fully comply with ADAAG may be taken. However, no measure shall be taken that poses a significant risk to the health or safety of individuals with disabilities or others.

## Key Stations

Existing rapid rail, light rail, and commuter rail transportation systems covered by Title II, Subtitle B of the ADA must identify "key stations", in accordance with requirements of 49 CFR 37.47 and 37.51. Generally, "key stations" must comply with ADAAG 10.3.2. Under some conditions, previously altered elements which conform to UFAS (when done by a public entity) or ANSI A117.1-1980 (when done by a private entity without Federal funds) may meet the key station requirements. This "grandfather" provision applies only to "key stations" and is discussed in 49 CFR 37.9(b) and the corresponding explanatory material in Appendix D to the Department of Transportation's regulations. All existing intercity rail stations must comply with ADAAG 10.3.2. The time frames for making "key stations" and existing intercity rail stations accessible are specified in the Department of Transportation's regulations at 49 CFR 37.47, 37.51, and 37.55.

## What Are "Places of Public Accommodation" and "Commercial Facilities"?

ADAAG applies to new construction and alterations of "places of public accommodation and commercial facilities". A "place of public accommodation" is a facility, operated by a private entity, who operations affect commerce and which falls within at least one of the twelve categories listed below:

1. An inn, hotel, motel, or other place of lodging, except for an establishment located within a building which contains not more than five rooms for rent or hire and that is actually occupied by the proprietor of the establishment as the residence of the proprietor;

2. A restaurant, bar or other establishment serving food or drink;

3. A motion picture house, theater, concert hall, stadium, or other place of exhibition or entertainment;

4. An auditorium, convention center, lecture hall, or other place of public gathering;

5. A bakery, grocery store, clothing store, hardware store, shopping center, or other sales or rental establishment;

6. A laundromat, dry cleaner, bank, barber shop, beauty shop, travel service, shoe repair service, funeral parlor, gas station, office of an accountant or lawyer, pharmacy, insurance office, professional office of a health care provider, hospital, or other service establishment;

7. A terminal, depot, or other station used for specified public transportation;

8. A museum, library, gallery, or other place of public display or collection;

9. A park, zoo, amusement park, or other place of recreation;

10. A nursery, elementary, secondary, undergraduate, or postgraduate private school, or other place of education;

11. A day care center, senior citizen center, homeless shelter, food bank, adoption agency, or other social service center establishment;

12. A gymnasium, health spa, bowling alley, golf course, or other place of exercise or recreation.

"Commercial facilities" are facilities whose operations will affect commerce and that are intended for nonresidential use by a private entity (e.g., factories and warehouses). "Commercial facilities" do not include facilities that are covered or expressly exempted from coverage under the Fair Housing Act of 1968, as amended; aircraft; and certain railroad equipment listed in 28 CFR 36.104.

**How the Checklist is Organized to Assist You**

This checklist presents the minimum scoping and technical requirements contained in ADAAG for newly constructed facilities in the logical progression of traveling to and through a building. The Minimum Requirements Summary Sheets tell you what to survey, such as an accessible route, an entry, or a bathroom. The Technical Requirements Survey Forms give you the specific features those elements must have. There are 29 survey forms to represent elements on the site and in the building. *(Nineteen of the 29 survey forms are contained in this Chapter.)* Many of ADAAG's general requirements are repeated on different forms because they apply to more than one element. Some survey forms may refer you to others for detailed provisions.

In general, the Minimum Requirements Summary Sheets and the Technical Requirements Survey Forms contain the ADAAG requirements for new construction. In alterations one must first attempt to meet the requirements for new construction unless it is technically infeasible or special provisions apply.

The survey process moves through a parallel structure in three steps using the following sheets and forms:

**Step 1: Building/Facility Identification and Data Sheet**

**Step 2: Minimum Requirements Summary Sheets[13]**

      Sheet A*:    Parking and Passenger Loading Zones
      Sheet B*:    Site Accessible Routes and Elements
      Sheet C*:    Entrances
      Sheet D*:    Building Accessible Route
      Sheet E*:    Rooms and Spaces (Including Assembly Areas and Dressing and Fitting Rooms)
      Sheet F*:    Toilet Rooms and Bathrooms

---

[13]The Sheets and Forms with an asterisk (*) after them are contained in this Appendix of the CIP.

| Sheet G*: | Special Features – Signage, Alarms, Detectable Warnings, and Automated Teller Machines (ATMs) |
| Sheet H*: | Special Types of Facilities |
| Sheet I*: | Accessible Buildings – Additions and Alterations |
| Sheet J*: | Accessible Buildings – Historic Preservation |

## Step 3: Technical Requirements Survey Forms

| Form 1*: | Parking |
| Form 2*: | Passenger Loading Zones |
| Form 3*: | Exterior Accessible Routes |
| Form 4*: | Curb Ramps |
| Form 5: | Drinking Fountains |
| Form 6*: | Telephones |
| Form 7*: | Ramps |
| Form 8: | Stairs |
| Form 9*: | Platform Lifts |
| Form 10*: | Entrances and Exits (Areas of Rescue Assistance) |
| Form 11*: | Doors and Gates |
| Form 12* | Building Lobbies and Corridors (Interior Accessible Route) |
| Form 13: | Elevators |
| Form 14*: | Rooms and Spaces |
| Form 15*: | Assembly Areas |
| Form 16*: | Toilet Rooms and Bathrooms |
| Form 17*: | Bathrooms and Showers |
| Form 18*: | Dressing and Fitting Rooms |
| Form 19: | Signage |
| Form 20: | Alarms |
| Form 21: | Detectable Warnings |
| Form 22: | Automated Teller Machines (ATMs) |

### Special Facility Types

| Form 23*: | Restaurants and Cafeterias |
| Form 24: | Medical Care Facilities |
| Form 25*: | Mercantile Facilities |
| Form 26*: | Libraries |
| Form 27: | Transient Lodging (Hotels, Motels, Inns, Boarding Houses, Dormitories, and other Similar Places) |
| Form 28: | Transient Lodging in Homeless Shelters, Halfway Houses, Transient Group Homes, and Other Social Service Establishments |
| Form 29: | Transportation |

## How Differences in Requirements for New Construction, Alterations, and Historic Properties are Addressed

Special provisions and exceptions allowed in alterations of buildings, including historic properties, are addressed in Minimum Requirements Summary Sheet I: Accessible Buildings – Additions and Alterations, and Sheet J: Accessible Buildings – Historic Preservation.

Special provisions and exceptions allowed in special facility types such as hotels, motels, hospitals, mercantile facilities, libraries, restaurants and cafeterias are addresses in Survey Forms 23 through 29.

212

# Survey Instructions

## Approach to Surveying

This checklist is designed to be used in full or in part, depending on the facility and our available time. If you are surveying a facility with which you are familiar, you may already know what the general access problems are and will want to use specific survey forms to check the details. If you are unfamiliar with the facility, it is helpful to make an initial tour through the building to orient yourself and to obtain information to help you compile your survey document.

Although this check list is structured for use on site, it can also be used by architects, facility managers, or others to review architectural plans.

## Preparing to Survey

Make contact with the building management and advise them that you will be surveying the building and that you will be glad to share your information with them. If you do not have a building plan, ask the management if they can provide you with one. A plan can be very helpful, particularly if you are surveying a large facility. You can assign numbers to areas or elements on the plan and use the same numbers to correlate the Survey Forms.

Take a copy of ADAAG with you when you do the survey. Since the Questions in this checklist are fairly brief, it is helpful to have the ADAAG with you to gain a thorough understanding of the full requirements of the Guidelines. Also, not every illustration in the ADAAG has been included in this survey. Illustrations are provided in the checklist only for those survey questions which cannot easily be stated or understood using words alone.

## Step 1: Identify the Type of Facility or Building Use

Complete the Building Identification and Data Sheet to document the name and address of the facility, dates of construction and alteration, type of facility or building use, number of stories and size of each, name of surveyor and date of survey.

Before surveying the facility it is essential to determine whether the provisions of ADAAG apply to the facility or portion of the facility and to identify certain attributes about the facility which might trigger or disallow certain exceptions contained in ADAAG. To determine which provisions of ADAAG apply, you must consult the Department of Justice regulations or Department of Transportation regulations as explained in the introduction. To determine the exceptions that apply you must also consult the DOJ or DOT regulations. Exceptions within ADAAG are noted on the Technical Requirements Survey Forms. An examples of an exception is the elevator exemption contained in ADAAG 4.3.1(5) Exception 1. Elevators are not required in places of public accommodation and commercial facilities that are less than three stories or that have less than 3,000 square feet per story unless the building is a shopping center or mall, the professional office of a health care provider, or a transportation facility.

## Step 2: Determine Minimum Requirements

The Minimum Requirements Summary Sheets tell you which elements are required to be accessible, such as a toilet room or an accessible route between the entrance and parking. Use the Summary Sheets to identify the specific elements of your facility which must be accessible.

With the Summary Sheets in hand, take a quick tour of the facility and/or look at the building plans. As you go through the facility, complete each Summary Sheet in the order in which it is presented. The Summary Sheets will ask you to inventory the elements of your facility which must be accessible.

The principle of an "accessible route" is key to the Summary Sheets. An "accessible route" is simply a path of travel which a person in a wheelchair, an elderly person, or someone with another mobility limitation would find safe and easy to use. (See ADAAG 3.5 Definitions. *These definitions are contained in the Glossary of the CIP*.) The Summary Sheets define where these accessible routes must be.

**Step 3: Copy and Assemble the Survey Forms**

Return to your workplace with the completed Summary Sheets. Using the completed Summary Sheets you can determine how many copies to make of each Technical Requirements Survey Form. Some forms will be needed more than once, others will not be needed at all. Some forms will reference other forms. Two forms that are referenced quite often are Form 11: Doors and Gate and Form 12: Building Lobbies and Corridors. Where forms are cross referenced you will always need to have a copy of the form for reference.

In some multi-story buildings, you will find certain elements required to be accessible are duplicated in the details of installation and you may be able to develop a "shorthand" method of surveying these elements. For instance, you might find that accessible drinking fountains are installed in the same location in a corridor and in the same way on the first through the tenth floor of a ten story building. It may be sufficient to use only one form (Form 5: Drinking Fountains) to assess compliance in detail for a typical fountain on the first floor, and then note that each fountain on the second through the tenth floor is the same. All elevators are required to be accessible but where there are three elevators in a bank, you will often find that the three elevators are the same. If this is true, you may be able to use a single form (Form 13: Elevators) to survey three elevators in the same bank.

Copy the necessary Survey Forms and attach them to the Summary Sheet which called for them. When you are finished, you will have a series of Survey Forms which progress logically through the facility and are divided by the Minimum Requirements Summary Sheets. If you are working with a team, you can give team members a complete section covered by a Summary Sheet. Cover the entire package with the Building Identification and Data Sheet. If you are surveying an alteration to a facility or an alteration which falls under historic preservation provisions, you will also need those Summary Sheets.

**Step 4: Survey**

Bring a copy of ADAAG, a clipboard, a pencil or a pen, a flexible measuring tape, and a stick of chalk for marking distances on surfaces. You may also want a line level or other device to measure ramp slopes, and a fish scale for determining door pull force.

Each Survey Form has a title block which allows you to identify the specific element you are inspecting. Be sure to fill in the location of the element and the facility name on each Survey Form.

Each survey question or series of questions has an ADAAG section number. Some questions have more than one ADAAG section number. If you do not understand the question, look up the section(s) in ADAAG. Illustrations referenced in the survey forms are printed on subsequent pages. If you have a question about a term, refer to ADAAG 3.5 (Definitions –*also found in the glossary of the CIP*).

Check off whether the element complies or not. If you cannot determine whether or not it complies, put a question mark in the box. Do not leave blank boxes because it will confuse someone who later reviews the forms. If the element does not exist, write "N/A" (Not Applicable).

Each Survey Form has boxes for you to check for each question, either "yes" or "no." Please also notice that extra space is provided for you to elaborate where a simple "yes" or "no" is insufficient. You should note as precisely as possible what the problem is; for example, "clear opening width only 29 inches," "hand rail diameter 4 inches," or "ramp slope 1:10." This information will assist those using the survey at a later date to make modifications and to evaluate which changes might be more critical in providing access.

# Building Identification and Data Sheet

**Facility Name:** _____

**Facility Address:** _____

_____

**Date(s) of Construction** _____

_____

**Date(s) of Alteration:** _____

_____

## Type of Facility of Building Use:

(In this space, provide information about the facility that will help you in applying the provisions of ADAAG and in using the survey data in the future. For example, is the building a place of public accommodation or commercial facility? Is it owned by a State or local government? Is it the professional office of a health care provider, a shopping center or a shopping mall, or a transportation facility?)

_____

_____

## Number of Stories and Size of Each:

_____

_____

**Name(s) of Surveyors:** _____

_____

_____

_____

**Date(s) of Survey:** _____

_____

_____

# A: Parking and Passenger Loading Zones

(Attach Needed Survey Forms to this Summary Sheet.)

**Parking – Minimum Number: 4.1.2(5)(a) and (b)**

**General Use Parking:** If self parking is provided for employees or visitors, each parking area/lot or structure is required to have accessible parking spaces complying with the following table and with 4.6.

**Note:** Spaces required by the table need not be provided in the particular area/lot or structure. They may be provided at a different location if equivalent or greater accessibility, in terms of distance from an accessible entrance, cost and convenience, is ensured.

**Total Parking in Area/Lot or Structure**    **Required Minimum Number of Accessible Spaces**

| Total Parking in Area/Lot or Structure | | | Required Minimum Number of Accessible Spaces |
|---|---|---|---|
| 1 | to | 25 | 1 |
| 26 | to | 50 | 2 |
| 51 | to | 75 | 3 |
| 76 | to | 100 | 4 |
| 101 | to | 150 | 5 |
| 151 | to | 200 | 6 |
| 201 | to | 300 | 7 |
| 301 | to | 400 | 8 |
| 401 | to | 500 | 9 |
| 501 | to | 1000 | 2% of total |
| 1001 | and | over | 20 plus 1 for each 100 over 1000 |

In addition, one in every eight accessible parking spaces (but not less than one) must be served by an access aisle at least 96 inches wide and must be designated "van accessible."

**Exception:** Provision of all required spaces in conformance with the "Universal Parking Space Design" which accommodates both cars and vans is permitted (See Appendix A4.6.3 of ADAAG).

**Parking at Health Care Facilities: 4.1.2(5)(a), (b) and (d)**

Employee and visitor parking at general health care facilities must comply with the table above, except as follows. At outpatient units and facilities, 10 percent of the total number of parking spaces provided serving each outpatient unit or facility must be accessible. At units and facilities specializing in treatment or services for people with mobility impairments, 20 percent of the total number of spaces provided serving each such unit or facility must be accessible.

**List parking areas/lots or structures to be surveyed:**

_____

_____

_____

*Survey each parking area/lot or structure with Form 1: Parking and Passenger Loading Zones and Form 3: Exterior Accessible Routes. For parking structures which have doors or gates, or elevators, use Form 11: Doors and Gates and Form 13: Elevators (Not in this CIP Chapter). If direct access is provided for pedestrians from an enclosed parking garage to a building, use Form 10: Entrances and Exits (Areas of Rescue Assistance). If the parking structure has public telephones or drinking fountains, use Form 5: Drinking Fountains (Not in this CIP Chapter) and Form 6: Telephones. If the parking structure has toilet rooms, use Minimum Requirements Summary Sheet F: Toilet Rooms and Bathrooms.*

Minimum Requirements Summary Sheet            A — 1

**Valet Parking: 4.1.2(5)(e)**

Valet parking facilities must provide a passenger loading zone complying with 4.6.6 located on an accessible route to the entrance of the facility.

**Note:** Valet parking facilities are <u>not</u> required to provide accessible parking spaces.

**List valet parking facilities to be surveyed:**                    ☐ **Not Applicable**

_____

_____

*Survey each valet parking facility with Form 2: Passenger Loading Zones. Survey the accessible route from the passenger loading zone to the entrance to the facility with Form 3: Exterior Accessible Routes, or Form 12: Building Lobbies and Corridors. You may also need Form 4: Curb Ramps and Form 21: Detectable Warnings (Not in this **CIP** Chapter).*

**Passenger Loading Zones: 4.1.2(5)(c)**

Where passenger loading zones are provided, at least one must be accessible. You can usually identify the accessible passenger loading zone by a sign bearing the International Symbol of Accessibility. If not sign is present, survey existing passenger loading zones to identify ones that may be accessible. Begin with the passenger loading zone closest to an accessible entrance.

List passenger loading zones to be surveyed:

_____

_____

_____

_____

*Survey each passenger loading zone with Form 2: Passenger Loading Zones. You may also need Form 4: Curb Ramps and Form 21: Detectable Warnings (Not in this **CIP** Chapter).*

<u>Number of Copies:</u>

| | | | |
|---|---|---|---|
| Form 1: | Parking | _____ | |
| Form 2: | Passenger Loading Zones | _____ | |
| Form 3: | Exterior Accessible Routes | _____ | |
| Form 4: | Curb Ramps | _____ | |
| Form 5: | Drinking Fountains | _____ | *(Not in this CIP Chapter)* |
| Form 6: | Telephones | _____ | |
| Form 10: | Entrances and Exits (Areas of Rescue Assistance) | _____ | |
| Form 11: | Doors and Gates | _____ | |
| Form 12: | Building Lobbies and Corridors | _____ | |
| Form 13: | Elevators | _____ | *(Not in this CIP Chapter)* |
| Form 21: | Detectable Warnings | _____ | *(Not in this CIP Chapter)* |

Minimum Requirements Summary Sheet                    A — 2

# B: Site Accessible Routes and Elements

(Attach Needed Survey Forms to this Summary Sheet)

**Site Accessible Routes and Elements: 4.1.2(1), 4.1.2(2), 4.1.2 (3), and 4.1.2(4)**

At least one accessible route must be provided within the boundary of the site connecting the following elements, where provided on the site, to an accessible building entrance.

| **From:** | **To:** |
|---|---|
| public transportation stops | accessible entrance |
| accessible parking spaces | accessible entrance |
| accessible passenger loading zones | accessible entrance |
| public streets and sidewalks | accessible entrance |

If you are using a plan drawing, you may want to mark each of these routes with a colored pencil.

In addition, at least one accessible route must connect accessible buildings, accessible facilities, accessible elements and accessible spaces that are on the same site.

Accessible routes must connect these elements. If they do exist, then the completed survey form will reveal their complying and non-complying features. The accessible route to an accessible entrance must, to the maximum extent feasible, coincide with the route for the general public.

All objects that protrude from surfaces or posts into circulation paths must comply with the requirements of 4.4; and the sidewalk, ramps and other walking surfaces that make up the accessible routes and spaces must comply with 4.5.

**List accessible routes to be surveyed:**

**From:**                                              **To:**

_____          _____

_____          _____

_____          _____

_____          _____

*Survey each accessible route with Form 3: Exterior Accessible Routes. You may also need Form 4: Curb Ramps; Form 7: Ramps; Form 8: Stairs (not in this CIP Chapter); Form 9: Platform Lifts\*; Form 13: Elevators (not in this CIP Chapter); Form 19: Signage (not in this CIP Chapter); and Form 21: Detectable Warnings (not in this CIP Chapter). If drinking fountains, public telephones, or automated teller machines are located on the site, use Form 5: Drinking Fountains (not in this CIP Chapter); Form 6: Telephones; and Form 22: Automated Teller Machines (ATMs) (not in this CIP Chapter). If a toilet facility or bathing facility is located on a site, use Minimum Requirements Summary Sheet F: Toilet Rooms and Bathrooms.*

**\*Note:** The use of stairs and platforms lifts to provide access is limited in new construction.

**Stairs: 4.1.3(4)**

Interior and exterior stairs connecting levels that are <u>not</u> connected by an elevator, ramp, or other accessible means of vertical access must comply with 4.9. In new construction, this condition may occur in facilities subject to the elevator exemption (see 4.1.3(5) Exception 1), or where mezzanines are exempt in restaurants (see 5.4).

**List stairs to be surveyed:**

_____

_____

*Survey stairs with Form 8: Stairs (not in this CIP Chapter) in those buildings and facilities only where the levels are not connected by an elevator, ramp, or other accessible means of vertical access.*

## Platform Lifts: 4.1.3(5) Exception 4

In new construction, platform lifts complying with 4.11 and applicable State or local codes may be used in place of an elevator only under the following conditions:

(a) To provide an accessible route to a performing area in an assembly occupancy.

(b) To comply with the wheelchair viewing position, line-of-sight, and dispersion requirements of 4.33.3.

(c) To provide access to incidental occupiable spaces and room which are not open to the general public and which house no more than five persons, including but not limited to equipment control rooms and projection booths.

(d) To provide access where existing site constraints or other constraints make use of a ramp to an elevator infeasible.

**List platform lifts to be surveyed:**

_____

_____

*Survey each platform lift with Form 9: Platform Lifts.*

<u>Number of Copies:</u>

| | | | |
|---|---|---|---|
| Form 3: | Exterior Accessible Routes | _____ | |
| Form 4: | Curb Ramps | _____ | |
| Form 5: | Drinking Fountains | _____ | (not in this CIP Chapter) |
| Form 6: | Telephones | _____ | |
| Form 7: | Ramps | _____ | |
| Form 8: | Stairs | _____ | (not in this CIP Chapter) |
| Form 9: | Platform Lifts | _____ | |
| Form 13: | Elevators | _____ | (not in this CIP Chapter) |
| Form 19: | Signage | _____ | (not in this CIP Chapter) |
| Form 21: | Detectable Warnings | _____ | (not in this CIP Chapter) |
| Form 22: | Automated Teller Machines (ATMs) | _____ | (not in this CIP Chapter) |

# C: Entrances

(Attach Needed Survey Forms to this Summary Sheet.)

**Entrances: 4.1.3(8)**

- At least 50% of all public entrances must be accessible.

- If the number of exits required by the applicable building/fire code is greater than 50% of public entrances, the number of accessible entrances must be at least equal to the number of required exits up to the total number of entrances planned. (See examples below.)

In addition:

- Each separate tenancy must have an accessible entrance.

- Where access is provided from a pedestrian tunnel or elevated walkway, an accessible entrance must be provided.

Examples:

- A facility has six (6) public entrances planned and four (4) fire exits are required. Four (4) of the six (6) public entrances must be accessible.

- A facility has one (1) public entrance planned, and two (2) fire exits are required. Only one (1) public entrance must be accessible.

- A facility has three (3) public entrances planned, and two (2) fire exits are required. Two (2) of the three (3) public entrances must be accessible.

**List accessible entrances to be surveyed:**

_____

_____

*Survey each accessible entrance with Form 10: Entrances and Exits (Areas of Rescue Assistance); Form 11: Doors and Gates; and Form 3: Exterior Accessible Routes. You may also need Form 7: Ramps; Form 8: Stairs\* (not in this **CIP** Chapter); Form 9: Platform Lifts\*; Form 13: Elevators (not in this **CIP** Chapter); and Form 19: Signage (not in this **CIP** Chapter), where these elements are part of the entrance.*

**\*Note:** Use of stairs and platform lifts to provide accessibility is limited in new construction. (See Minimum Requirements Summary Sheet B: Site Accessible Routes and Elements.)

<u>Number of Copies</u>

| | | | |
|---|---|---|---|
| Form 3: | Exterior Accessible Routes | _____ | |
| Form 7: | Ramps | _____ | |
| Form 8: | Stairs | _____ | (not in this CIP Chapter) |
| Form 9: | Platform Lifts | _____ | |
| Form 10: | Entrances | _____ | |
| Form 11: | Doors and Gates | _____ | |
| Form 13: | Elevators | _____ | (not in this CIP Chapter) |
| Form 19: | Signage | _____ | (not in this CIP Chapter) |

# D: Building Accessible Route

(Attach Needed Survey Forms to this Summary Sheet.)

**Building Accessible Route: 4.1.3(1), 4.1.3(3), 4.1.3(4), and 4.1.3(5)**

At least one accessible route complying with 4.3 must connect accessible building or facility entrances with all accessible spaces and elements within the building or facility.

In a multi-story building, an accessible elevator must provide access to each level unless a ramp complying with 4.8 is provided. Use of stairs or platform lifts to provide access in new construction is limited. If the building is less than three stories, or has less than 3,000 square feet per story, an elevator is not required unless the building is the professional office of a health care provider, a shopping center, or shopping mall, or a transportation facility. There terms are defined in 36 CFR §36.401(d.).

All objects that overhang or protrude into circulation paths must comply with 4.4; and ground and floor surfaces along accessible routes must comply with 4.5.

**List building lobbies and corridors to be surveyed:**

_____

_____

_____

_____

*Survey each building lobby and corridor with Form 12: Building Lobbies and Corridors. You may also need Form 19: Signage (not in this **CIP** Chapter) and Form 20: Alarms (not in this **CIP** Chapter). If a door or gate is across an accessible route, use Form 11: Doors and Gates. If drinking fountains, public telephones, or automated teller machines are located in a building lobby or corridor, use Form 5: Drinking Fountains (not in this **CIP** Chapter); Form 6: Telephones; and Form 22: Automated Teller Machines (ATMs) (not in this **CIP** Chapter).*

**List ramps to be surveyed:**

_____

_____

*Survey each ramp with Form 7: Ramps.*

**Stairs: 4.1.3(4)**

Interior and exterior stairs connecting levels that are not connected by an elevator, ramp, or other accessible means of vertical access must comply with 4.9. In new construction, this condition may occur in facilities subject to the elevator exemption (see 4.1.3(5) Exception 1), or where mezzanines are exempt in restaurants (see 5.4).

**List stairs to be surveyed:**

_____

_____

*Survey stairs with Form 8: Stairs (not in this **CIP** Chapter) in those buildings and facilities only where the levels are not connected by an elevator, ramp, or other accessible means of vertical access.*

Minimum Requirements Summary Sheet

D — 1

**Platform Lifts: 4.1.3(5) Exception 4**

In new construction, platform lifts complying with 4.11 and applicable State or local codes may be used in lieu of an elevator only under the following conditions:

(a) To provide an accessible route to a performing area in an assembly occupancy.

(b) To comply with the wheelchair viewing position, line-of-sight, and dispersion requirements of 4.33.3.

(c) To provide access to incidental occupiable spaces and room which are not open to the general public and which house no more than five persons, including but not limited to equipment control rooms and projection booths.

(d) To provide access where existing site constraints or other constraints make use of a ramp or an elevator infeasible.

**List platform lifts to be surveyed:**

_____

_____

**Survey each platform lift with Form 9: Platform Lifts.**

<u>Number of Copies:</u>

| | | | |
|---|---|---|---|
| Form 5: | Drinking Fountains | _____ | (not in this **CIP** Chapter) |
| Form 6: | Telephones | _____ | |
| Form 7: | Ramps | _____ | |
| Form 8: | Stairs | _____ | (not in this **CIP** Chapter) |
| Form 9: | Platform Lifts | _____ | |
| Form 11: | Doors and Gates | _____ | |
| Form 12: | Building Lobbies and Corridors | _____ | |
| Form 13: | Elevators | _____ | (not in this **CIP** Chapter) |
| Form 19: | Signage | _____ | (not in this **CIP** Chapter) |
| Form 20: | Alarms | _____ | (not in this **CIP** Chapter) |
| Form 22: | Automated Teller Machines (ATMs) | _____ | (not in this **CIP** Chapter) |

Minimum Requirements Summary Sheet

D — 2

# E: Rooms and Spaces (Including Assembly Areas and Dressing and Fitting Rooms)

(Attach Needed Survey Forms to this Summary Sheet.)

**Public and Common Use Areas: 4.1.1**

Rooms and spaces which are not specifically exempt or which are not used solely as work areas must be fully accessible.

**Note:** Accessibility is not required to: (i) observation galleries used primarily for security purposes; or (ii) non-occupiable spaces accessed only by ladders, catwalks, crawl spaces, very narrow passageways, or freight (non-passenger) elevators and frequented only by service personnel for repair purposes (e.g., elevator pits, elevator penthouses, piping or equipment catwalks).

**Work Areas: 4.1.1(3)**

Areas that are used only by employees as work areas must be designed and constructed so that individuals with disabilities can approach, enter, and exit the areas. The guidelines do not require that areas used only by employees as work areas be constructed to permit maneuvering within the work area or be constructed or equipped (i.e., with racks or shelves) to be accessible.

**List rooms and spaces which must be accessible:**

_____
_____
_____
_____

*Survey each room and space with Form 14: Rooms and Spaces. You may also need Form 11: Doors and Gates; Form 19: Signage (not in this **CIP** Chapter); and Form 20: Alarms (not in this **CIP** Chapter). If ramps, stairs\*, or lifts\* are part of a room or space, use Form 7: Ramps, Form 8: Stairs\* (not in this **CIP** Chapter), and Form 9: Platform Lifts\*. If drinking fountains or public telephones are located in a room or space, use Form 5: Drinking Fountains (not in this **CIP** Chapter) and Form 6: Telephones.*

**\*Note:** Use of stairs and platform lifts to provide accessibility is limited in new construction. (See Minimum Requirements Summary Sheet D: Building Accessible Route.)

**List rooms and spaces that are used solely as work areas:**

_____
_____
_____
_____

*Survey the door to each area with Form 11: Doors and Gates and survey the accessible route with Form 12: Building Lobbies and Corridors.*

Minimum Requirements Summary Sheet

E — 1

**Assembly Areas:**

An assembly area is defined as a room or space accommodating a group of individuals for recreational, educational, political, social, or amusement purposes, or for the consumption of food and drink.

**List assembly areas to be surveyed:**

_____

_____

_____

_____

*Survey each assembly area with Form 15: Assembly Areas.*

**Dressing and Fitting Rooms: 4.1.3(21)**

Where dressing and fitting rooms are provided for use by the general public, patients, customers, or employees, 5% (but not less than one) of dressing rooms for each type of use in each cluster of dressing and fitting rooms must comply with 4.35.

**List dressing rooms to be surveyed:**

_____

_____

_____

_____

*Survey each dressing room with Form 18: Dressing and Fitting Rooms.*

<u>Number of Copies:</u>

| | | | |
|---|---|---|---|
| Form 5: | Drinking Fountains | _____ | (not in this **CIP** Chapter) |
| Form 6: | Telephones | _____ | |
| Form 7: | Ramps | _____ | |
| Form 8: | Stairs | _____ | (not in this **CIP** Chapter) |
| Form 9: | Platform Lifts | _____ | |
| Form 11: | Doors and Gates | _____ | |
| Form 12: | Building Lobbies and Corridors | _____ | |
| Form 14: | Rooms and Space | _____ | |
| Form 15: | Assembly Areas | _____ | |
| Form 18: | Dressing and Fitting Rooms | _____ | |
| Form 19: | Signage | _____ | (not in this **CIP** Chapter) |
| Form 20: | Alarms | _____ | (not in this **CIP** Chapter) |

# F: Toilet Rooms and Bathrooms

(Attach Needed Survey Forms to this Summary Sheet.)

**Toilet Rooms/Facilities and Bathrooms/Bathing Facilities: 4.1.2(6) and 4.1.3(11)**

In a building or facility, each public and common use toilet room/facility, and bathroom/bathing facility must be accessible, Employee toilet rooms are considered to be "common use" toilet rooms. Other toilet rooms and bathrooms must be adaptable in that all space and door requirements must be satisfied.

For single user portable toilet or bathing units clustered at a single location (where not associated with construction sites), at least 5% (but not less than one) accessible toilet units or bathing units must be installed at each cluster whenever typical inaccessible units are provided. Accessible units must be identified by the International Symbol of Accessibility.

**List the toilet rooms/facilities and bathrooms/bathing facilities to be surveyed (include portable units on a site):**

_____
_____
_____
_____

*Survey each toilet room/facility with Form 16: Toilet Rooms and Bathrooms and Form 19: Signage (not in this **CIP** Chapter). Survey each bathroom/bathing facility with Form 16: Toilet Rooms and Bathrooms; Form 17: Bathtubs and Showers, and Form 19: Signage (not in this **CIP** Chapter). You may also need Form 11: Doors and Gates and Form 20: Alarms (not in this **CIP** Chapter). If a drinking fountain is located in the toilet room/facility or bathroom/bathing facility, use Form 5: Drinking Fountains (not in this **CIP** Chapter).*

Number of Copies:

| | | | |
|---|---|---|---|
| Form 5: | Drinking Fountains | _____ | (not in this **CIP** Chapter) |
| Form 11: | Doors and Gates | _____ | |
| Form 16: | Toilet Rooms and Bathrooms | _____ | |
| Form 17: | Bathtubs and Showers | _____ | |
| Form 19: | Signage | _____ | (not in this **CIP** Chapter) |
| Form 20: | Alarms | _____ | (not in this **CIP** Chapter) |

# G: Special Features – Signage, Alarms, Detectable Warnings, and Automated Teller Machines

(Attach Needed Survey Forms to this Summary Sheet.)

**Signage: 4.1.2(7) and 4.1.3(16)**

Signs which designate permanent rooms and spaces must comply with 4.30.1, 4.30.4, and 4.39.6. Other signs which provide direction to, or information about, functional spaces of the building must comply with 4.30.1, 4.30.2, 4.30.3, and 4.30.5.

Exception: Building directories, menus, and all other signs which are temporary are not required to comply.

**List signs to be surveyed:**

_____

_____

*Survey each sign with Form 19: Signage (not in this **CIP** Chapter). Form 19: Signage is also used with Form 3: Exterior Accessible Routes; Form 6: Telephones; Form 10: Entrances and Exits (Areas of Rescue Assistance); Form 12: Building Lobbies and Corridors; Form 14: Rooms and Spaces; Form 16: Toilet Rooms and Bathrooms; and Form 29: Transportation Facilities.*

**Alarms: 4.1.3(14)**

If emergency warning systems are provided, then they must include both audible alarms and visual alarms complying with 4.28. Sleeping accommodations required to comply with 9.3 must have an auxiliary visual alarm complying with 4.28.4. Emergency warning systems in medical care facilities may be modified to suit standard health care alarm design practice.

**List alarms to be surveyed:**

_____

_____

*Survey each alarm with Form 20: Alarms (not in this **CIP** Chapter). Form 20: Alarms is also used with Form 12: Building Lobbies and Corridors; Form 14: Rooms and Spaces: Form 15: Assembly Areas; and Form 16: Toilet Rooms and Bathrooms.*

**Detectable Warnings: 4.1.3(15)**

Detectable warnings must be provided at reflecting pools that are not protected by railings, walks, or curbs. At hazardous vehicular areas on a site, if a walk crosses or adjoins a vehicular way, and the walking surfaces are not separated by curbs, railings, or other elements between the pedestrian areas and vehicular areas, then the boundary between the areas must be defined by a continuous detectable warning. Detectable warnings must also be provided on curb ramps on a site.

List detectable warnings to be surveyed:

_____

_____

*Survey each detectable warning with Form 21: Detectable Warnings (Not in this **CIP** Chapter). Detectable warnings on curb ramps are included on Form 4: Curb Ramps. Form 21: Detectable Warnings is also used with Form 2: Passenger Loading Zones and Form 3: Accessible Routes.*

Minimum Requirements Summary Sheet

G — 1

**Automated Teller Machines (ATMs): 4.1.3(20)**

Where one or more automated teller machines is provided at a location, at least one ATM at that location must comply with 4.34.

Exception: Drive-up-only automated teller machines are not required to comply with 4.27.2, 4.27.3 and 4.34.3.

**List ATMs to be surveyed:**

_____

_____

*Survey each ATM with Form 22: Automated Teller Machine (ATMs) (not in this **CIP** Chapter). Form 22: Automated Teller Machines (ATMs) is also used with Form 3: Exterior Accessible Routes and Form 12: Building Lobbies and Corridors.*

Number of Copies:

| | | | |
|---|---|---|---|
| Form 19: | Signage | _____ | (not in this **CIP** Chapter) |
| Form 20: | Alarms | _____ | (not in this **CIP** Chapter) |
| Form 21: | Detectable Warnings | _____ | (not in this **CIP** Chapter) |
| Form 22: | Automated Teller Machines | _____ | (not in this **CIP** Chapter) |

Minimum Requirements Summary Sheet                                   G — 2

# H. Special Types of Facilities

(Attach Needed Survey Forms to this Summary Sheet.)

The facilities listed below have further specific requirements in addition to those of 4.1 to 4.35. If you are surveying one of these special facilities, you will also need the appropriate form for the type of facility. For instance, if you are surveying a hotel or motel, use Minimum Requirements Summary Sheets A - G to identify which Forms (1 - 22) are needed to survey the facility for compliance with 9.0. If the facility also has a gift shop and a restaurant, you will also need Form 25: Mercantile Facilities to survey for compliance with 7.0 and Form 23: Restaurants and Cafeterias to survey for compliance with 5.0.

Special Facilities:

Form 23:    Restaurants and Cafeterias
Form 24:    Medical Care Facilities (not in this **CIP** Chapter)
Form 25:    Mercantile Facilities
Form 26:    Libraries
Form 27:    Transient Lodging (Hotels, Motels, Inns, Boarding Houses, Dormitories, Resorts, and Other Similar Places) (not in this **CIP** Chapter)
Form 28:    Transient Lodging in Homeless Shelters, Halfway Houses, Transient Group Homes, and other Social Service Establishments (not in this **CIP** Chapter)
Form 29:    Transportation Facilities

# I: Accessible Buildings – Additions & Alterations

**Additions 4.1.5:**

Additions must meet the applicable minimum requirements for new construction in 4.1.1 to 4.1.3 and the applicable technical provisions in 4.2 through 4.35 and 5.0 through 10.0 for each space or element added to the existing building or facility. Use the applicable survey forms for new construction for each altered element or space.

Additions to an existing building or facility also are regarded as alterations. An addition that affects an area of primary function must also comply with 4.1.6(2) and 28 CFR §36.403.

**Alterations 4.1.6(1):**

No alteration may decrease accessibility below the requirements for new construction. Alterations are not required to provide greater accessibility than that in new construction. In existing buildings or facilities, alterations must comply with the following:

- Each element, space, feature, or area that is altered must comply with the applicable minimum requirements for new construction in 4.1.1 through 4.1.3 and the applicable technical provisions in 4.2 through 4.35 and 5.0 through 10.0. (Use Forms 1-29.) If the applicable requirements for new construction require that an element, space, feature, or area be on an accessible route, an accessible route is not required except as provided in 4.1.6(2) (Alterations to an Area containing Primary Function).

- When alterations of single elements amount to an alteration of a room or space, the entire space must be made accessible.

- If full compliance with the technical provisions (4.2 through 4.35 and 5.0 through 10.0) of an altered element, space, feature, or area is technically infeasible, the special technical provision in 4.1.6(3) may be utilized. If there is not special technical provision in 4.1.6(3) for an altered element, space, feature, or area, or if full compliance with the special technical provision is technically infeasible, the alteration must provide accessibility to the maximum extent feasible. Any elements or features of the building of facility that are being altered and can be made accessible, must be made accessible within the scope of the alteration.

**Special Technical Provisions 4.1.6(3): The following elements may be modified only as described below.**

- **Curb Ramps and Ramps – Slope and Rise:** Where space limitations prohibit the use of a 1:12 slope, a slope between 1:10 and 1:12 is allowed for a maximum rise of 6 inches; and a slope between 1:8 and 1:10 is allowed for a maximum rise of 3 inches.

- **Stairs – Handrail Extensions:** Where handrail extensions would be hazardous (e.g., protruding into pedestrian traffic perpendicular to the stair) or impossible due to plan configuration, full extension of handrails is not required.

- **Elevators – Safety Edges and Car Dimensions:** If safety edges are provided in an existing automatic elevator, automatic door opening devices may be omitted. Where existing shaft configuration or technical infeasibility prohibits full compliance with 4.10.9, the car plan dimensions may be reduced by the minimum amount necessary, but in no case shall the inside car area be less than 48 inches by 48 inches. Equivalent facilitation may be provided with an elevator car of different dimensions when usability can be demonstrated and when all other accessible elements comply with 4.10.

- **Doors – Clear Opening and Thresholds:** Where it is technically infeasible to comply with the 32 inch clear opening width requirement, a maximum projection of 5/8 inch will be permitted for the latch side stop. If existing thresholds are no more than 3/4 inch high, and have (or are modified to have) a beveled edge on each side, they may remain.

- **Toilet/Bathrooms – Unisex, Alternate Stall, Directional Signage:** Where it is technically infeasible to modify both men's and women's toilets/bath rooms in compliance with 4.22 or 4.23, a unisex toilet/bath room is permitted. Each unisex toilet room must contain one water closet complying with 4.16 and one lavatory complying with 4.19, and the door must have a privacy latch. Where it is technically infeasible to install a required standard stall (Fig. 30(a)), or where other codes prohibit reduction of the fixture count, either alternate stall (Fig. 30(b)) may be provided. where existing toilet/bath rooms are not altered to be accessible, signage must be provided indicating the location of the nearest accessible toilet/bath room within the facility.

- **Assembly Areas – Dispersal of Seating and Performing Areas:** Where it is technically infeasible to meet dispersal requirements, accessible seating may be clustered. Each accessible seating area must have provisions for companion seating and must be located on an accessible route usable as a means of emergency egress. Where it is technically infeasible to alter all performing areas to be on an accessible route, at least one of each type of performing area must be made accessible.

- **Lifts – Conditions for Use:** In alterations, the use of lifts is not limited to the four conditions in 4.1.3(5) Exception 4. Lifts must comply with 4.11 and applicable State and local codes.

- **Dressing/Fitting Rooms – Minimum Number:** Where technically infeasible to provide the minimum number of dressing/fitting rooms required in 4.1.3(21), one dressing room for each sex (or one unisex if typical) on each level must be made accessible.

## Additional Requirements and Exceptions (4.1.6(1)):

- **Text Telephones –** At least one interior public text telephone complying with 4.31.9 must be provided where:
  (1) Alterations to existing buildings or facilities with fewer than four exterior or interior public pay telephones would increase the total number to four or more telephones with at least one in an interior location; or

  (2) Alterations to one or more exterior or interior public pay telephones occur in an existing building or facility with four or more public telephones with at least one in an interior location.

- **Accessible Vertical Access –** If an escalator or stairs planned or installed where none existed previously and major structural modifications are necessary for such installation, then a means of accessible vertical access must be provided that complies with the applicable provisions of 4.7 Curb Ramps, 4.8 Ramps, 4.10 Elevators, or 4.11 Lifts.

- **Areas of Rescue Assistance –** In alterations, areas of rescue assistance are not required because the new construction requirements of 4.1.3(9), 4.3.10, and 4.3.11 do not apply.

- **Entrances –** If a planned alteration entails alterations to an entrance, and the building has an accessible entrance, the entrance being altered is not required to comply with 4.1.3(8), except to the extent required by 4.1.6(2). If a particular entrance is not made accessible, appropriate accessible signage indicating the location of the nearest accessible entrance(s) must be installed at or near the inaccessible entrance such that a person with a disability will not be required to retrace the approach route from the inaccessible entrance.

- **Alterations Not Affecting Accessibility –** If the alteration work is limited solely to the electrical, mechanical, or plumbing system, or to hazardous material abatement, or automatic sprinkler retrofitting, and does not involve the alteration of any elements or spaces required to be accessible under ADAAG then 4.1.6(2) does not apply.

- **Elevator Exception –** If a building is less than three stories or has less than 3,000 square fee per story, an elevator is not required unless the building is a shopping center or shopping mall, the professional office of a health care provider, or a transportation facility. These terms are defined in 28 CFR §36.404(a).

## Alterations to an Area Containing a Primary Function (4.1.6(2)):

In addition to the requirements of 4.1.6(1), an alteration that affects or could affect the usability of or access to an area containing a primary function must be made so as to ensure that, to the maximum extent feasible, the path of travel to the altered area and the restrooms, telephones, and drinking fountains serving the altered area, are readily accessible to and usable by individuals with disabilities, unless such alterations are disproportionate to the overall alternation in terms of cost and scope (as determined under criteria established by the Attorney General.) These terms are further defined in 28 CFR §36.403.

# J: Accessible Buildings – Historic Preservation

Alterations to a qualified historic building or facility must comply with the minimum requirements for alterations in 4.1.6. Use the applicable survey forms for new construction for each altered element or space.

If it is determined, in accordance with the required procedures in 4.1.7(2), that the proposed alterations would threaten or destroy the historic significance of the building or facility, the following alternative requirements in 4.1.7(3) may be utilized:

- **Site Accessible Route – Minimum Number:** At least one accessible route complying with 4.3 must be provided from a site access point to an accessible entrance.

- **Ramps – Slope and Rise:** A ramp with a slope no steeper than 1:6 may be used as part of an accessible route to an entrance but the run must not exceed 2 feet.

- **Entrances – Minimum Number and Primary Entrance:** At least one accessible entrance complying with 4.14 and which is used by the public must be provided. If no public entrance can be made accessible, then access may be provided at any entrance which is open (unlocked) when directional signage is provided at the primary public entrance. The alternative accessible entrance must have a notification system, and where security is a concern, remote monitoring may be used.

- **Building Accessible Route –Access to Other Floors:** Accessible routes from an accessible entrance to all publicly used spaces must be provided at least on the accessible entrance level. Access must be provided in compliance with 4.1 to all levels of a building and facility whenever practicable.

- **Toilet Rooms – Unisex:** If toilets are provided, then at least one toilet facility, which may be unisex in design, complying with 4.22 and 4.1.6, must be provided on an accessible route.

- **Displays:** Displays and written information should be located so as to be seen by a seated person.

If it is determined, in accordance with the required procedures in 4.1.7(2), that it is not feasible to provide physical access to a qualified historic building or facility using the alternative requirements in 4.1.7(3) without threatening or destroying the historic significance of the building or facility, alternative methods of access must be provided. See 36 CFR §36.405(b).

# Survey Form 1: Parking

Use with the Minimum Requirements Summary Sheets and ADAAG.

**Facility Name:** _____ **Parking Area/Lot Location:** _____

See minimum Requirements Summary Sheets I and J for special requirements and exceptions which may be allowed in alterations and historic preservation. See Also ADAAG 4.1.6 and 4.1.7.

|  | Total Parking Spaces in Area/Lot | Number Accessible | Number Van Accessible |
|---|---|---|---|
| ❑ General Use: (Use table in 4.1.2(5)(a) | _____ | _____ | _____ |
| ❑ Outpatient Unit/Facility: (10% required) | _____ | _____ | _____ |
| ❑ Specialized Unit/Facility Serving or Treating Persons with Mobility Impairments (20% required) | _____ | _____ | _____ |

| Section | Item | Technical Requirements | Comments | Yes | No |
|---|---|---|---|---|---|
| 4.1.2(5) 4.6.1 | **Number –** Accessible Parking Spaces | Where parking spaces are provided for self-parking by employees or visitors or both, are the required number of accessible parking spaces complying with 4.6 (see below) provided? (See Minimum Requirements Summary Sheet A)<br><br>(All or some of the accessible parking spaces may be in a different location if equivalent or greater accessibility is ensured.) |  |  |  |
|  | Each Area/Lot | Are the accessible parking spaces located in each specific area/lot?<br>OR<br>If the accessible parking spaces are in a different location, is equivalent or greater accessibility provided in terms of distance from the accessible entrance, cost and convenience? |  |  |  |
|  | Van Accessible Spaces | Is one in every eight accessible parking spaces (but not less than one) designated "van accessible?" |  |  |  |
| 4.6.2 | **Location –** Serving Accessible Entrance | Are accessible parking spaces which serve a particular building on the shortest accessible route of travel from adjacent parking to the building's accessible entrance? |  |  |  |
|  | Serving Multiple Accessible Entrances | If the building has multiple accessible entrances with adjacent parking, are the accessible parking spaces on the shortest accessible route of travel to the parking facility's accessible pedestrian entrance? |  |  |  |

| | Item | Technical Requirements | Comments | Yes | No |
|---|---|---|---|---|---|
| | Separate Parking Facility | Where a parking facility does not serve a particular building, are the accessible parking spaces on the shortest accessible route of travel to the parking facility's accessible pedestrian entrance? | | | |
| 4.6.3 | **Parking Spaces and Access Aisles** Width of Parking Space | Acre accessible parking spaces, including van spaces, at least 96 inches wide with a demarcated access aisle? Two spaces may share a common aisle. (See Figure 9) | | | |
| 4.1.2(5)(a) | Width of Car Access Aisles | Are all other access aisles at least 60 inches wide? | | | |
| 4.1.2(5)(b) | Width of Van Accessible Access Aisle | If the parking space is designated as "van accessible," is the adjacent access aisle at least 96 inches wide? | | | |
| 4.6.3 | Level | Are the accessible parking spaces and access aisles level with no slope greater than 1:50 in all directions? | | | |
| 4.6.3 4.3.6 4.5.1 | Surface | Are access aisles stable, firm, and slip resistant? | | | |
| **4.6.3 4.3** | **Access Aisle and Accessible Route** | Does each access aisle connect directly to an accessible route complying with 4.3? (Use Form 3: Exterior Accessible Route.) | | | |
| 4.3.3 | | Is the accessible route a full 36 inches wide and not reduced in width by vehicles overhanging parking space? | | | |
| **4.6.4** | **Signs –** Accessible Parking Spaces | Does each accessible parking space have a vertical sign, which is unobscured by a parked vehicle, showing the International Symbol of Accessibility? | | | |
| 4.6.4 | Van Accessible Spaces | Do van accessible spaces have a vertical sign, which is unobscured by a parked vehicle, showing the International Symbol of Accessibility with an additional sign "Van-Accessible" mounted below the symbol of accessibility? Exception: "Van-Accessible" sign is not required if all accessible parking spaces are Universal Parking Design. (See Figure A5) | | | |
| **4.6.5** | **Van Accessible Spaces –** Vertical Clearance | Do van accessible spaces have a vertical clearance of at least 98 inches? | | | |
| | | Does one vehicular access route to and from van accessible spaces have a vertical clearance of at least 98 inches? (Van accessible spaces may be grouped on one level of a parking structure.) | | | |

Survey Form

1 — 2

234

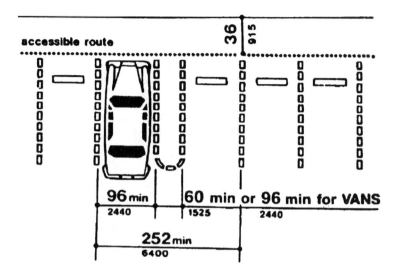

**Figure 9: Dimensions of Parking Spaces**

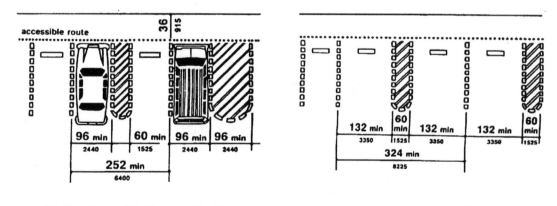

(a) Van Accessible Space at End Row

(b) Universal Parking Space Design

**Figure A5: Parking Space Alternatives**

Parking: 1 — 3

235

# Survey Form 2: Passenger Loading Zone

Use with the Minimum Requirement Summary Sheets and ADAAG.

Facility Name: _____ Passenger Zone Location: _____

See Minimum Requirements Summary Sheets I and J for special requirements and exceptions which may be allowed in alterations and historic preservation. See also ADAAG 4.1.6 and 4.1.7.

| Section | Item | Technical Requirements | Comments | Yes | No |
|---|---|---|---|---|---|
| 4.1.2(5)(c) | **Loading Zones** | Are passenger loading zones provided? If so, at least one must meet all of the following requirements: | | | |
| 4.6.6 | Access Aisle | Is there an access aisle adjacent and parallel to the vehicle pull-up space? | | | |
| | Aisle Size | Is the access aisle at least 60 inches wide by 20 feet long? | | | |
| | Level Aisle | Is the vehicle pull-up space level, with no slope greater than 1:50 in all directions? | | | |
| | Level Space | Is the vehicle pull-up space level, with no slope greater than 1:50 in all directions? | | | |
| 4.6.6 4.3.6 4.5.1 | Aisle Surface | Is the access aisle surface stable, firm and slip-resistant? | | | |
| 4.6.6 4.7 | Curbs | If there are curbs between the access aisle and the vehicle pull-up space, is there a curb ramp complying with 4.7? (Use Form 4: Curb Ramps) | | | |
| 4.29.5 | **Hazardous Vehicular Area–** Detectable Warnings | If a walk crosses or adjoins the vehicular way and the walking surface is not separated by curbs, railings, or other elements between the pedestrian areas and vehicular areas, is the boundary between the areas defined by a continuous detectable warning at least 36 inches wide complying with 4.29.2? (Use Form 21: Detectable Warnings (Not in this **CIP** Chapter.)) | | | |
| 4.6.5 | **Vertical Clearance** | Is there at least 114 inches vertical clearance along the vehicle route to the vehicle pull-up space of the accessible passenger loading zone from site entrance(s) and exit(s)? | | | |
| | | Is there at least 114 inches vertical clearance at the accessible passenger loading zone (including vehicle pull-up space and access aisle)? | | | |
| 4.1.2(7)(b) | **Sign** | Is there a sign displaying the International Symbol of Accessibility at the accessible passenger loading zone? | | | |

# Survey Form 3: Exterior Accessible Routes

Use with the Minimum Requirements Summary Sheets and ADAAG.

**Facility Name:** _____ **Access Route to be Surveyed:** _____

**From:** _____ **To:** _____

See Minimum Requirements Summary Sheets I and J for special requirements and exceptions which may be allowed in alterations and historic preservation. See also ADAAG 4.1.6 and 4.1.7.

| Section | Item | Technical Requirements | Comments | Yes | No |
|---------|------|------------------------|----------|-----|-----|
| **4.1.2(1)** **4.3.2(1)** | **Accessible Route Site–** Public Transportation | Is there an accessible route within the boundary of the site linking an accessible building entrance with the following, if provided: public transportation stops; passenger loading zones; public streets and sidewalks? | | | |
| | Route for General Public | Does the accessible route generally coincide with the route for the general public, to the maximum extent feasible? | | | |
| **4.1.2(2)** **4.3.2(2)** | Buildings Connected | Is there an accessible route connecting accessible buildings, facilities, elements, and spaces on the same site? | | | |
| **4.3.3** | **Accessible Route Size –** Width | Is the accessible route at least 36 inches wide except at doorways or gates? | | | |
| | U-turn | Where the accessible route makes a U-turn around an obstacle less than 48 inches wide, is the pathway width at least 42 inches on approaches and 48 inches in the turn? (See Figure 7(b)) | | | |
| 4.3.4 | Passing Spaces | If the accessible route is less than 60 inches wide, are there passing spaces at least 60 inches wide and 60 inches long or intersecting walkways allowing passing at reasonable intervals not exceeding 200 feet? | | | |
| **4.3.5** **4.4.2** | **Provisions for Persons Who are Blind –** Head Room | Is there at least 80 inches clear head room on an accessible route? | | | |
| 4.4.2 | Cane Detectable Barrier Where Head Room is Less Than 80 Inches | If there is less than 80 inches clear head room in an area adjoining an accessible route, is there a cane detectable barrier within 27 inches of the floor? (See Figure 8(c-1) | | | |
| 4.4.1 | Protruding Objects | If objects mounted to the wall have leading edges between 27 and 80 inches from the floor, do they project less than 4 inches into the pathway? (Wall mounted objects with leading edges at or below 27 inches may project any amount so long as the required clear width of an accessible route is not reduced.) | | | |

Survey Form

3 — 1

| Section | Item | Technical Requirements | Comments | Yes | No |
|---------|------|------------------------|----------|-----|-----|
| | | Do free standing objects mounted on posts with leading edges between 27 and 80 inches high (such as a sign or telephone) project less than 12 inches into the perpendicular route of travel? | | | |
| | | Is there an accessible path at least 36 inches clear alongside the protruding object? | | | |
| 4.3.7 | Slopes – Cross Slope | Is the cross slope of the accessible route no greater than 1:50? | | | |
| | Walkway Slope | Is the slope of the accessible route no greater than 1:20? | | | |
| 4.8.1 | | Where the slope is greater than 1:20, does it comply with the requirements for ramp? (Use Form 7: Ramps) | | | |
| 4.3.8 4.5.2 | Changes in Level | When walkway levels change, is the vertical difference between them less than 1/4 inch? OR Are changes in level between 1/4 inch and 1/2 inch beveled with a slope no greater than 1:2? | | | |
| | | Are curb ramps, ramps, or elevators used for changes in level greater than 1/2 inch? (Lifts may only be used in certain limited situations in new construction. See Minimum Requirements Summary Sheet B and ADAAG 4.1.3(5)) | | | |
| | | Does the curb ramp, ramp, or elevator comply with 4.7, 4.8, or 4.10? (Use Form 4: Curb Ramps; Form 7: Ramps; or Form 13: Elevators (not in this **CIP** Chapter) | | | |
| 4.3.6 4.5.1 | Surface | Are accessible route surfaces stable, firm, and slip-resistant? | | | |
| 4.5.4 | Grates | Is the smaller dimension of grate openings no more than 1/2 inch, and are long dimensions of rectangular gaps placed perpendicular to the usual direction of travel? | | | |
| 4.1.2(7) 4.30.1 | Directional and Informational Signs | Do signs which provide direction to, or information about, functional spaces of the building, comply with 4.30.2, 4.30.3, and 4.30.5? (Use Form 19: Signage) (Not in this **CIP** Chapter) | | | |
| 4.1.2(7) 4.30.1 | Room Identification Signs | Do signs which designate permanent rooms and spaces comply with 4.30.4, 4.30.5, and 4.30.6? (Use Form 19: Signage) (Not in this **CIP** Chapter) | | | |

| Section | Item | Technical Requirements | Comments | Yes | No |
|---------|------|------------------------|----------|-----|-----|
| 4.1.2 | Symbols | If provided, are the following elements identified by the International Symbol of Accessibility?<br>(a) accessible parking spaces;<br>(b) accessible passenger loading zones;<br>(c) accessible entrances when not all are accessible;<br>(d) accessible toilet and bathing facilities when not all are accessible | | | |
| 4.1.3(8)(d) | Directions to Accessible Entrance | When not all entrances are accessible, is there directional signage indicating the accessible route to an accessible entrance? | | | |
| 4.29.5 | Hazardous Vehicular Areas – Detectable Warnings | If a walk crosses or adjoins the vehicular way and the walking surface is not separated by curbs, railings, or other elements between the pedestrian areas and vehicular areas, is the boundary between the areas defined by a continuous detectable warning at least 36 inches wide complying with 4.29.2? (Use Form 21: Detectable Warnings) (Not in this **CIP** Chapter.) | | | |

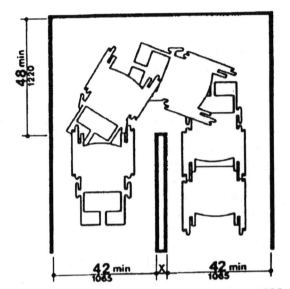

NOTE: Dimensions shown apply when x < 48 in (1220 mm).

**Figure 7 (b) Accessible Route – Turns Around an Obstruction**

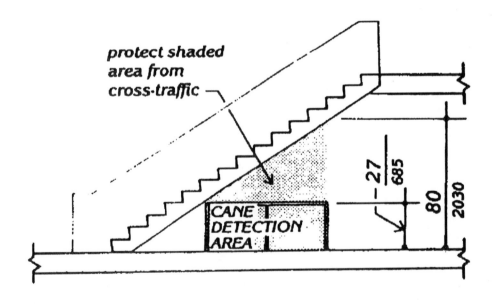

**Figure 8 (c-1) Protruding Object – Overhead Hazards**

# Survey Form 4: Curb Ramps

Use with the Minimum Requirements Summary Sheets and ADAAG

**Facility Name:** _____ **Curb Ramp Location:** _____

See Minimum Requirements Summary Sheets I and J for special requirements and exceptions which may be allowed in alterations and historic preservation. See also ADAAG 4.1.6 and 4.1.7.

| Section | Item | Technical Requirements | Comments | Yes | No |
|---------|------|------------------------|----------|-----|-----|
| **4.7.1** | **Curb Ramp –** Location | Is there a curb ramp wherever an accessible route crosses a curb? | | | |
| 4.7.2 4.8.2 | Slope | Is the slope of the curb ramp 1:12 or less in new construction? | | | |
| 4.7.2 | Transition | Is the transition from the curb ramp to the walkway and to the road or gutter flush and free of abrupt changes? | | | |
| | Counter Slope | Are the running slopes of the road, gutter, or accessible route adjoining the ramp no greater than 1:20? | | | |
| 4.7.3 | Width | Is the width of the curb ramp, not including the flared sides, at least 36 inches? | | | |
| 4.7.4 4.5.1 | Surface | Is the surface of the curb ramp stable, firm, and slip-resistant? | | | |
| **4.7.5** | **Side Flares** | If the curb ramp is located where pedestrians must walk across it or where it is not protected by handrails or guard rails, does it have flared sides? | | | |
| | Side Flare Slope | Do these flared sides have a slope of 1:10 or less? | | | |
| | | Where the space at the top of the ramp is less than 48 inches and wheelchair users must use the side flares for access, do the flared sides have a slope of 1:12 or less? (See Figure 12(a) | | | |
| **4.7.5** | **Returned Curbs** | If sharp return curb cuts are present, is pedestrian cross traffic prohibited by walls, guardrails, shrubbery, or other elements? (See Figure 12(b)) | | | |
| **4.7.6 4.6.3** | **Built-up Curb Ramps** | Are built-up curb ramps located so that they do not project into vehicular traffic lanes or parking access aisles? | | | |
| 4.7.7 | Detectable Warnings | Does the curb ramp have a detectable warning? | | | |
| 4.29.2 | Domes | Does the detectable warning consist of raised truncated domes? | | | |
| | Size and Spacing | Are the truncated domes 0.9 inches in diameter and 0.2 inches in height with a center-to-center spacing of 2.35 inches? All measurements are nominal. (see Figures below) | | | |
| | Visual Contrast | Does the detectable warning contrast visually with adjoining surfaces (light-on-dark or dark-on-light)? | | | |

Survey Form

4 — 1

| Section | Item | Technical Requirements | Comments | Yes | No |
|---------|------|------------------------|----------|-----|-----|
| | | Is the material used to provide contrast an integral part of the walking surface? | | | |
| 4.7.8 | **Parked Vehicles** | Are curb ramps located or protected so that they will not be obstructed by parked vehicles? | | | |
| 4.7.9 | **Curb Ramps at Crosswalks** | Are curb ramps at crosswalks wholly contained within the crosswalk lines, except for the flared sides? | | | |
| 4.7.10 | **Diagonal Curb Ramps** | If diagonal (or corner-type) curb ramps have returned curbs or other well-defined edges, are these edges parallel to the direction of the pedestrian traffic flow? | | | |
| | Bottom of Diagonal | Is there at least 48 inches clear space within the crosswalk lines at the bottom of a diagonal curb ramp? | | | |
| | Straight Curb | If the diagonal curb ramp has flared sides, is there at least a 24 inch segment of straight curb located on each side of the curb ramp within the crosswalk lines? | | | |
| 4.7.11 | **Island** | Where an accessible pathway crosses an island, is the island cut through at street level? OR Are there curb ramps on both side and a level area at least 48 inches long between them? (With a 6 inch high curb, the island will be at least 16 feet wide.) | | | |

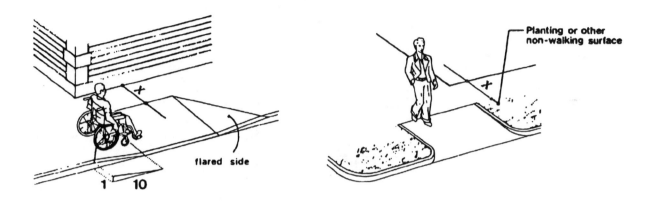

If X less than 48 inches,
then the slope of the flared side
shall not exceed 1:12

(a) Flared Sides

(b) Returned Curve

**Figure 12 Sides of Curb Ramps**

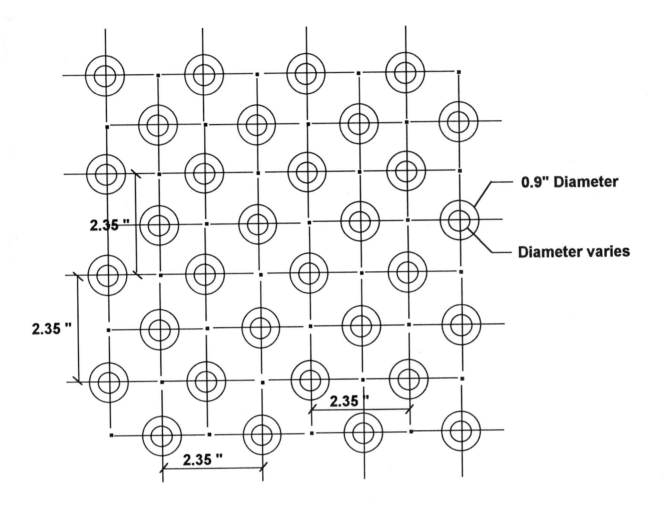

**0.9" Diameter**

**Diameter varies**

2.35 "

2.35 "

2.35 "

2.35 "

## Detectable Warning: Pattern

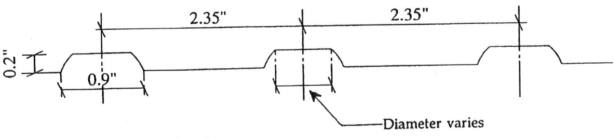

**Detectable Warning: Section**
NTS

# Survey Form 6: Telephones

Use with the Minimum Requirements Summary Sheets and ADAAG

**Facility Name:** _____ **Telephone Location:** _____

See Minimum Requirements Summary Sheets I and J for special requirements and exceptions which may be allowed in alterations and historic preservation. See also ADAAG 4.1.6 and 4.1.7.

| Section | Item | Technical Requirements | Comments | Yes | No |
|---|---|---|---|---|---|
| **4.1.3(17)(a)** **4.31.1** | **Telephones** | At each bank of public pay telephones, is there at least one telephone per bank accessible to wheelchair users complying with 4.31.2 through 4.31.8 (See below)? If there is only one public pay telephone per floor, does it comply with 4.31.2 through 4.31.8? | | | |
| | | Where two or more banks of public pay telephones are provided on a floor, does at least one telephone per floor provide for a forward reach complying with 4.2.5 (See below)? (For exterior installations only, if dial tone first service is available, a side reach telephone may be installed instead of a forward reach telephone.) | | | |
| **4.1.17(a)** **4.31.2** **4.2.4** | Clear Floor Space | Does the accessible telephone have at least 30 by 48 inches clear floor space that allows either a forward or parallel approach by wheelchair users? (Where two or more banks of public telephones are provided on a floor, at least one telephone per floor must allow a forward approach and be mounted so the highest operable part is no higher than 48 inches.) | | | |
| | Accessible Route | Is there an accessible route at least 36 inches wide adjoining or overlapping the clear floor space? | | | |
| 4.31.3 4.2.5 | Forward Reach Telephone | If the clear floor space allows only a forward approach, is the highest operable part of the telephone no more than 48 inches from the floor? | | | |
| 4.31.3 4.2.6 | Side Reach Telephone | If the clear floor space allows only a parallel approach, is the highest operable part of the telephone no more than 54 inches from the floor? | | | |
| 4.31.7 | Directories | Are telephone books also within these reach ranges? | | | |
| 4.31.6 | Controls | Does the telephone have pushbutton controls unless such service is unavailable? | | | |
| 4.31.8 | Cord | Is the cord from the telephone to the handset at least 29 inches long? | | | |
| **4.1.3(17)(b)** | **Volume Controls** | Is each accessible telephone equipped with a volume control? | | | |

Survey Form

6 — 1

| Section | Item | Technical Requirements | Comments | Yes | No |
|---------|------|------------------------|----------|-----|-----|
| | | Are 25% of all other public telephones equipped with volume controls and dispersed among all types of public telephones? (Public telephones include public pay telephones and public closed-circuit telephones.) | | | |
| 4.30.7(2) | Signs | Are volume controlled telephones identified by a sign showing a handset with radiating sound waves? | | | |
| 4.31.5 | Amplification | Are volume controls capable of amplification between 12 dbA and 18 dbA above normal? (If an automatic reset button is provided, the maximum of 18 dbA may be exceeded.) | | | |
| | Hearing Aid Compatible | Are telephones hearing aid compatible? | | | |
| **4.1.3(17)(c)** | **Text Telephones/TDD — General** | If there are 4 or more public pay telephones (with at least one in an interior location), is there at least one interior public text telephone? | | | |
| | Specific Facilities | If an interior public pay telephone is provided in a stadium or arena, convention center, a hotel with a convention center, or a covered mall, is there at least one interior public text telephone in the facility? | | | |
| | Hospitals | If there is a public pay telephone in or adjacent to a hospital emergency room, a hospital recovery room, or a hospital waiting room, is there a public text telephone in each such location? | | | |
| 4.31.9(3) | Equivalent Facilitation | If a required text telephone is not provided, is equivalent facilitation provided? (e.g., A portable text telephone may be made available in a hotel at the registration desk if it is available on a 24-hour basis for use with nearby public pay telephones. In this instance, at least one public pay telephone must have a shelf and outlet complying with 4.31.9(2) (see below) to accommodate a portable text telephone. In addition, if an acoustic coupler is used, the telephone handset cord must be sufficiently long so as to allow connection of the text telephone and the telephone receiver. Directional signage must be provided in compliance with 4.30.7) (See below) | | | |
| 4.31.9 | Mounting Location | Is a required text telephone permanently mounted within, or adjacent to, the telephone enclosure? | | | |
| | Cord Length | If an acoustic coupler is used, is the telephone cord sufficiently long enough to allow connection of the text telephone to the telephone receiver? | | | |

| Section | Item | Technical Requirements | Comments | Yes | No |
|---------|------|------------------------|----------|-----|-----|
| 4.30.7(3) | TDD Symbol | Are required text telephones identified by the international TDD symbol? | | | |
| 4.1.3(16) 4.30.1 4.30.7 | Directional Signs | Is the directional signage complying with 4.30.2, 4.30.3, and 4.30.5 provided to indicate the location of the text telephone? (See Form: 19: Signage (Not in this **CIP** Chapter)) | | | |
| | | Is the directional signage placed adjacent to all telephone banks which do not contain a text telephone? (If the facility does not have any telephone banks, the directional signage must be provided at the entrance (e.g., in a building directory.)) | | | |
| **4.1.3(17)(d) 4.31.9(2)** | **Text Telephone, Shelves and Outlets** | If there are 3 or more telephones in an interior bank of telephones, does at least one telephone have a shelf and electrical outlet for use with a portable text telephone? | | | |
| | | Is the shelf large enough to accommodate a text telephone and does it provide at least 6 inches of vertical clearance? | | | |
| | | Is the telephone handset capable of being placed flush on the surface of the shelf? | | | |
| | | Is the directional signage placed adjacent to all telephone banks which do not contain a text telephone? (If the facility does not have any telephone banks, the directional signage must be provided at the entrance (e.g., in a building directory.)) | | | |
| 4.31.4 | Protruding Objects | If a wall-mounted telephone has leading edges between 27 and 80 inches from the floor, does it project less than 4 inches into the pathway? (Wall mounted telephones or their enclosures with leading edges at or below 27 inches may project any amount so long as the required clear width of an accessible route is not reduced.) | | | |
| | | If a telephone is mounted on a post with leading edges between 27 and 80 inches high, does it project less than 12 inches into a perpendicular route of travel? | | | |
| | | Is there an accessible route at least 36 inches wide alongside the telephone? | | | |

# Survey Form 7: Ramps

Use with the Minimum Requirements Summary Sheets and ADAAG

**Facility Name:** _____  **Ramp Location:** _____

See Minimum Requirements Summary Sheets I and J for special requirements and exceptions which may be allowed in alterations and historic preservation. See also ADAAG 4.1.6 and 4.1.7.

| Section | Item | Technical Requirements | Comments | yes | No |
|---------|------|------------------------|----------|-----|-----|
| 4.8.1 | **Ramps** | Does each part of an accessible route with a slope greater than 1:20 comply with 4.8 (See below)? (For curb ramps use Form 4: Curb Ramps) | | | |
| 4.8.2 | Running Slope | Is the ramp slope 1:12 or less? | | | |
| | Maximum Rise | Is the rise for any run a maximum of 30 inches? | | | |
| 4.8.6 | Gross Slope | Is the cross slope of the ramp surface no greater than 1:50? | | | |
| 4.8.6 4.5 | Surface | Is the ramp surface stable, firm, and slip-resistant? | | | |
| | Grates | Is the smaller dimension of grate openings no more than 1/2 inch, and are long dimensions of rectangular gaps placed perpendicular to the usual direction of travel? | | | |
| 4.8.3 | Clear Width | Is the clear width (between handrails) of the ramp at least 36 inches? | | | |
| 4.8.4 | **Landings** | Is there a level landing at the top and bottom of each ramp and each ramp run? | | | |
| | Size | Is each landing at least as wide as the ramp and at least 60 inches long? | | | |
| | | Where the ramp changes direction, is there a landing of at least 60 by 60 inches? | | | |
| | Landings and Doors | If a doorway is located on a landing, does the area in front of the door comply with the maneuvering space requirements for doors? (Use Form 11: Door and Gates) | | | |
| 4.8.7 | **Edge Protection** | If a ramp or landing has a drop off, does it have a minimum 2 inch curb, a wall, railings, or projecting surfaces which prevent people from falling off? | | | |
| 4.8.8 | **Drainage** | Are outside ramps and their approaches designed so that water will not accumulate on walking surfaces? | | | |
| 4.8.5 | **Handrails** | If the ramp rises more than 6 inches or is longer than 72 inches, does it have a handrail on each side? (Handrails are not required on curb ramps or adjacent to seating in assembly areas.) | | | |
| | | On dogleg or switchback ramps, is the inside handrail continuous? | | | |

| Section | Item | Technical Requirements | Comments | Yes | No |
|---------|------|------------------------|----------|-----|-----|
| | Gripping Surface | Are the gripping surfaces continuous? | | | |
| | Mounting | Are handrails fixed so that they do not rotate within their fittings? | | | |
| | Height | Is the top of the handrail between 34 and 38 inches above the ramp surface? | | | |
| | Handrail Extension | At ends of handrails, are there at least 12 inches of handrail, parallel to the floor or ground surface, extending beyond the top and bottom of the ramp segment? | | | |
| | Ends of Handrails | Are the ends of handrails rounded or returned smoothly to the floor, wall, or post? | | | |
| 4.85 4.26.2 | Diameter | Is the diameter of the handrail between 1-1/4 and 1-1/2 inches? OR Does the shape provide an equivalent gripping surface? Note: Standard pipe sizes designated by the industry as 1-1/4 to 1-1/2 inches are acceptable for purposes of this section. | | | |
| 4.8.5 4.26.2 | Clearance | Is the clear space between handrails and walls exactly 1-1/2 inches? | | | |
| 4.8.5 4.26.2 | Clearance in Recess | If a handrail is located in a recess, is the recess no more than 3 inches deep extending at least 18 inches above the top of the rail? | | | |
| 4.8.5 4.26.3 | Structural Strength | Do the handrails meet the structural strength requirements for bending stress and shear stress? (See 4.26.3) | | | |
| 4.8.5 4.26.3 | | Do the fasteners meet the structural strength requirements for shear force and tensile force? | | | |
| 4.8.5 4.25.4 | Hazards | Are handrail edges free of sharp or abrasive elements and do they have edges with minimum radius of 1/8 inch? | | | |

# Survey Form 9: Platform Lifts

Use with the Minimum Requirements Summary Sheets and ADAAG.

**Facility Name:** _____ **Lift Location:** _____

See Minimum Requirements Summary Sheets I and J for special requirements and exceptions which may be allowed in alterations and historic preservation. See also ADAAG 4.1.6 and 4.1.7

4.1.3(5) Exception 4: — In new construction, platform lifts may be used in lieu of an elevator only under the following conditions and where State and local codes permit.

- To provide an accessible route to a performing area in an assembly occupancy.
- To comply with the wheelchair viewing position, line-of-sight, and dispersion requirements in assembly areas with fixed seating.
- To provide access to incidental occupiable rooms and spaces that are not open to the general public and which house no more than five persons. (This includes, but is not limited to, equipment control rooms and projection booths.)
- To provide access where existing site constrains or other constraints make use of a ramp or elevator infeasible.

4.1.6(3)(g): — In alterations, the use of platform lifts is not limited to the above conditions. Platform lifts may be used as part of an accessible route in alterations.

| Section | Item | Technical Requirements | Comments | Yes | No |
|---|---|---|---|---|---|
| **4.1.3(5) Exception 4** | **Lifts** | In new construction, if a lift is installed in lieu of an elevator or ramp, was it installed consistent with 4.1.3(5) Exception 4 (above) and in compliance with applicable State and local codes? | | | |
| 4.11.3 | Independent Use | Can the lift be entered, operated, and exited without assistance? | | | |
| 4.11.2 4.2.4 | Platform Size | Is the lift platform at least 30 by 48 inches? | | | |
| 4.11.2 4.2.4 | Clear Space Outside Lift | Is there at least a 30 by 48 inch clear space outside the lift positioned for a wheelchair user to reach the controls from a parallel or forward approach and to enter the lift? | | | |
| **4.11.2 4.27.3 4.2.5** | **Controls - Forward Reach** | Where a forward reach is provided, is the height of the lift control no more than 48 inches? | | | |
| 4.11.2 4.27.3 4.2.6 | Side Reach | Where a side reach is provided, is the height of the lift control no more than 54 inches? | | | |
| 4.11.2 4.27.4 | Operation | Are the controls operable with one hand and without tight grasping, pinching, or twisting of the wrist? | | | |
| | | Is the force required to operate the controls no greater than 5 lb.? | | | |
| **4.1.2(1) 4.3.2** | **Accessible Route** | Is the lift on an accessible route? | | | |

| Section | Item | Technical Requirements | Comments | Yes | No |
|---|---|---|---|---|---|
| 4.11.2<br>4.3.6<br>4.5.1 | Surface | Is the surface of the lift, as well as the accessible route to which it connects, stable, firm, and slip-resistant? | | | |
| 4.11.2<br>4.5.2 | Edge Bevel | If there is a change in the level of between 1/4 and 1/2 inch, is the edge beveled with a slope of 1:2 or less? | | | |
| **4.11.2** | **Safety Code** | Does the lift meet the ASME A17.1 Safety Code for Elevators and Escalators, Section XX, 1990? | | | |

# Survey Form 10: Entrances and Exits (Areas of Rescue Assistance)

Use with the Minimum Requirements Summary Sheets and ADAAG

Facility Name: _____    Entrance and Exit Location: _____

Area of Rescue Assistance Location: _____

See Minimum Requirements Summary Sheets I and J for special requirements and exceptions which may be allowed in alterations and historic preservation. See also ADAAG 4.1.6 and 4.1.7.

Total Number of Entrances: _____

Number of Accessible Entrances: _____

Number of Exits Required by
Building/Fire Code: _____

| Section | Item | Technical Requirements | Comments | Yes | No |
|---|---|---|---|---|---|
| 4.1.3(8)(a) | Entrances – Number Accessible | Are at least 50% of all public entrances accessible? | | | |
| | Ground Floor Entrances | Is at least one accessible entrance on the ground floor? | | | |
| | Separate Tenant Entrances | Does each separate tenancy have an accessible entrance? | | | |
| | Equivalent to Required Exits | Is the number of accessible entrances at least equivalent to the number of exits required by the applicable building/fire codes? (Use Minimum Requirements Summary Sheet C: Entrances)<br><br>(This does not require an increase in the total number of entrances planned for the facility.) | | | |
| | Primary Entrance | Where feasible, are the accessible entrances the entrances used by the majority of the people visiting or working in the building? | | | |
| 4.1.3(8)(b) | Pedestrian Tunnels and Elevated Walkways | If access is provided for pedestrians through a pedestrian tunnel or elevated walkway, is one entrance to the building from each tunnel or walkway accessible? | | | |
| | Direct Entrance From Parking Garage | If direct access is provided for pedestrians from an enclosed parking garage to the building, is at least one direct entrance from the garage to the building accessible? | | | |
| 4.1.3(8)(c)<br>4.14.2 | Public Entrance | If the only entrance is a service entrance, is it accessible? | | | |
| 4.1.2(7)<br>4.30.1 | Directional Signs | If an entrance is not accessible, are there directional signs indicating the location of the nearest accessible entrance? | | | |

| Section | Item | Technical Requirements | Comments | Yes | No |
|---------|------|------------------------|----------|-----|-----|
| | | Do the directional signs comply with 4.30.2, 4.30.3, and 4.30.5? (Use Form 19: Signage) (Not in this **CIP** Chapter) | | | |
| 4.14.1 4.3.2(1) 4.3 | Accessible Route | Within the boundaries of the site, is the accessible entrance connected by an accessible route to existing public transportation stops, accessible parking and passenger loading zones, and to public streets or sidewalks? (Use Form 3: Exterior Accessible Routes) | | | |
| | | Is the accessible entrance connected by an accessible route to all accessible elements or spaces within the building or facility? (Use Form 12: Building Lobbies and Corridors) | | | |
| 4.14.1 4.3.8 | Level Change | If there is a vertical level change between 1/4 inch and 1/2 inch at or along the route to the entrance, is the edge beveled with a slope of 1:2 or less? | | | |
| | | If there is a vertical level change greater than 1/2 inch at the entrance, is a curb ramp, ramp, or elevator complying with 4.7, 4.8, or 4.10 provided? (Use Form 4: Curb Ramps; Form 7: Ramps; or Form 13: Elevators (Not in this **CIP** Chapter)) (Lifts may be used in certain limited situations in new construction. See Minimum Requirements Summary Sheet D and ADAAG 4.1.3(5) Exception 4) | | | |
| 4.1.3(7)(a) 4.13.1 | Doors | At each accessible entrance to a building or facility, is there at least one accessible door meeting the requirements of 4.13? (Use Form 11: Doors and Gates) | | | |
| 4.13.2 | Turnstiles | If turnstiles or revolving doors are used on an accessible route, is there an accessible gate or door provided adjacent to the turnstile or revolving door to facilitate the same use pattern? | | | |
| 4.13.3 | Gates | Do all gates, including ticket gates, comply with the applicable specifications of 4.13? (Use Form 11: Doors and Gates) | | | |
| **4.1.3(9)** | **Exits and Areas of Rescue Assistance** | Does each occupiable level of a building or facility which is required to be accessible have accessible means of egress equal to the number of exits required by local building/life safety regulations? OR Is there a horizontal exit complying with local building/life safety regulations provided in lieu of an area of rescue assistance? OR Does the building or facility have a supervised automatic sprinkler system? | | | |

Survey Form

| Section | Item | Technical Requirements | Comments | Yes | No |
|---|---|---|---|---|---|
| 4.1.3(16)<br>4.30.1 | Exit Door Signs | Do signs which designate exit doors comply with 4.30.4, 4.30.5, and 4.30.6? (Use Form 19: Signage – Not in this **CIP** Chapter) | | | |
| 4.3.11.1 | Location and Construction of Areas of Rescue Assistance | Are each of the required areas of rescue assistance located and constructed in compliance with one of the following:<br>*A portion of a stairway landing in a smoke proof enclosure complying with the local building requirements?<br>*A portion of an exterior exit balcony, complying with local requirements, immediately adjacent to an exit stairway? Openings to the interior of the building located within 20 feet of the area of rescue assistance must have fire assemblies with 3/4 hour fire protection rating.<br>*A portion of a one-hour fire-resistive corridor, complying with local requirements for fire-resistive construction and for openings, immediately adjacent to an exit enclosure?<br>*A vestibule immediately adjacent to an exit enclosure constructed to the same fire-resistive standards required for corridors and openings?<br>*A portion of a stairway landing within an exit enclosure which is vented to the exterior and is separated from the interior of the building with not less than one hour fire resistive doors?<br>*When approved by local authorities, an area or room separated by a smoke barrier from other portions of the building, and which has an exit directly into an exit enclosure, where smoke barriers completely enclose the area or room and have a fire resistive rating of not less than one hour? Doors in the smoke barrier must be tight-fitting smoke-and-draft-control assemblies with a fire rating of not less than 20 minutes, and must also be self-closing or automatic closing. Where the room or area exits into an exit enclosure which is required to be of more than one hour fire-resistive construction, the room or area must have the same fire-resistive construction, including the same opening protection, as required for the adjacent exit enclosure.<br>*An elevator lobby when elevator shafts and adjacent lobbies are pressurized as required for a smoke proof enclosure by local regulations and when complying with the requirements in 4.3.11 (see below) for size, communication, and signage? The pressurization system and its duct work must be separated from other portions of the building by a minimum two hour fire resistive construction. | | | |
| 4.3.11.2 | Wheelchair Spaces in Areas of Rescue Assistance –Size | Does each area of rescue assistance provide at least 2 spaces no less than 30 by 48 inches which do not encroach on any required exit width? | | | |

| Section | Item | Technical Requirements | Comments | Yes | No |
|---------|------|------------------------|----------|-----|-----|
| | Required Number of Wheelchair Spaces | Is the total number of wheelchair spaces per story at least equal to one for every 200 persons of calculated load served by the area of rescue assistance?<br>**Exception: The appropriate local authority may reduce the minimum number of such spaces to one for each area of rescue assistance on floors where the occupant load is less than 200.** | | | |
| 4.3.11.3 | Stairway Width | Is each stairway serving an area of rescue assistance at least 48 inches wide between handrails? | | | |
| 4.3.11.4 | Two-Way Communication | Is there a method of two-way communication (using both visible and audible signals) between each area of rescue assistance and the primary entry?<br>(The fire department or other local authority may approve a location other than a primary entry.) | | | |
| 4.3.11.5 | Instructions for Use | Are there instructions for the use of the area of rescue assistance during an emergency posted adjacent to the communication system? | | | |
| 4.3.11.5 | Identification Signs | Is each area of rescue assistance identified by a sign which states "Area of Rescue Assistance," and which also displays the International Symbol of Accessibility? | | | |
| 4.3.11.5 | | Is the sign illuminated when/where exit signs are required to be illuminated? | | | |
| 4.3.11.5 | Directional Signs | Is there directional signage posted at all inaccessible exits indicating the direction to areas of rescue assistance? | | | |
| 4.1.3(16)<br>4.30.1 | | Does the directional signage comply with 4.30.2, 4.30.3, and 4.30.5? (Use Form 19: Signage (Not in this **CIP** Chapter) | | | |
| 4.3.10 | Accessible Routes | Do accessible routes also serve as a means of egress or connect to areas of rescue assistance? | | | |
| 4.1.3(7)(d) | Doors | Is each door along a means of egress an accessible door meeting the requirements of 4.13? (Use Form 11: Doors and Gates) | | | |

# Survey Form 11: Doors and Gates

Use with the Minimum Requirements Summary Sheets and ADAAG

**Facility Name:** _____  **Door Location:** _____

See Minimum Requirements Summary Sheets I and J for special requirements and exceptions which may be allowed in alterations and historic preservation. See also ADAAG 4.1.6 and 4.1.7.

| Section | Item | Technical Requirements | Comments | Yes | No |
|---------|------|------------------------|----------|-----|-----|
| 4.1.3(7) 4.13.1 | **Doors – Accessible Entrances** | Is there at least one accessible door complying with 4.13 (see below) at each accessible entrance to the building or facility? | | | |
| | Accessible Spaces | Is there at least one accessible door complying with 4.13 (see below) at each accessible space in the facility? | | | |
| | Accessible Routes | Does each door that is an element of an accessible route comply with 4.13 (See below)? | | | |
| | Egress Door and Areas of Rescue Assistance | Does each door that is an element of an accessible means of egress or that connects to an area of rescue assistance comply with 4.13 (See below)? | | | |
| 4.13.2 | **Revolving Doors and Turnstiles** | If a revolving door or turnstile is used on an accessible route, is an accessible door or gate provided adjacent to the turnstile or revolving door to facilitate the same use pattern? | | | |
| 4.13.3 | **Gates** | Do gates, including ticket gates, meet the applicable specifications of 4.13 (See below)? | | | |
| 4.13.5 | **Clear Opening** | When the door is open 90 degrees, is there a clear opening width at least 32 inches measured between the face of the door and the door stop on the latch side? | | | |
| | Closets | If the door does not require full-user passage, such as that to a shallow closet, is the clear opening width at least 20 inches? | | | |
| 4.13.4 | Double Leaf Doors | If the doorway has two independently operated door leaves, does at least one active leaf provide at least a 32 inch clear opening width? | | | |
| 4.13.6 | **Maneuvering Space** | If the door is not automatic or power assisted, does it have maneuvering space relative to the direction of approach as shown in Figure 25? Exception: Entry doors to acute care hospital bedrooms are exempt from the requirement for the 18 inch space at the latch side of the door if the door is at least 44 inches wide. | | | |
| | | Is the floor level and clear within the required maneuvering space? | | | |

Survey Form

11 — 1

256

| 4.13.7 | **Vestibules** – Doors in Series | If there are two door in a series, is the clear space between door in a vestibule at least 48 inches plus the width of any door swinging into the space (See Figure 26) | | | |
| --- | --- | --- | --- | --- | --- |
| | | Do doors in a series swing in the same direction?<br>  OR<br>Do they swing away from the space between the doors? | | | |
| 4.13.8 | **Thresholds** | Is the threshold at doorways no higher than 3/4 inch in height for exterior sliding doors? | | | |
| | | Is the threshold no higher than 1/2 inch for other doors? | | | |
| | | If there is a raised threshold, is it beveled at 1:2 or less? | | | |
| 4.13.9 | **Hardware** | Are all handles, locks, and latches or other operative devices operable with one hand? | | | |
| | | Are they operable without tight grasping, pinching, or twisting of the wrist? (U-shaped handles, levers, and punch type mechanisms are acceptable designs.) | | | |
| | | If there are sliding doors, is the operating hardware exposed and usable from both sides when the doors are fully open? | | | |
| | | Is the force required to operate the controls no greater than 5 lbf? (This does not apply to the force required to retract latch bolts or to disengage other devices that only hold the door in a closed position.) | | | |
| | | Is the operating hardware mounted no higher than 48 inches above the floor? | | | |
| 4.13.10 | **Door Closers** | If the door has a closer, is the closer adjusted so that from an open position of 70 degrees, the door will take at least 3 seconds to move to a point 3 inches from the latch (measured to the leading edge of the door)? | | | |
| 4.13.11 | **Opening Force**<br>Fire Doors | Do fire doors have the minimum opening force allowable by the appropriate local authority? | | | |
| | Interior Doors | Do interior hinged doors, and sliding or folding doors, have an opening force of 5 lbf or less? | | | |
| 4.13.12 | **Automatic Doors** | If an automatic door is used, does it comply with ANSI/BHMA A156.10-1985? | | | |

| Section | Item | Technical Requirements | Comments | Yes | No |
|---------|------|------------------------|----------|-----|-----|
| | Low Powered Doors | If there is a slow-opening, low-powered automatic door, does it comply with ANSI A156.19-1984 and does it take at least 3 seconds to open to back check? | | | |
| | | Do such doors require no more than 15 lbf to stop door movement? | | | |
| | Power Assisted Doors | If a power assisted door is used, does it have an opening force of 5 lbf or less and does its closing conform to the requirements in ANSI A156.19-1984? | | | |

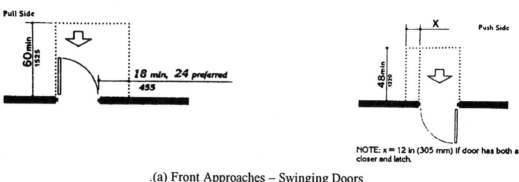

(a) Front Approaches – Swinging Doors

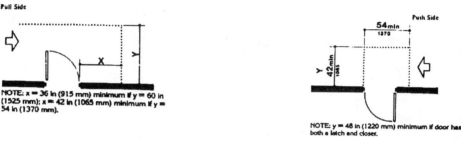

(b) Hinge Side Approaches – Swinging Doors

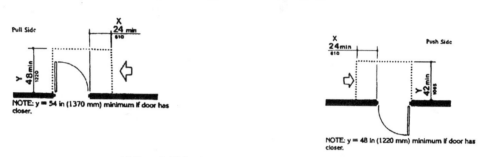

(c) Latch Side Approaches – Swinging Doors

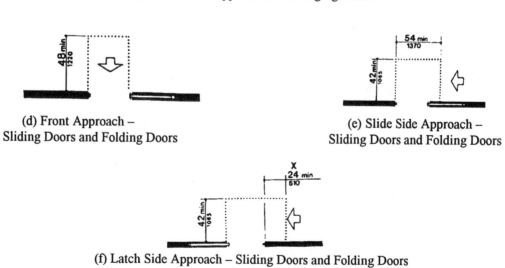

(d) Front Approach –
Sliding Doors and Folding Doors

(e) Slide Side Approach –
Sliding Doors and Folding Doors

(f) Latch Side Approach – Sliding Doors and Folding Doors

NOTE: All doors in alcoves shall comply with the clearances for front approaches.

**Figure 25 – Maneuvering Clearances at Doors**

259

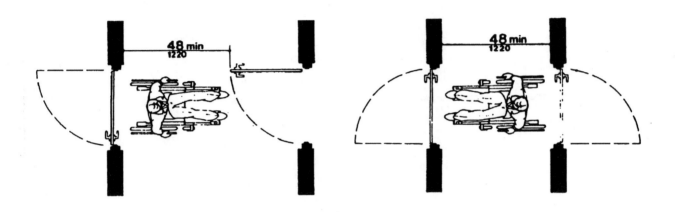

Figure 26 Two Hinged Doors in Series

# Survey Form 12: Building Lobbies and Corridors (Interior Accessible Route)

Use with the Minimum Requirements Summary sheets and ADAAG.

Facility Name: _____ Lobby or Corridor Location: _____

See Minimum Requirements Summary Sheets I and J for special requirements and exceptions which may be allowed in alterations and historic preservation. See also **ADAAG** 4.1.6 and 4.1.7

| Section | Item | Technical Requirements | Comments | Yes | No |
|---------|------|------------------------|----------|-----|-----|
| 4.1.3(1) | **Accessible Route** | Is there an accessible route connecting accessible entrances with all accessible elements and spaces within the building? | | | |
| 4.3.3 | **Width –** General | Is the accessible route at least 36 inches wide except at doorways? | | | |
| | U-Turn | Where the accessible route makes a U-turn around an obstacle which is less than 48 inches wide, does the pathway width increase to at least 42 inches on the approaches and 48 inches in the turn? (See Figure 7(b)) | | | |
| 4.3.4 | **Passing Spaces** | If the accessible route is less than 60 inches wide, are there passing spaces at least 60 inches wide and 60 inches long or intersecting corridors allowing passing at reasonable intervals not exceeding 200 feet? | | | |
| 4.3.5 4.4.1 | **Provisions for Persons Who are Blind** <br><br> Protruding Objects | If objects mounted to the wall have leading edges between 27 and 80 inches from the floor, do they project less than 4 inches into the pathway? (Wall mounted objects with leading edges at or below 27 inches may project any amount so long as the required clear width of an accessible route is not reduced.) | | | |
| | | Do free-standing objects mounted on posts with leading edges between 27 and 80 inches high project less than 12 inches into the perpendicular route of travel? | | | |
| | | Is there an accessible path at least 36 inches clear alongside the protruding object? | | | |
| 4.4.2 | Headroom | Is there at least 80 inches clear head room on an accessible route? | | | |
| | | If there is less than 80 inches clear head room in an area adjoining an accessible route, is there a cane detectable barrier within 27 inches of the floor? (See Figure 8(c-1)) | | | |

Survey Form

12–1

261

| Section | Item | Technical Requirements | Comments | Yes | No |
|---------|------|------------------------|----------|-----|-----|
| **4.5.1** | **Floor Surface** | Are the floor surfaces on accessible routes stable, firm, and slip-resistant? | | | |
| 4.3.7<br>4.8.1 | Slope | Is the slope of the accessible route no greater than 1:20?<br>OR<br>Where the slope is greater than 1:20, does it comply with the requirements for ramps? (Use Form 7: Ramps) | | | |
| 4.3.7<br>4.8.1 | Cross Slope | Is the cross slope no greater than 1:50? | | | |
| **4.3.8**<br>**4.5.2** | **Changes in Level** | Are ramps or elevators used for changes in level greater than 1/2 inch? (Lifts may only be used in certain limited situations in new construction. See Minimum Requirements Summary Sheet D and ADAAG 4.1.3(5) Exception 4.) | | | |
| | | Does the ramp or elevator comply with 4.8 or 4.10? (Use Form 7: Ramps or Form 13: Elevators (Not in this CIP chapter.)) | | | |
| | | When walkway levels change, is the vertical difference less than 1/4 inch?<br>OR<br>Are changes in level between 1/2 inch and 1/2 inch beveled with a slope no greater than 1:2? | | | |
| | | When floor materials change, does the vertical difference between them meet the above requirements? | | | |
| **4.5.3** | **Carpet** | If carpet or carpet tile is used on the floor, is it securely attached? | | | |
| | | Are exposed edges of carpet fastened to the floor and have trim along their entire length? | | | |
| | | Is it a low pile type of carpet (1/2 inch maximum) with a firm pad or no pad underneath it? | | | |
| **4.1.3(7)(e)**<br>**4.13** | **Doors** | Does each door that is an element of an accessible route comply with 4.13? (Use Form 11: Doors and Gates) | | | |
| 4.13.2 | Revolving Door | If a revolving door or turnstile is used on an accessible route, is an accessible door or gate provided adjacent to the revolving door or turnstile to facilitate the same use pattern? | | | |

| Section | Item | Technical Requirements | Comments | Yes | No |
|---------|------|------------------------|----------|-----|-----|
| 4.13.3 | Gates | Do gates, including ticket gates, meet all the applicable specifications of 4.13? (Use Form 11: Doors and Gates) | | | |
| **4.1.3(16)** **4.30.1** | **Directional and Informational Signs** | Do signs which identify permanent rooms and spaces comply with 4.30.4, 4.30.5, and 4.30.5? (Use Form 19: Signage (Not in this CIP chapter.))<br><br>**Exception: Building directories, menus, and all other signs which are temporary are not required to comply.** | | | |
| **4.1.3(16)** **4.30.1** | **Room Identification Signs** | Do signs which identify permanent rooms and spaces comply with 4.30.4, 4.30.5, and 4.30.6? (Use Form 19: Signage (Not in this CIP chapter.)) | | | |
| **4.1.3(14)** **4.28** | **Alarms** | If emergency warning systems are provided, do they include both audible alarms and visual alarms complying with 4.25? (Use Form 20: Alarms (Not in this CIP chapter.)) | | | |

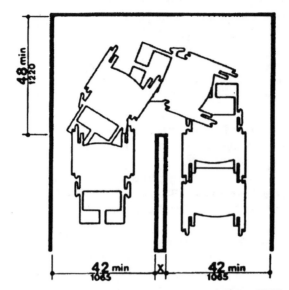

NOTE: Dimensions shown apply when x < 48 in (1220 mm).

**Figure 7 (b) Accessible Route – Turns Around an Obstruction**

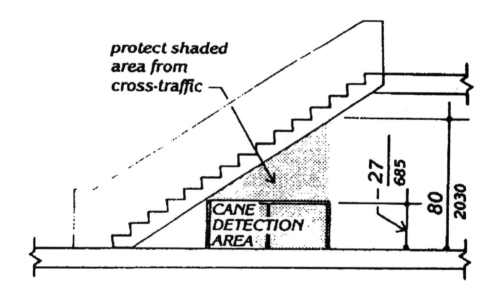

**Figure 8 (c-1) Protruding Object – Overhead Hazards**

# Survey Form 14: Rooms and Spaces

Use with the Minimum Requirements Summary sheets and ADAAG.

**Facility Name:** _____ **Room or Space Location:** _____

See Minimum Requirements Summary Sheets I and J for special requirements and exceptions which may be allowed in alterations and historic preservation. See also **ADAAG** 4.1.6 and 4.1.7

| Section | Item | Technical Requirements | Comments | Yes | No |
|---------|------|------------------------|----------|-----|-----|
| 4.1.3(7)(b) | **Doors** | Do doors comply with 4.13? (Use Form 11: Doors and Gates) | | | |
| 4.3.3 | **Aisles** | Are aisles between permanently built-in case work or partitions at least 36 inches wide (or at least 32 inches wide for a length not to exceed 24 inches)? (See Figure 8(e)) | | | |
| | | Where the aisle makes a U-turn around an obstacle which is less than 48 inches wide, is the pathway width at least 48 inches in the turn? (See Figure 7(b)) | | | |
| 4.3.4 | Passing Spaces | If the aisles between permanently built-in casework or partitions are less than 60 inches wide, are there passing spaces at least 60 inches wide and 60 inches long or intersecting aisles allowing passing at reasonable intervals not exceeding 200 feet? | | | |
| 4.3.5 4.4.2 | **Headroom** | Is there at least 80 inches clear head room in the accessible space? | | | |
| | | If there is less than 80 inches clear head room in part of an accessible space, is there a cane detectable barrier within 27 inches of the floor? (See Figure 8(c-1)) | | | |
| 4.4.1 | **Protruding Objects** | If objects mounted to the wall have leading edges between 27 and 80 inches from the floor, do they project less than 4 inches into the accessible space? (Wall mounted objects with leading edges at or below 27 inches may project any amount so long as they do not reduce the required clear width of an accessible route.) | | | |
| | | Do free-standing objects, mounted on posts with leading edges between 27 and 80 inches high (such as drinking fountains or telephones) project less than 12 inches into the perpendicular route of travel? | | | |
| | | Is there an accessible route at least 36 inches clear alongside the protruding object? | | | |

| Section | Item | Technical Requirements | Comments | Yes | No |
|---|---|---|---|---|---|
| 4.5.1 | Floors | Are the floor surfaces in all accessible rooms and spaces stable, firm, and slip-resistant? | | | |
| 4.1.3(5) 4.3.8 4.5.2 | Level Changes | Are ramps or elevators used for any change in level greater than 1/2 inch? (Lifts may only be used in certain limited situations in new construction See Minimum Requirements Summary Sheet D and ADAAG 4.1.3(5) Exception 4) | | | |
| | | Do the ramps or elevators comply with 4.8 or 4.10? (Use Form 7: Ramps or Form 13: Elevators (Not in this CIP chapter.)) | | | |
| | | When walkway levels change, is the vertical difference less than 1/4 inch? OR Are changes in level between 1/4 and 1/2 inch beveled with a slope no greater than 1:2? | | | |
| | | When floor materials change, does the vertical difference between them meet the above requirement? | | | |
| 4.5.3 | Carpet | If carpet or carpet tile is used on the floor, is it securely attached? | | | |
| | | Is it low pile type of carpet (1/2 inch or less) with a firm pad or no pad underneath? | | | |
| 4.1.3(16) 4.30.1 | Directional and Informational Signage | Do signs which provide direction to, or information about, functional spaces of the building comply with 4.30.2, 4.30.3, and 4.30.5? (Use Form 19: Signage (Not in this CIP chapter.)) | | | |
| 4.1.3(16) 4.30.1 | Room Identification Signage | Do signs which designate permanent rooms and spaces comply with 4.30.4, 4.30.5, and 4.30.6? (Use Form 19: Signage (Not in this CIP chapter.)) | | | |
| 4.13.3(12) 4.25.1 | Storage | Does at least one of each type of fixed or built-in storage facilities (e.g., cabinets, shelves, closets, and drawers) comply with 4.25 (See below)? (Additional storage may be provided outside the dimensions required by 4.25. Accessible reach range requirements do not apply to shelves or display units allowing self-service by customers in mercantile occupancies but they must be located on an accessible route.) | | | |
| 4.25.2 4.2.4 | Clear Floor Space | Is there a clear floor space at least 30 by 48 inches at fixed or built-in storage facilities which allows for either a forward or parallel approach? | | | |

| Section | Item | Technical Requirements | Comments | Yes | No |
|---------|------|------------------------|----------|-----|-----|
| 4.25.3<br>4.2.5<br>4.2.6 | Side Reach | If a parallel approach is provided, are clothes rods and shelves between 9 and 54 inches from the floor? | | | |
| 4.25.3 | | Where the distance between a wheelchair and clothes rod or shelve is between 10 - 21 inches (e.g., closets without accessible doors) is the accessible shelf no more than 48 inches from the floor and the reach no more than 21 inches? (See Figure 38) | | | |
| | Forward Reach | If a front approach is provided, are clothes rods and shelves between 15 and 48 inches from the floor? | | | |
| 4.13.5 | Closet Doors | Where passage is not required to access storage, does the door have at least 20 inches clear opening width? | | | |
| 4.25.4<br>4.27.4 | Hardware | Is the hardware on the storage space doors operable with one hand, and without tight grasping, pinching, or twisting of the wrist? | | | |
| | | Is the force required to activate the hardware less the 5 lbf? | | | |
| **4.1.3(18)**<br>**4.32.1** | Fixed/Built-In Seating, Tables or Counters | Do 5% (but not less than one) of fixed or built-in seating, tables, or counters (e.g., study carrels and student laboratory stations) comply with 4.32 (See below)? (For specific requirements for restaurants and cafeterias, use Form 23: Restaurants and Cafeterias.) | | | |
| **4.32.2**<br>**4.2.4** | Clear Space – Seating | Do seating spaces which are provided for wheelchair users have a 30 by 48 inch clear space which overlaps an accessible route? | | | |
| | Knee Space | Is no more than 19 inches if the 30 by 48 inch clear space measured under the table? (See figure 45) | | | |
| 4.32.3 | | Is the knee space at least 27 inches high, 30 inches wide, and 19 inches deep? (See Figure 45) | | | |
| 4.32.4 | | Is the top of the table or counter between 28 and 34 inches from the floor? | | | |
| 4.3.3 | Aisles | Are the aisles leading up to and between tables at least 36 inches wide? | | | |
| **4.1.3(13)**<br>**4.27.1**<br>**4.27.2**<br>**4.27.3**<br>**4.2.5**<br>**4.2.6** | **Controls** | Are light switches, controls, dispensers, and similar devices between 9 and 54 inches from the floor when the clear floor space allows a parallel approach?<br>OR<br>Are they between 15 and 48 inches from the floor when the clear floor space allows only a forward approach? | | | |

| Section | Item | Technical Requirements | Comments | Yes | No |
|---|---|---|---|---|---|
| | | Are all electrical and communications receptacles used by building occupants at least 15 inches above the floor? | | | |
| 4.27.4 | | Are controls operable with one hand, and without tight grasping, pinching, or twisting of the wrist? | | | |
| | | Is the force required to activate controls less than 5 lbf? | | | |
| 4.1.3(14) 4.15.1 | **Alarms** | Where alarms are provided, do they comply with 4.28? (Use Form 20: Alarms (Not in this CIP chapter.)) | | | |
| 4.1.3(10) 4.15.1 | **Drinking Fountains** | If drinking fountains are located in a room or space, do they comply with 4.15? (Use Form 5: Drinking Fountains (Not in this CIP chapter.)) | | | |
| 4.1.3(17) 4.31.1 | **Public Telephones** | If public telephones are located in a room or space, do they comply with 4.31? (Use Form 6: Telephones) | | | |

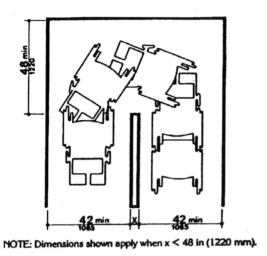

NOTE: Dimensions shown apply when x < 48 in (1220 mm).

**Figure 7 (b) Accessible Route – Turns Around an Obstruction**

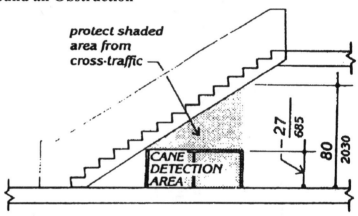

**Figure 8 (c-1) Protruding Object – Overhead Hazards**

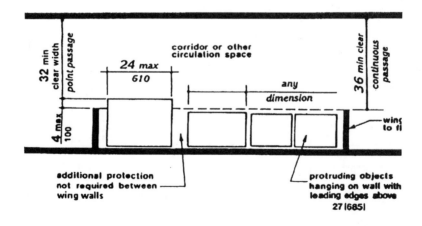

**Figure 8 (e): Protruding Objects – Example of Protection Around Wall-Mounted Objects and Measurements of Clear Widths**

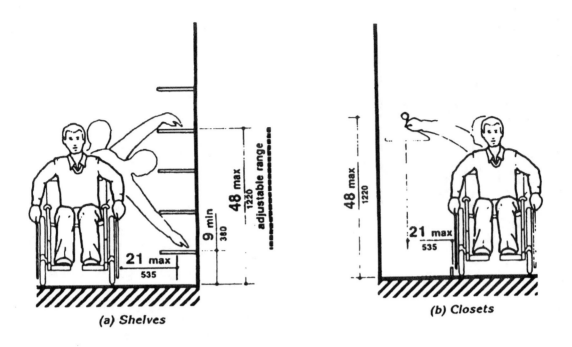

**Figure 38: Storage Shelves and Closets**

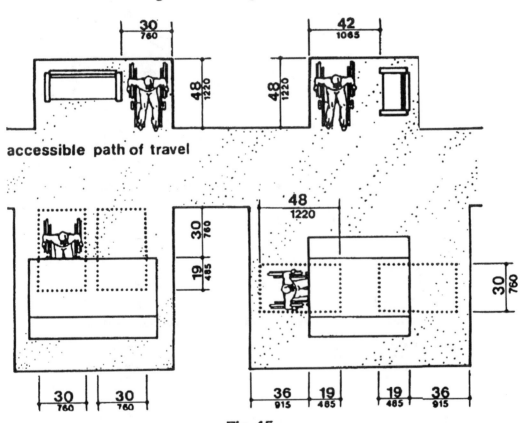

accessible path of travel

**Fig. 45
Minimum Clearances for Seating and Tables**

# Survey Form 15: Assembly Areas

Use with the Minimum Requirements Summary sheets and ADAAG.

**Facility Name:** _____  **Assembly Room Location:** _____

See Minimum Requirements Summary Sheets I and J for special requirements and exceptions which may be allowed in alterations and historic preservation. See also **ADAAG** 4.1.6 and 4.1.7

| Capacity of Seating in Assembly Areas | Number of Required Wheelchair Locations |
|---|---|
| 4 to 25 | 1 |
| 26 to 50 | 2 |
| 51 to 300 | 4 |
| 301 to 500 | 6 |
| over 500 | 6, plus 1 additional space for each total seating capacity increase of 100 |

| Section | Item | Technical Requirements | Comments | Yes | No |
|---|---|---|---|---|---|
| **4.1.3(19)(a) 4.33.1** | **Wheelchair Seating** | In assembly areas with fixed seating, is the required number of wheelchair locations provided (See Table above)? | | | |
| | Aisle Seating | In addition, are one percent (but not less than one) of all fixed seats, aisle seats with no armrests on the aisle side, or removable or folding armrests on the aisle side? | | | |
| | Identification | Is each such aisle seat identified by a sign or marker? | | | |
| | | Is there a sign posted at the ticket office notifying patrons of such aisle eats? | | | |
| | | Do the wheelchair locations comply with 4.33.2, 4.33.3 and 4.33.4 (See below) | | | |
| **4.33.2** | **Wheelchair Seating Size – Width** | Do paired wheelchair spaces total 66 inches in width? (It is not required that all wheelchair spaces be paired.) | | | |
| | Depth | If wheelchair users enter the space from the side, is the space at least 60 inches deep? | | | |
| | | If wheelchair users enter the space from the front or back, is the space at least 48 inches deep? | | | |
| **4.33.3** | **Placement of Wheelchair Areas** | Are the wheelchair areas an integral part of the fixed seating plan with a choice of admission prices and lines of sight comparable to those for the general public? (Readily removable seats may be installed in wheelchair spaces when the spaces are not required to accommodate wheelchair users.) | | | |

| Section | Item | Technical Requirements | Comments | Yes | No |
|---|---|---|---|---|---|
| | Multiple Locations | If the seating capacity exceeds 300, are the wheelchair spaces provided in more than one location?<br><br>**Exception: Accessible viewing positions may be clustered for bleachers, balconies, and other areas having sight lines which require slopes greater than 5%.** | | | |
| | Companion Seating | Is there at least one companion fixed seat provided next to each wheelchair seating area? | | | |
| | Accessible Route | Do wheelchair spaces adjoin an accessible route that also serves as a means of egress in an emergency? | | | |
| 4.33.4<br>4.5 | **Surfaces** | Are the floor surfaces at wheelchair areas level, stable, firm, and slip-resistant? | | | |
| 4.1.3(5)<br>4.3.8<br>4.5.2 | **Level Changes** | Are ramps or elevators used for changes in level greater than 1/2 inch? (Lifts may only be used in certain limited situations in new construction. See Minimum requirements Summary Sheet D and ADAAG 4.1.3(5) Exception 4) | | | |
| | | Do the ramps or elevators comply with 4.8 or 4.10? (Use Form 7: Ramps or Form 13: Elevators (Not in this CIP chapter.)) | | | |
| | | When walkway levels change, is the vertical difference less than 1/4 inch?<br>OR<br>Are changes in level between 1/4 and 1/2 inch beveled with a maximum slope of 1:2? | | | |
| | | Where floor materials change, does the vertical difference between them meet the above requirements? | | | |
| 4.5.3 | **Carpet** | If carpet or carpet tile is used on the floor, is it securely attached? | | | |
| | | Is it low pile type of carpet (1/2 inch thick or less) with a firm pad or no pad underneath? | | | |
| 4.33.5 | **Performing Areas** | Is there an accessible route connecting wheelchair seating locations and performance areas including stages, arena floors, dressing rooms, locker rooms, and other spaces used by performers? (Use Form 12: Building Lobbies and Corridors) | | | |
| 4.1.3(19)(b) | **Assistive Listening Systems** – Permanently Installed | In assembly areas where audible communications are integral to the use of the space, is there a permanently installed assistive listening system if (1) the assembly area accommodates 50 or more persons or has an audio-amplification system and (2) it has fixed seats? | | | |

| Section | Item | Technical Requirements | Comments | Yes | No |
|---|---|---|---|---|---|
| | Portable Systems | For other assembly areas, is there a permanently installed assistive listening system or adequate number of outlets/wiring to permit use of a portable assistive listening system? | | | |
| | Receivers | Is the minimum number of receivers provided equal to 4% of the total number of seats, but not less than two? | | | |
| 4.30.7(4) | Signage | Where a permanently installed Assistive listening system is provided, is there signage installed to notify patrons of the availability of such a system? | | | |
| | | Does the signage include the International Symbol for hearing loss? | | | |
| 4.33.6 | Placement of Assistive Listening Systems | If the Assistive listening system serves individual fixed seats, are these seats located within a 50-foot viewing distance of the stage or playing area? | | | |
| | | Do these seats have a complete view of the stage or playing area? | | | |

# Survey Form 16: Toilet Rooms and Bathrooms

Use with the Minimum Requirements Summary sheets and ADAAG.

Facility Name: _____ Toilet Room Location: _____

See Minimum Requirements Summary Sheets I and J for special requirements and exceptions which may be allowed in alterations and historic preservation. See also **ADAAG** 4.1.6 and 4.1.7

| Section | Item | Technical Requirements | Comments | Yes | No |
|---------|------|------------------------|----------|-----|-----|
| 4.1.26(6) 4.1.3(11) 4.22.1 | **Public and Common Use Toilet Rooms** | If toilet rooms are provided, does each public and common use toilet room comply with 4.22 (See below)? (A common use toilet room is one used for a restricted group of people such as occupants of a building or employees of a company). | | | |
| | Private Use Toilet Rooms | If other toilet rooms are provided for the use of an occupant of a specific space, (such as a private toilet room for a company president) is each toilet room adaptable (e.g., door clearance, clear floor space at fixtures and maneuvering space)? | | | |
| 4.1.2(6) 4.1.3(11) .4.23.1 | **Public and Common Use Bathing Facilities** | If bathrooms or bathing facilities are provided, does each public and common use bathroom or bathing facility comply with 4.23 (See below)? | | | |
| 4.1.3(5) **Exception 1** | **Toilet/Bath Rooms in Buildings Eligible for Elevator Exemption** | In buildings eligible for the elevator exception, if toilet/bath rooms are provided on a level not served by an elevator, is a toilet/bath room complying with 1.22 or 4.23 provided on the accessible ground floor? If toilet or bathing facilities are also provided on floors above or below ground level, they must be accessible. | | | |
| 4.22.1 | **Accessible Route** | Are the toilet/bath rooms located on an accessible route? (Use Form 12: Building Lobbies and Corridors) | | | |
| 4.22.3 4.23.3 | | If provided, are each of the following accessible fixtures and controls located on an accessible route? (Use Form 12: Building Lobbies and Corridors)<br>• 4.22.4 & 4.23.4 Water closets<br>• 4.22.5 & 4.23.5 Urinals<br>• 4.22.6 & 4.23.6 Lavatories and Mirrors<br>• 4.22.7 & 4.23.7 Controls and Dispensers<br>• 4.23.8 Bathing and Shower Facilities<br>• 4.23.9 Medicine Cabinets | | | |

| Section | Item | Technical Requirements | Comments | Yes | No |
|---------|------|------------------------|----------|-----|-----|
| 4.22.3<br>4.23.3 | **Maneuvering Space** | Is there an unobstructed turning space (a 60-inch diameter circle or T-shaped space) in the toilet/bath room? (See Figure 3.) (The clear floor space of fixtures and controls, the accessible route, and the turning space may overlap.) | | | |
| 4.22.3<br>4.23.3 | **Doors** | Do the doors comply with 4.13? (Use Form 11: Doors and Gates) | | | |
| | | Does the door swing not intrude into the clear floor space at any fixture. | | | |
| 4.1.3(16)<br>4.30.1 | **Room Identification Signage** | Do signs which designate toilet/bath rooms comply with 4.30.4, 4.30.5, and 4.30.6? (Use Form 19: Signage (Not in this CIP chapter.)) | | | |
| 4.22.4<br>4.23.4 | **Toilet Stalls – Standard Stall** | If toilet stalls are provided, is at lest one a standard stall at least 60 inches wide complying with 4.17 (See below)? | | | |
| 4.17.3 | Size and Arrangement | Does the size and arrangement of the standard toilet stall comply with Figure 30(a)? (Arrangements may be reversed.) | | | |
| | Stall Width | Is the stall at least 60 inches wide? | | | |
| | Stall Depth | If the toilet is wall mounted, is the stall at least 56 inches deep? | | | |
| | | If the toilet is a floor mounted model, is the stall at least 59 inches deep? | | | |
| | Door location | Is the stall door located at the "open" side of the toilet stall? | | | |
| 4.17.4 | Toe Clearance | If the stall is less than 60 inches deep, does the front partition and at least one side partition have toe clearance of at least 9 inches above the floor? | | | |
| 4.17.5<br>4.13.5 | Stall Door Width | When the stall is open 90 degrees, is there a clear opening of at least 32 inches measured between the face of the door and the edge of the partition on the latch side? | | | |
| | Door Swing | If the stall door swings into the stall, is there at least 36 inches additional depth in the stall so that it does not encroach on the clear floor space required at the toilet and is there at least 18 inches of maneuvering space at the latch side of the door? (See Figure 30 (a-1)) | | | |
| | Approach Aisle | If the stall door swings out and the approach is from the latch side, is the aisle approaching the stall at least 42 inches wide?<br>OR<br>If the stall door swings out and the approach is from the hinge side, is the aisle approaching the stall at least 49 inches wide? | | | |

| Section | Item | Technical Requirements | Comments | Yes | No |
|---|---|---|---|---|---|
| 4.17.5<br>4.13.6 | Maneuvering Space | If the stall door opens out at the end of an aisle, is there at least 18 inches of maneuvering space at the latch side of the stall door? | | | |
| 4.17.6 | Grab Bars in Standard Stall | Are the grab bars in the standard stall placed as shown in Figure 30 (a), (c), and (d)? | | | |
| | | Do the grab bars comply with 4.26.2, 4.26.3, 4.26.4 (See below)? | | | |
| **4.22.4**<br>**4.23.4** | **Additional Toilet Stall** | Where 6 or more toilet stalls are provided, in addition to the 60 inch wide standard stall, is at least one stall 36 inches wide with an outward swinging, self-closing door provided? | | | |
| | Grab Bars in Additional Stall | Do the parallel grab bars in the 36 inch wide stall comply with Figure 30(d)? | | | |
| | | Do the grab bars comply with 4.26.2, 4.26.3 and 4.26.4 (See below)? | | | |
| **4.16.2** | **Toilets Not in Stalls–**<br>Front Approach | If the toilet is not in a stall and is approached from the **front** and there is a lavatory alongside the toilet, is there a clear floor space at least 48 inches wide by 66 inches long? (See Figure 28) | | | |
| | Side Approach | If the toilet is not in a stall and is approached from the **side** and there is a lavatory alongside the toilet, is there a clear floor space at least 48 inches wide by 56 inches long? (See Figure 28) | | | |
| | Lateral Transfer | If the toilet is not in a stall and there is provision for a lateral transfer (no lavatory alongside the toilet), is there a clear floor space at least 60 inches wide by 56 inches long? (See Figure 28) | | | |
| **4.16.4** | Grab Bars for Toilets Not in Stalls | If the toilet is not in a stall, is the back grab bar at least 36 inches long with the end closer to the side wall mounted at least 12 inches from the centerline of the toilet? (See Figure 29) | | | |
| | | Is the side grab bar at least 42 inches long and mounted a maximum 12 inches from the back wall? (See Figure 29) | | | |
| | | Are the grab bars horizontal and mounted between 33 and 36 inches above the floor? | | | |
| | | Do the grab bars comply with 4.26.2, 4.26.3, or 4.26.4 (See below)? | | | |
| **4.26.2** | **Grab Bars for All Accessible Toilets –**<br>Diameter | Is the outside diameter of the grab bar between 1-1/4 and 1-1/2 inch?<br>OR<br>Does the shape provide an equivalent gripping surface?<br><br>Note: Standard pipe sizes designated by the industry ad 1-1/4 to 1-1/2 inches are acceptable for purposes of this section. | | | |

| Section | Item | Technical Requirements | Comments | Yes | No |
|---------|------|------------------------|----------|-----|-----|
| 4.26.2 | Wall Clearance | Is the space between the grab bar and the wall exactly 1-1/2 inches? | | | |
| 4.26.3(5) | Fixed | Are the grab bars secured so that they do not rotate within their fittings? | | | |
| 4.26.2 | Clearance in Recess | If a grab bar is located in a recess, is the recess a maximum of 3 inches deep extending at least 18 inches above the rail? (See Figure 39(d)) | | | |
| 4.26.3 | Structural Strength | Do the grab bars meet the structural strength requirements for bending stress and shear stress? (See 4.26.3(1) and (2)) | | | |
| | | Do the fasteners meet structural strength requirements for shear force and tensile force? (See 4.26.3(3) and (4)) | | | |
| 4.26.4 | Hazards | Are grab bars and adjacent walls free of sharp or abrasive elements? | | | |
| | | Do grab bars have edges with a minimum radius of 1/8 inch? | | | |
| **4.22.4** **4.23.4** | **Accessible Toilets** | Is the centerline of the toilet 18 inches from a wall or partition? | | | |
| 4.16.3 | Toilet Seat | Is the top of the toilet seat between 17 and 19 inches from the floor? | | | |
| | | Is the seat a type that does not automatically spring back to a lifted position? | | | |
| 4.16.5 4.27.4 | Toilet Flush Controls | Are flush controls automatic or operable with one hand without tight grasping, pinching or twisting of the wrist? | | | |
| | | Is the force required to operate the controls no greater than 5 lbf? | | | |
| | | Are they mounted on the wide side of the toilet where the clear floor space is provided? | | | |
| | | Are the controls no higher than 44 inches above the floor? | | | |
| 4.16.6 | Toilet Paper Dispenser | Is the paper dispenser mounted below the grab bar no more than 36 inches from the back wall and least 19 inches from the floor? | | | |
| | | Is the dispenser located so that it does not obstruct the use of the grab bar? | | | |
| | | Does the dispenser allow continuous paper delivery? | | | |
| **4.22.5** **4.23.5** | **Urinals** | Where urinals are provided, does at least one comply with 4.18 (See below)? | | | |
| | Rim Height | Does the urinal have an elongated rim no more than 17 inches above the floor? | | | |
| 4.18.3 4.2.4 | Clear Floor Space | Is there a clear floor space at least 30 by 48 inches which allows a forward approach to the urinal? | | | |
| | | Does the clear floor space adjoin or overlap an accessible route? | | | |

| Section | Item | Technical Requirements | Comments | Yes | No |
|---------|------|------------------------|----------|-----|-----|
| 4.2.4.3 | Surface | Is the surface of the clear floor space stable, firm and slip resistant? | | | |
| | Width Between Shields | If urinal shields are provided and they do not extend beyond the front edge of the urinal rim, is there at least 29 inches between the two panels? | | | |
| 4.18.4<br>4.27.4 | Urinal Flush Controls | Are the flush controls automatic or operable with one hand without tight grasping, pinching, or twisting of the wrist? | | | |
| | | Is the force required to operate the controls no greater than 5 lbf? | | | |
| | | Are the controls mounted no more than 44 inches above the floor? | | | |
| **4.22.6**<br>**4.23.6** | **Lavatories** | If lavatories are provided, does at least one lavatory meet the following requirements? | | | |
| 4.19.2 | Rim Height | Is the lavatory rim or counter surface no higher than 34 inches above the finish floor? | | | |
| | Knee Clearance | Is there a clearance of at least 29 inches from the floor to the bottom of the apron? (See Figure 31) | | | |
| | Wall Projection | Does the front edge of the lavatory project at least 17 inches from the wall? | | | |
| | | Do the toe and knee clearances comply with Figure 31? | | | |
| 4.19.3<br>4.2.4 | Clear Floor Space | Is there a clear floor space at least 30 by 48 inches in front of the lavatory allowing a forward approach? | | | |
| | | Is no more than 19 inches of this clear floor space measured underneath the lavatory? | | | |
| | | Does the clear floor space adjoin or overlap an accessible route? | | | |
| 4.2.4.3 | Surface | Is the surface of the clear floor space stable, firm and slip resistant? | | | |
| 4.19.4 | Pipe Shielding | Are hot water pipes and drain pipes insulated or otherwise configured to protect against contact? | | | |
| | Smooth Surfaces | Is the area below the lavatory free of sharp or abrasive surfaces? | | ✓ | |
| 4.19.5<br>4.27.4 | Faucet Operation | Can the faucet be operated with one hand without tight grasping, pinching, or twisting of the wrist? | | | |
| | | Is the force required to operate controls no greater than 5 lbf? | | | |
| | | If the valve is self-closing, does it remain open for at least 10 seconds? | | | |
| **4.22.6**<br>**4.23.6**<br>**4.19.6** | **Mirrors** | Where mirrors are provided, does at least one mirror have a bottom edge of the reflecting surface no higher than 40 inches from the floor? | | | |

| Section | Item | Technical Requirements | Comments | Yes | No |
|---|---|---|---|---|---|
| **4.22.7**<br>**4.23.7** | **Dispensers –**<br>Location | Is at least one of each dispenser type accessible and on an accessible route? | | | |
| 4.27.2<br>4.2.4 | Floor Space | Is there a clear floor space at least 30 by 48 inches in front of the dispenser allowing either a forward or a parallel approach to the dispenser? | | | |
| 4.2.4.3 | Surface | Is the surface of the clear floor space stable, firm and slip resistant? | | | |
| 4.27.3 | Dispenser Height | If a forward approach is provided, is the highest operable part no higher than 48 inches? | | | |
| | | If a parallel approach is provided, is the highest operable part no higher than 54 inches? | | | |
| 4.27.4 | Dispenser Operation | Can the dispenser be operated with one hand without tight grasping, pinching, or twisting of the wrist? | | | |
| **4.23.9** | **Medicine Cabinet** | If medicine cabinets are provided, does at least one have a usable shelf no higher than 44 inches from the floor? | | | |
| 4.2.4 | Clear Floor Space | Is there a clear floor space at least 30 by 48 inches in front of the medicine cabinet allowing either a forward or parallel approach to the medicine cabinet? | | | |
| 4.2.4.3 | Surface | Is the surface of the clear floor space stable, firm and slip resistant? | | | |
| **4.25.2**<br>**4.2.4** | **Storage** | If fixed or built-in storage facilities are provided, does at least one of each type have a clear floor space 30 by 48 inches allowing either a forward or parallel approach? | | | |
| 4.25.3<br>4.2.5<br>4.2.6 | | If a parallel approach is provided, are clothes rods and shelves between 9 and 54 inches from the floor? | | | |
| 4.25.3 | Shelf Height | Where the distance between a wheelchair and clothes rod or shelf is between 10 - 21 inches (e.g., closets without accessible doors) is the accessible shelf no more than 48 inches from the floor and the reach no more than 21 inches? (See Figure 38) | | | |
| 4.25.3 | | If a front approach is provided, are clothes rods and shelves between 15 and 48 inches from the floor? | | | |
| **4.23.8** | **Bathtubs and Showers** | Where bathtubs or showers are provided, does at least one comply with 4.20 or 4.21? (Use Form 17: Bathtubs and Showers) | | | |
| **4.1.3(14)**<br>**4.28.1** | **Alarms** | Where alarms are provided, do they comply with 4.28? (Use Form 20: Alarms (Not in this **CIP** chapter)) | | | |

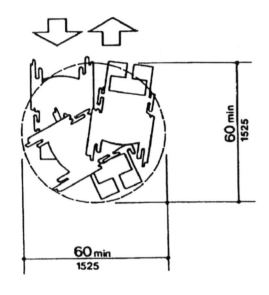

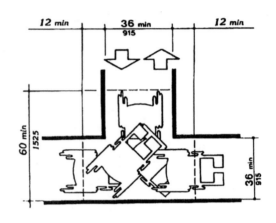

(a) 60-in (1525 mm) Diameter Space        (b) T-Shaped Space for 180° turns

**Figure 3: Wheelchair Turning Space**

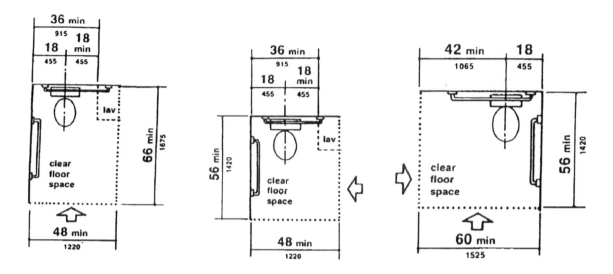

**Figure 28: Clear Floor Space in Water Closets**

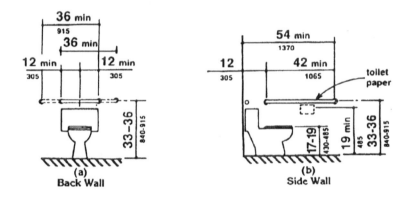

**Figure 29: Grab Bars at Water Closets**

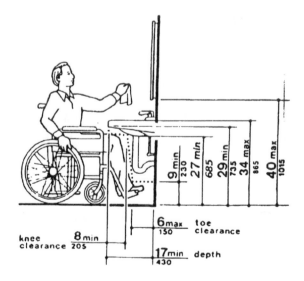

**Figure 31: Lavatory Clearances**

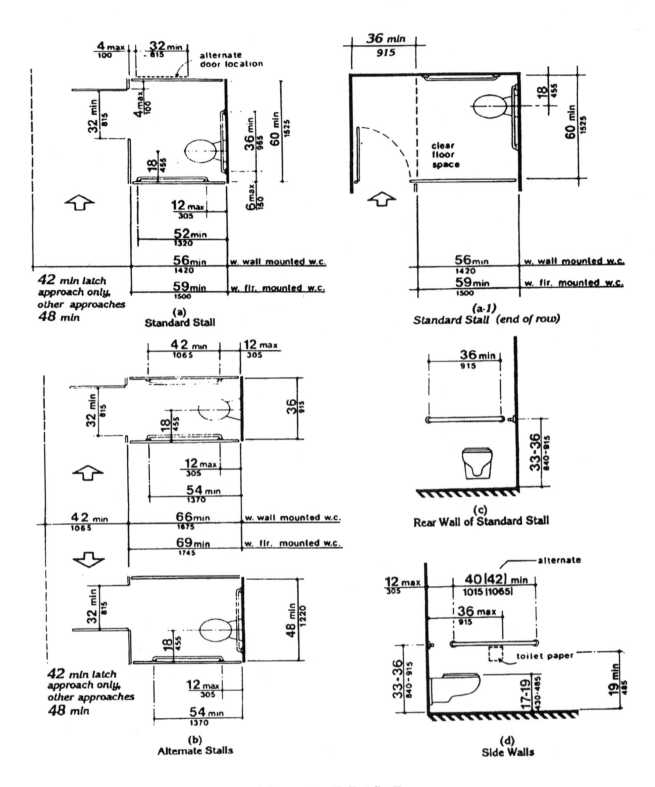

**Figure 30: Toilet Stalls**

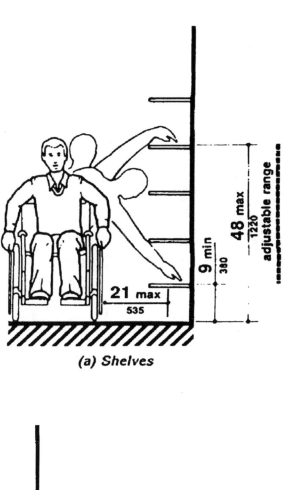

(a) Shelves

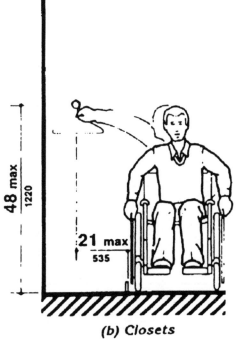

(b) Closets

**Figure 38: Storage Shelves and Closets**

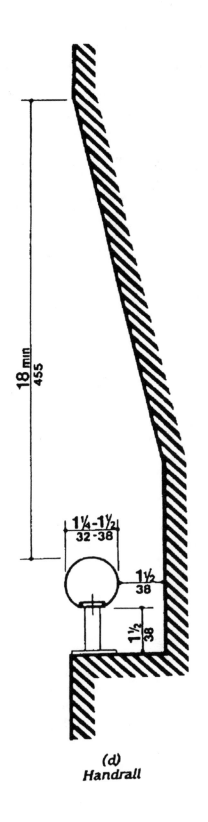

(d)
Handrall

**Figure 39: Size and Spacing of
Handrails and Grab Bars**

283

# Survey Form 17: Bathtubs and Showers

Use with the Minimum Requirements Summary sheets and ADAAG.

**Facility Name:** _____ **Bathroom Location:** _____

See Minimum Requirements Summary Sheets I and J for special requirements and exceptions which may be allowed in alterations and historic preservation. See also **ADAAG** 4.1.6 and 4.1.7

| Section | Item | Technical Requirements | Comments | Yes | No |
|---|---|---|---|---|---|
| **4.23.1** | **Accessible Route** | Are the bathing facilities located on an accessible route? | | | |
| **4.23.2** | **Doors** | Do the doors comply with 4.13? (Use Form 11: Doors and Gates) | | | |
| | | Does the door swing not intrude into the clear floor space at any time? | | | |
| **4.23.8** **4.20.1** | **Bathtubs** | Where bathtubs are provided, does at least one comply 4.20 (See below)? | | | |
| 4.20.2 | Clear Space | Does the clear floor space comply with both the dimensions and approach shown in Figure 33? | | | |
| 4.20.3 | Seat | Is a securely mounted in-tub seat or built-in seat provided at the head of the tub? | | | |
| 4.20.4 | Grab Bar Placement | Are grab dimensions and locations as shown in Figure 34? | | | |
| 4.20.5 4.27.4 | Controls | Can faucets and other controls be operated with one hand and without tight grasping, pinching, or twisting of the wrist? | | | |
| | | Is the force required to operate the controls no greater than 5 lbf? | | | |
| 4.20.5 | | Are controls located within the area shown in Figure 34? | | | |
| 4.20.6 | Spray Unit | Is there a shower spray unit with a hose at least 60 inches long? | | | |
| | | Can the shower spray unit be used as a hand-held and as a fixed shower head? | | | |
| 4.20.7 | Enclosures | If provided, are bathtub enclosures designed so that they do not obstruct the controls or transfer from a wheelchair onto the bathtub seat or into the bathtub? | | | |
| | | If an enclosure is provided on the bathtub, is there no track mounted on the bathtub rim? | | | |
| **4.23.8** **4.21.1** | **Showers** | Where showers are provided, does at least one comply with 4.21 (See below)? | | | |

| Section | Item | Technical Requirements | Comments | Yes | No |
|---|---|---|---|---|---|
| 4.21.2<br>9.1.2 | | On public and common use bathing facilities with showers, does the shower stall size and clear floor space comply with either Figure 35(a) for a transfer type shower or figure 35(b) for a roll-in shower?<br>OR<br>In guest rooms in transient lodging required to have roll-in showers, does the shower stall size and clear floor space comply with Figure 57(a) or 57(b)? | | | |
| **4.21.2** | **Transfer Type Showers** | If the shower stall is transfer type shown in Figure 35(a), is it exactly 36 by 36 inches? | | | |
| | Clear Floor Space | In a transfer type shower, is there a clear floor space at least 36 by 48 inches outside the stall with 12 inches extending beyond the seat wall? (See Figure 35(a)) | | | |
| 4.21.3 | Seat | In a transfer type shower, is there a seat mounted between 17 and 19 inches from the floor? | | | |
| | | Does the seat extend the full depth of the stall? | | | |
| | | Is the seat L-shaped and as shown in figure 36? | | | |
| | | Is the seat on the wall opposite the controls? | | | |
| 4.21.4 | Grab Bars | In a transfer type shower, are grab bars provided between 33 and 36 inches above the floor along the control wall and half the back wall (but not behind the seat) as shown in figure 37(a)? | | | |
| 4.21.7 | Curbs | If curbs are provided in a transfer type shower, are they no higher than 1/2 inch? | | | |
| 4.21.5 | Faucets | In a transfer type shower, are the faucets and other controls located within the area shown in Figure 37(a)? | | | |
| **4.21.2** | **Roll-in Showers –** Public and Common Use | In public or common use bathing facilities, if the shower stall is a roll-in type shown in Figure 35(b), is it at least 30 by 60 inches? | | | |
| 4.21.2 | | Is there at least a 36 by 60 inch clear floor space alongside the roll-in shower as shown in figure 35(b)? | | | |
| 4.21.4 | Grab Bars | In a roll-in shower, does a grab bar extend around three sides as shown in Figures 35(b) and 37(b)? | | | |
| 4.21.7 | Curbs | Is there no curb at the roll-in shower? | | | |
| 4.21.5 | Faucets | In a roll-in shower, are the faucets and other controls located on the back wall within the area shown in Figure 37(b) or on a side wall as shown in figure 37(a)? | | | |

Survey Form

17 — 2

| Section | Item | Technical Requirements | Comments | Yes | No |
|---|---|---|---|---|---|
| **9.1.2**<br>**4.21.2** | **Roll-in Showers –**<br>Transient Lodging | In accessible guest rooms in transient lodging required to have roll-in showers, is there a shower complying with Figure 57(a)?<br>OR<br>Is there a shower complying with figure 57(b)? | | | |
| 4.21.3 | Seat | In a roll-in shower required in accessible guest rooms in transient lodging, is there a folding seat affixed to the wall adjacent to the controls as shown in figure 57(a) or 57(b)? | | | |
| 4.21.4 | Grab Bars | In a roll-in shower required in accessible guest rooms in transient lodging, are grab bars provided between 33 and 36 inches above the floor around two sides as shown in figure 57(a) or 57(b)? | | | |
| 4.21.7 | Curbs | Is there no curb at the roll-in shower? | | | |
| 4.21.5 | Faucets | In a roll-in shower required in accessible guest rooms in transient lodging, are the faucets and other controls located within the area shown in figure 57(a) or 57(b)? | | | |
| **4.21.5**<br>**4.27.4** | **Faucets – All**<br>Accessible<br>Showers | In all accessible showers, can faucets and other controls be operated with one hand and without tight grasping, pinching, or twisting of the wrist? | | | |
| | | Is the force required to operate the controls no greater than 5 lbf? | | | |
| **4.21.6** | **Spray Unit –**<br>All Accessible<br>Showers | In all accessible showers, does the shower spray unit have a hose at least 60 inches long?<br><br>**Exception: In unmonitored facilities where vandalism is a consideration, a fixed shower head mounted at 48 inches above the shower floor may be used in lieu of a hand-held shower head.** | | | |
| | | Can the shower spray unit be used both as a hand-held and as a fixed shower head? | | | |
| **4.20.4**<br>**4.21.4**<br>**4.26.1** | **Grab Bars** | Do all grab bars for accessible bathtubs and showers comply with 4.26 (See below)? | | | |
| 4.26.2 | Diameter | Is the outside diameter of the grab bar between 1-1/4 inch and 1-1/2 inch?<br>OR<br>Does the shape provide an equivalent gripping surface?<br><br>Note: Standard pipe sizes designated by the industry as 1-1/4 to 1-1/2 inches are acceptable for purposes of this section. | | | |

| Section | Item | Technical Requirements | Comments | Yes | No |
|---|---|---|---|---|---|
| | | In the space between grab bars and walls exactly 1-1/2 inches? | | | |
| 4.26.3 | | Are the grab bars secured so that they do not rotate within the fittings? | | | |
| 4.26.2 | Clearance in Recess | If a grab bar is located in a recess, is the recess a maximum of 3 inches deep extending at least 18 inches above the rail? | | | |
| 4.26.3 | Structural Strength | Do the grab bars meet the structural strength requirements for bending stress and shear stress in 4.26.3? | | | |
| 4.26.3 | | Do the fasteners meet the structural strength requirements for shear force and tensile force in 4.26.3? | | | |
| 4.26.4 | Hazards | Are the grab bar edges free of sharp of sharp or abrasive elements and do edges have a minimum radius of 1/8 inch? | | | |
| 4.20.3 4.21.3 4.26.3 | Seats | Do all seats for accessible bathtubs and showers meet the structural strength requirements for bending stress and shear stress in 4.26.3? | | | |
| | | Do the fasteners meet the structural strength requirements for shear force and tensile force in 4.26.3? | | | |
| 4.21.8 | **Shower Stall Enclosures** | If a shower stall enclosure is provided for an accessible shower, is it located so that it does not obstruct the controls or obstruct transfer from a wheelchair into shower seat? | | | |

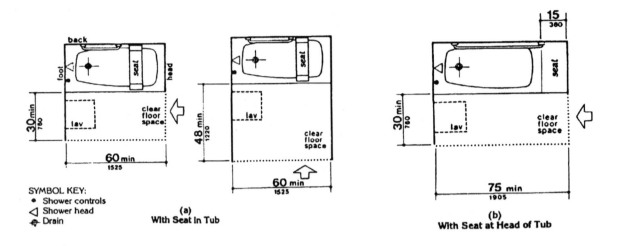

**Figure 33: Clear Floor Space at Bathtubs**

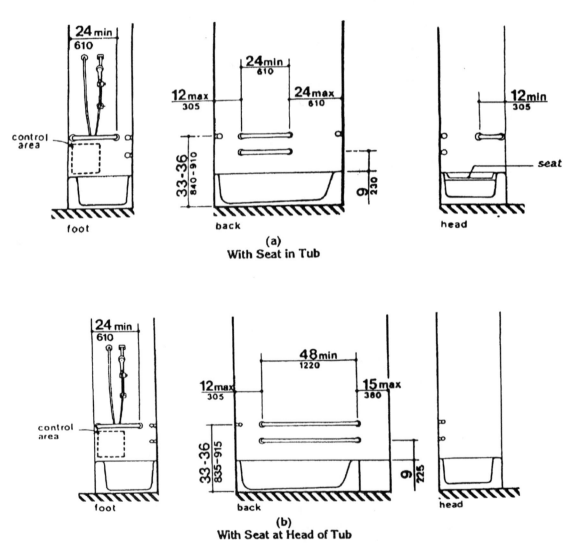

**Figure 34: Grab Bars at Bathtubs**

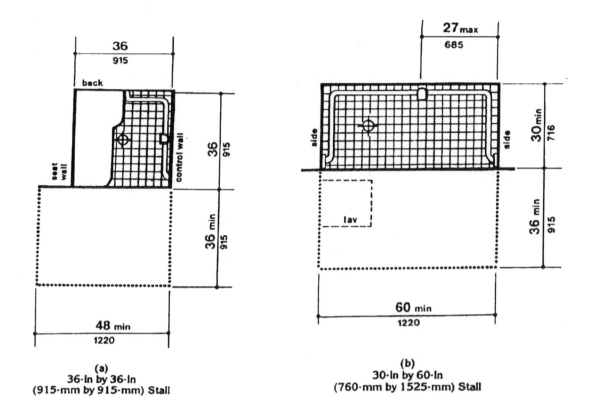

(a)
36-In by 36-In
(915-mm by 915-mm) Stall

(b)
30-In by 60-In
(760-mm by 1525-mm) Stall

**Figure 35: Shower Sizes and Clearances**

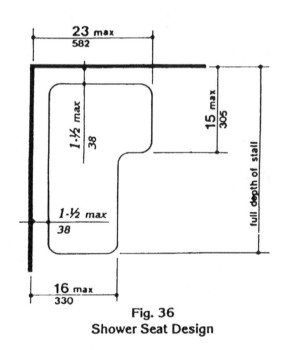

Fig. 36
Shower Seat Design

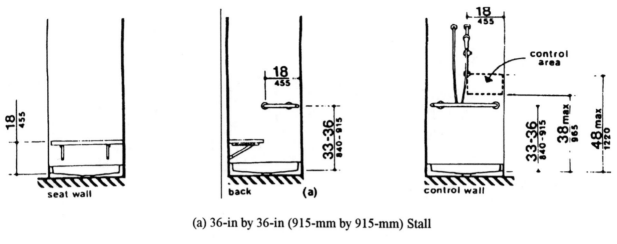

(a) 36-in by 36-in (915-mm by 915-mm) Stall

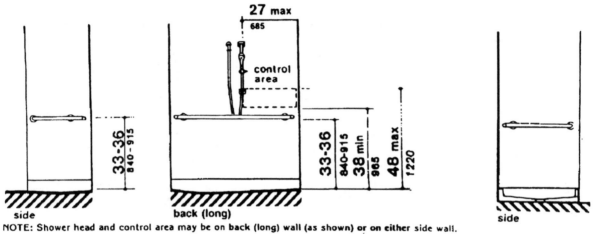

NOTE: Shower head and control area may be on back (long) wall (as shown) or on either side wall.

(b)

30-in by 60-in (760-mm by 1525-mm) Stall

**Figure 37: Grab Bars at Shower Stalls**

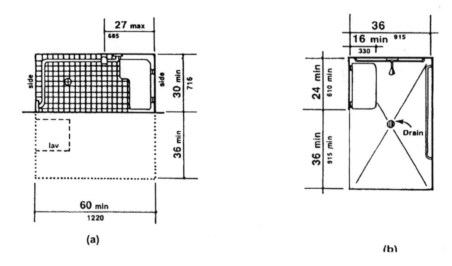

(a)

(b)

**Figure 57: Roll-In Shower with Folding Seat**

# Survey Form 18: Dressing and Fitting Rooms

Use with the Minimum Requirements Summary sheets and ADAAG.

**Facility Name:** _____ **Bathroom Location:** _____

See Minimum Requirements Summary Sheets I and J for special requirements and exceptions which may be allowed in alterations and historic preservation. See also **ADAAG** 4.1.6 and 4.1.7

| Section | Item | Technical Requirements | Comments | Yes | No |
|---------|------|------------------------|----------|-----|-----|
| 4.1.3(21) 4.35.1 | **Dressing and Fitting Rooms** | Where dressing and fitting rooms are provided for use by the general public, patients, customers or employees, does 5 percent (but not less than one) of dressing and fitting rooms for each type of use in each cluster of dressing and fitting rooms comply with 4.35 (See below)? | | | |
| 4.35.1 | **Accessible Route** | Are dressing and fitting rooms that are required to be accessible located on an accessible route? (Use Form 12: Building Lobbies and Corridors) | | | |
| 4.35.2 | **Clear Floor Space** | In a dressing and fitting room with a swinging or sliding door, is there clear floor space at least 60 inches in diameter (or a 60 by 60 inch T-shape allowing a wheelchair user to make a 180 degree turn? | | | |
| | Door Swing | Is the clear turning space not obstructed by the door swing? | | | |
| 4.35.3 4.13 | **Doors** | Do all doors to accessible dressing and fitting rooms comply with 4.13? (Use Form 11: Doors and Gates) | | | |
| | Curtained Openings | If the dressing or fitting room is private and entered through a curtained opening, is the opening at least 32 inches wide? | | | |
| | | Is there adequate clear floor space in the dressing or fitting room and immediately adjacent to the curtained opening so that the dressing room is usable by a wheelchair user? | | | |
| 4.35.4 | **Bench Affixed to Wall** | Does every accessible dressing and fitting room have a 24 by 48 inch (minimum) bench fixed to the wall along the longer dimension? (The bench may be a folding type.) | | | |
| | Bench Height | Is the bench mounted 17 to 19 inches above the finished floor? | | | |
| | | Is there clear floor space at least 30 inches by 48 inches provided alongside of the bench to allow a person using a wheelchair to make a parallel transfer onto the bench? | | | |

| Section | Item | Technical Requirements | Comments | Yes | No |
|---------|------|------------------------|----------|-----|-----|
| 4.35.4<br>4.26.3 | Bench Strength | Does the structural strength of the bench and attachments comply with 4.26.3? | | | |
| 4.35.4 | Bench in Wet Areas | Where installed in conjunction with showers, swimming pools, or other wet locations, does the surface of the bench have a slip-resistant surface? | | | |
| | | Is the bench in a wet location constructed so that water does not accumulate on the surface? | | | |
| **4.35.5** | **Mirror** | If there is a mirror, is it a full-length mirror at least 18 inches wide by 54 inches high? | | | |
| | | Is the mirror mounted in a position affording a view to a person on the bench as well as to a person in a standing position? | | | |

# Survey Form 23: Restaurants and Cafeterias

Use with the Minimum Requirements Summary sheets and ADAAG.

Facility Name: _____ Restaurant Location: _____

See Minimum Requirements Summary Sheets I and J for special requirements and exceptions which may be allowed in alterations and historic preservation. See also **ADAAG** 4.1.6 and 4.1.7

| Section | Item | Technical Requirements | Comments | Yes | No |
|---------|------|------------------------|----------|-----|-----|
| **5.1** **4.1.3(18)** | **Accessible Tables and Dining Counters** | Does at least 5% (but not less than 1) of all fixed tables comply with 4.32 (See below?) OR Where food is consumed at a dining counter but there is no service, does a portion of the dining counter comply with 4.32 (See below)? | | | |
| 4.32.2 4.2.4 | Clear Floor Space – Seating | do seating spaces provided for wheelchair users have at least a 30 by 48 inches clear space which adjoins or overlaps an accessible route? | | | |
| | | Is no more than 19 inches of the 30 by 48 inch clear space measured under the table? (See Figure 45) | | | |
| 4.32.3 | Knee Space | Is the knee space at least 27 inches high, 30 inches wide, and 10 inches deep? (See Figure 45) | | | |
| 4.32.4 | Table/Counter Height | Is the top of the table or counter between 28 and 34 inches above the floor? | | | |
| 5.1 | Distribution | Where separate areas are designated for smoking and non-smoking patrons, are accessible tables or counters proportionally distributed between smoking and non-smoking areas? | | | |
| | | In new construction, and where practicable in alterations, are the accessible tables or counters distributed throughout the space? | | | |
| **5.7** | **Raised Platforms** | In banquet rooms or spaces where a head table or speaker's lectern is located on a raised platform, is the platform accessible by means of a ramp or platform lift complying with 4.8 or 4.11? (Use Form 7: Ramps or Form 9: Platform Lifts.) (Lifts may only be used in certain limited situations in new construction. See Minimum Requirements Summary Sheets D and ADAAG 4.1.3(5) Exception 4) | | | |
| | | Are the open edges of a raised platform protected by placement of tables or by a curb? | | | |
| **5.8** **4.2** | **Vending Machines** | Are spaces for vending machines located on an accessible route? (Use Form 12: Building Lobbies and Corridors) | | | |

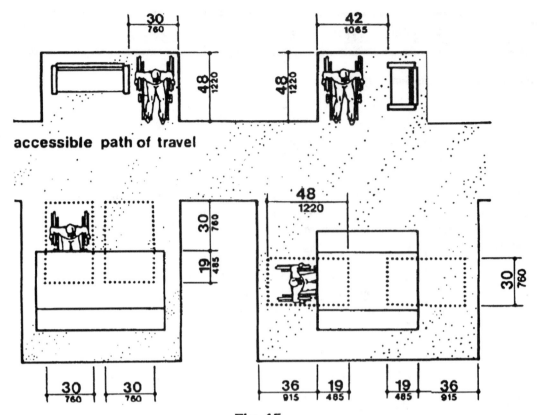

**accessible path of travel**

**Fig. 45**
**Minimum Clearances for Seating and Tables**

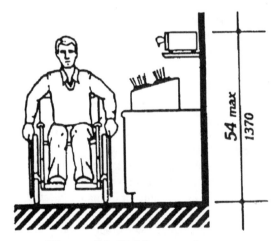

**Figure 54: Tableware Areas**

# Survey Form 25: Mercantile Facilities

Use with the Minimum Requirements Summary sheets and ADAAG.

**Facility Name:** _____  **Facility Location:** _____

See Minimum Requirements Summary Sheets and **ADAAG.** Use Survey Forms 1 to 22, as applicable, as well as this form.

| Total Check-Out Aisles of Each Design | Minimum Number of Accessible Check-Out Aisles of Each Design |
|---|---|
| 1 - 4 | 1 |
| 5 - 8 | 2 |
| 9 - 15 | 3 |
| over 15 | 3, plus 20% of additional aisles |

**Exception:** In new construction, where the selling space is under 5,000 square feet, only one check-out aisle is required to be accessible.

**Exception:** In alterations, at least one check-out aisle shall be accessible in facilities under 5,000 square feet of selling space. In facilities of 5,000 or more square feet of selling space, at least one of each design of check-out aisle shall be made accessible when altered until the number of accessible check-out aisles of each design equals the number required in new construction.

| Section | Item | Technical Requirements | Comments | Yes | No |
|---|---|---|---|---|---|
| 7.1 | **General** | Are all areas used for business transactions with the public accessible as required below? | | | |
| 7.2(1) | **Sales/Service Counters – With Cash Registers** | In department stores and miscellaneous retail stores where counters have cash registers, is there at least one of each type of counter where a portion of the counter is at least 36 inches high? OR In alterations, where it is technically infeasible to provide an accessible counter, is an auxiliary counter meeting the above requirements provided? | | | |
| | | Are the accessible counters dispersed throughout the building? | | | |
| 7.2(2) | **Sales/Service Counters – Without Cash Register** | At ticketing counters, teller stations, registration counters and other counters which may not have cash registers, is there a portion of the main counter at least 36 inches long and no more than 36 inches high? | | | |

| Section | Item | Technical Requirements | Comments | Yes | No |
|---|---|---|---|---|---|
| | | OR Is there an auxiliary counter at least 36 inches high near the main counter? OR Is equivalent facilitation provided? (e.g., at a hotel registration desk, equivalent facilitation might consist of : (1) the provision of a folding shelf attached to the main counter on which a person with a disability can write, and (2) use of the space at the side of the counter for handing materials back and forth.) | | | |
| | | Do all accessible counters on an accessible route comply with 4.3? (Use Form 12: Building Corridors and Lobbies) | | | |
| 7.3(1) | **Check-Out Aisles** – New Construction | In new construction, does the number of accessible check-out aisles comply with the table above? OR In new construction where the selling space is under 5,000 square feet, is at least one check-out aisle accessible? | | | |
| | Alterations | In alterations, is at least one check-out aisle of each design made accessible when altered until the number of accessible check-out aisles equals the number required in the table above? OR In alterations of facilities that have under 5,000 square feet of selling space, is there at least one check-out aisle accessible? | | | |
| 7.3(2) 4.2.1 | Aisle Width | Is the clear aisle width of accessible check-out aisles at least 36 inches wide for lengths greater than 24 inches long and at least 32 inches wide for lengths 24 inches or less? | | | |
| | | If there is a lip in the edge of the counter adjoining the aisle, is the top of the lip no more than 40 inches above the floor? | | | |
| | Height | Is the adjoining counter/belt height no more than 38 inches above the floor? | | | |
| 7.3(3) | Signs | Is there a sign identifying each accessible check-out aisle which is mounted above the check-out aisle? | | | |
| | | Does the sign include the International Symbol of Accessibility? | | | |
| 7.4 | **Security Bollards** | Are security bollards or other such devices installed so that access and egress for wheelchair users is provided? OR Is there an alternate accessible entry that is equally convenient as that provided for the general public? | | | |

# Survey Form 26: Libraries

Use with the Minimum Requirements Summary sheets and ADAAG. Use Survey Forms 1 to 22 as applicable, as well as this form.

**Facility Name:** _____  **Library Location:** _____

In addition to the requirements of ADAAG 4.1 through 4.35, libraries must comply with ADAAG 8.

| Section | Item | Technical Requirements | Comments | Yes | No |
|---|---|---|---|---|---|
| **8.2** | **Reading and Study Areas** | Do at least 5% (but not less than one) of fixed seating, tables, or study carrels comply with 4.2 and 4.3.2 (See below)? | | | |
| 4.2.4 4.32.2 | Seating Clear Floor Space | Do spaces provided for wheelchair users have a 30 by 48 inch clear space which overlaps an accessible route? | | | |
| | | Is no more than 19 inches of the 30 by 48 inch clear space measured under the table? (See Figure 45) | | | |
| 4.32.3 | Knee Space | Is the knee space under the table at least 27 inches high, 30 inches wide, and 19 inches deep? (See Figure 45) | | | |
| 4.32.4 | Height | Is the top of the table between 28 and 34 inches from the floor? | | | |
| 4.3.3 | Aisles | Are the aisles leading up to and between the tables or study carrels at lest 36 inches wide? | | | |
| **8.3** 7.2(1) | **Check-Out Areas** | Is there at least one lane at each check-out areas where a portion of the counter is at least 36 inches long and no more than 36 inches high? | | | |
| **8.3** **4.13** | **Security Gates** | Do security gates or turnstiles comply with 4.13? (Use Form 11: Doors and Gates) OR Is there an accessible gate or door next to a turnstile or security device? | | | |
| 8.4 | **Card Catalogs and Magazine Displays** | Is the aisle between card catalogs and magazine displays at least 36 inches wide? (See Figure 55) | | | |
| | Reach | Are the card catalogs between 18 and 54 inches from the floor? (A height of 48 inches is preferred.) | | | |
| **8.5** **4.2** | **Stacks** | Is the minimum clear aisles width between the stacks at least 36 inches? (See Figure 56) (A minimum clear aisle width of 42 inches is preferred where possible. Shelf height in stack areas is unrestricted.) | | | |

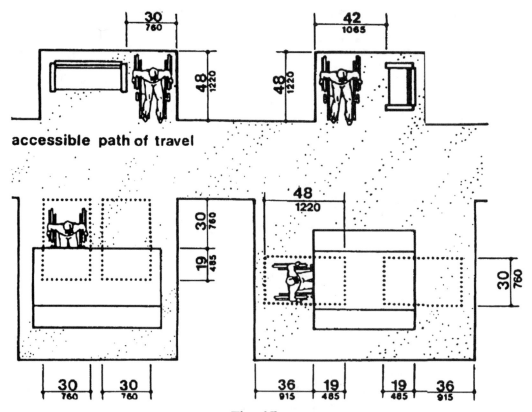

**Fig. 45**
**Minimum Clearances for Seating and Tables**

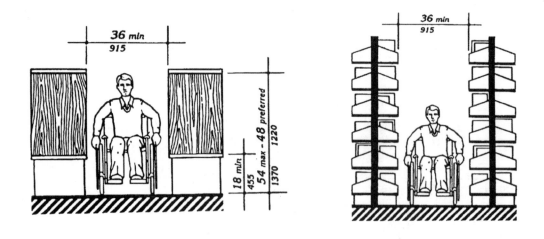

**Figure 55: Card Catalog**

**Figure 56: Stacks**

# 18. Transticket Safety

*Purpose: The purpose of this chapter is to provide the therapist with the technical information needed to provide and teach safe transportation for patients.*

Many years of research and millions of dollars have been spent to test the effectiveness of passenger restraint systems in motor vehicles. Beyond a doubt, seatbelts save lives. However, only limited studies have been done to test the effectiveness of passenger restraint systems for people who ride in their wheelchairs. The University of Michigan Transportation Research Institute, notably Lawrence W. Schneider, BSE, MSE, PhD, has been striving to determine the correct (safe) and incorrect (unsafe) ways to restrain passengers who are traveling in their wheelchairs. Using crash test dummies they have established some basic guidelines:

1. A passenger should ride in his/her wheelchair only if s/he cannot sit in a regular passenger seat and use that seat's restraining system(s).

2. If the passenger must ride in his/her own wheelchair, then two restraint systems are required: one to restrain the passenger to the wheelchair and a second, totally separate restraint system, to secure the wheelchair to the vehicle.

3. The rivets that attach seatbelts to wheelchairs usually will fail at impact of 25 mph. They come will right off the wheelchair, providing the passenger with no restraint. A seatbelt/cargo strap may be placed low over the passengers hip, around the frame of the wheelchair, and secured in back of the wheelchair.

4. Most wheelchair back hardware and fabric will fail at impact of 25 mph. The momentum of the impact could force the passenger's head to hit the floor *behind the wheelchair*. While the upper frame of most wheelchairs are not adequate to stay undamaged (unbent) during an impact, they would still be able to provide moderate support if a seat belt strap/cargo strap were placed across the passenger's chest, around both handlebars, and then buckled behind the wheelchair seat. This strap would be in addition to one around the passenger's hips.

5. The way that wheelchairs are constructed makes the wheels a poor choice for use in tie downs. Always tie down (restrain) the wheelchair to the floor using the frame, not the wheels, of the wheelchair.

6. Do not secure passengers so that they face the side of the vehicle. Crash tests have shown that side facing passengers sustain far greater injuries than passengers who face forward (preferable) or backwards.

7. Remember, many individuals who use wheelchairs are at risk for skin breakdowns (pressure sores). Their restraint system should be snug and yet still allow a shifting of weight from side to side.

As a result of the Americans with Disabilities Act (ADA) individuals who live in the United States of America now have minimum standards for securement and other adaptive devices (e.g., ramps and lifts) for passenger vehicles. These standards only apply to vehicles built after October 7, 1991.

The reader will find the technical standards for vehicle ramps, securement devices, and lifts in this chapter. This information is part of the publication **Buses, Vans, and Systems Technical Assistance Manual**, October 1992 by the United States Architectural and Transportation Barriers Compliance Board.

### Ramps (Vehicle Ramps)

The ADA specifies minimum standards in eight areas related to the design of ramps used to load and unload individuals with disabilities into and out of vehicles:

- *Design load* - Ramps 30 inches or longer will need to be able to support a load of 600 pounds, placed at the centroid of the ramp distributed over an area of 26 inches by 26 inches, with a safety factor of at least three times that based on the ultimate strength of the material. Ramps shorter than 30 inches will need to support a load of 300 pounds.

- *Ramp surface* - The ramp surface will need to be continuous and slip resistant; it will not have protrusions from the surface greater than ¼ inch high; the surface will have a clear width of 30 inches and will be able to accommodate both four-wheel and three-wheel mobility aids.

- *Ramp threshold* - The transition from roadway or sidewalk and the transition from vehicle floor to the ramp may be vertical without edge treatment up to ¼ inch. Changes in level between ¼ inch and ½ inch will be beveled with a slope no greater than 1:2.

- *Ramp barriers* - Each side of the ramp will need to have barriers at least 2 inches high to prevent mobility aid wheels from slipping off.

- *Slope* - Ramps will have the least slope practicable and will not exceed 1:4 when deployed to ground level.

| Height of Vehicle Floor Above 6 inch Curb | Maximum Ramp Slope |
|---|---|
| 3 inches or less | 1:4 |
| 6 inches or less but more than 3 inches | 1:6 |
| 9 inches or less but more than 6 inches | 1:8 |
| more than 9 inches | 1:12 |

- *Attachment* - When in use for boarding or alighting, the ramp will need to be firmly attached to the vehicle so that it is not subject to displacement when loading or unloading a heavy power mobility aid and that no gap between the vehicle and ramp exceeds 5/8 inches.

- *Stowage* - A compartment, securement system, or other appropriate method will need to be provided to ensure that stowed ramps, including portable ramps stowed in the passenger area, do not impede on a passenger's wheelchair or mobility aid or pose any hazard to passengers in the event of a sudden stop or maneuver.

- *Handrails* - If provided, handrails will need to allow people with disabilities to grasp them from the outside of the vehicle while starting to board, and to continue to use them throughout the boarding process, and will need to have the top between 30 inches and 38 inches above the ramp surface. The handrails will need to be capable of withstanding a force of 100 pounds concentrated at any point on the handrail without permanent deformation of the rail or its supporting structure. The handrail will need to have a cross-sectional diameter between 1¼ inches and 1½ inches or will need to provide an equivalent grasping surface, and have eased edges with corner radii of not less than 1/8 inch. Handrails will not interfere with wheelchair or mobility aid maneuverability when entering or leaving the vehicle.

## Securement Devices

A securement device is a mechanical object which ties the wheelchair or the mobility device to the vehicle. A securement device is not a seatbelt and should never be used to tie the passenger to his/her mobility device! The ADA has seven parts to the regulations concerning the securement of mobility devices to the inside of the vehicle:

- *Design load* - Securement systems on vehicles with GVWRs of 30,000 pounds or above, and their attachments to such vehicles, will need to be able to restrain a force in the forward longitudinal direction of up to 2,000 pounds per securement leg or clamping mechanism and a minimum of 4,000 pounds for each mobility aid. Securement systems on vehicles with GVWRs of up to 30,000 pounds, and their attachments to such vehicles, will need to restrain a force in the forward longitudinal direction of up to 2,500 pounds per securement leg or clamping mechanism and a minimum of 5,000 pounds for each mobility aid. (The force requirement for different weight vehicles is based on research on the g-forces experienced by various vehicles and their crash profiles. Smaller vehicles generally experience higher g-forces than large buses.) The significant forces during collision are imposed primarily on the rear securement legs (for a forward facing securement). Four-point securement systems are common, with the two forward straps being primarily designed to provide containment and reduce or prevent rebound. Therefore, the front straps are not subjected to the same forces. Most securement devices consist of two straps or clamping devices, one attached to each side of the wheelchair or mobility aid frame. As such, each leg accounts for about half of the force of restraint. At least one device in current use has a metal bracket which has a hook on each side that attaches to the wheel axles, both of which are secured to the vehicle floor through a single belt. In this case, the single belt must accommodate all of the 4,000 or 5,000 pounds of force, depending on the vehicle size. The more securement straps or devices used for each wheelchair or mobility aid, the less force each one must accommodate individually. To be effective, the securement devices must be attached to the wheelchair or mobility aid frame, not the wheels.

- *Location and size* - The securement system will need to be placed as near to the accessible entrance as practicable and will need to have a clear floor area of 30 inches by 48 inches. Such space will need to adjoin, and may overlap, an access path. Not more than 6 inches of the required clear floor space may be accommodated for footrests under another seat provided there is a minimum of 9 inches from the floor to the lowest part of the seat overhanging the space. Securement areas may have fold-down seats to accommodate other passengers when a wheelchair or mobility aid is not occupying the area, provided the seats, when folded up, do not obstruct the clear floor space required.

- *Mobility aids accommodated* - The securement system must secure common wheelchairs and mobility aids and will need to either be automatic or easily attached by a person familiar with the system and mobility aid having average dexterity.

- *Orientation* - In vehicles in excess of 22 feet in length, at least one securement device or system will secure the wheelchair or mobility aid facing toward the front of the vehicle. In vehicles 22 feet in length or less, the required securement device may secure the wheelchair or mobility aid either facing toward the front of the vehicle or rearward. Additional securement devices or systems need to also secure the wheelchair or mobility aid facing forward or rearward. Where the wheelchair or mobility aid is secured facing the rear of the vehicle, a padded barrier must be provided. The padded barrier must extend from a height of 38 inches from the vehicle floor to a height of 56 inches from the vehicle floor with a width of 18 inches, laterally centered immediately in back of the seated individual. Such barriers need not be solid provided equivalent protection is afforded. It used to be that many vehicles secured the passengers in so that they faced the side of the vehicle. While it may save some space, it does not provide the passenger safety. There is overwhelming support through research for permitting only forward or rearward facing securement.

**Vehicle Lift**

The ADA outlines minimum size, function, and weight bearing ability of vehicle lifts used to help individuals access the vehicle.

- The weight that a lift can carry is called "the design load". The design load required by ADA is 600 pounds. This does not mean that a lift will break if 700 pounds of weight is loaded onto it. (An obese patient who is respirator dependent and who uses an electric wheelchair may exceed 600 pounds.) The design load is a maximum safety limit which allows for some wear of the equipment. The working parts of the lift, such as cables, pulleys, and shafts, which can be expected to wear, and upon which the lift depends for support, must have a safety capability of at least six times that, based on the ultimate strength of the material. The non working parts, such as the platform, frame, and attachment hardware, which would not be expected to wear, is required to have a safety factor of at least three. None the less, the CTRS should be aware of the 600 pound load limit and work with both the patient and the team to ensure that the weight being loaded upon a lift does not exceed 600 pounds. The CTRS should also visually inspect the vehicle lift prior to each outing to ensure that all of the parts are in working condition.

- The lift and the platform on the vehicle must have sufficient clearance to permit a wheelchair or other mobility aid user to reach the securement location or the exit. The lift platform itself must be at least 28½ inches wide, with a minimum clearance of 30 inches measured from 2 inches above the platform surface to 30 inches above the platform, and a minimum clear length of 48 inches measured from 2 inches above the surface of the platform to 30 inches above the surface of the platform.

- The controls which activate the lift must be interlocked with the vehicle brakes, transmission, or door, or otherwise ensure that the vehicle cannot move without the lift being fully stowed. These controls must also be controlled by a mechanism that requires constant pressure to be activated. This type of switch is called a "momentary contact type". These switches require the person activating the lift to be purposefully working the switch. This allows an extra bit of safety for the lift rider over those lifts which automatically ascend or descend to a predetermined level. The only exceptions to this regulation are platform rotary lifts. With these lifts the individual in the mobility device completes the entire trip with his/her device secured to a platform which rotates into the vehicle. In no case, (even with a power or equipment failure) may the lift allow the rider to drop more than 12 inches a second. Each lift will need to have such a safety built into it.

- The platform barrier of the lift must be built so that a wheelchair or mobility aid is prevented from rolling off the platform during its operation. There must be a minimum of a 1½ inch lip around the platform while it is being operated. This lip is not allowed to interfere with the lift user's ability to access the vehicle, so the design must allow for this rule. The CTRS must ensure that this lip is in place any time the lift is occupied and is 3 inches or more off the ground.

- The surface of the platform must not have openings which exceed 5/8 inch in width.

- The platform may not list (tilt) more than 3° (exclusive of vehicle roll or pitch) in any direction between its unloaded position and its position when loaded with 600 pounds applied through a 26 inch by 26 inch test pallet at the centroid of the platform.

- The lift platform must allow the occupant to face both inboard or outboard while loading.

- The lift needs to accommodate both those individuals who ride on their mobility device and those who stand. The platform may be marked to indicate standing positions. The platforms on lifts shall be equipped with handrails on two sides, which move in tandem with the lift, and which shall be graspable and provide support to standees throughout the entire lift operation. Handrails shall have a usable component at least 8 inches long with the lowest portion a minimum 30 inches above the platform and the highest portion a maximum of 38 inches above the platform. The handrails will need to be capable of withstanding a force of 100 pounds concentrated at any point on the handrail without permanent deformation of the rail or its supporting structure. The handrail will need to have a cross section diameter between 1¼ inches and 1½ inches or will need to provide an equivalent grasping surface, and have eased edges with corner radii of not less than 1/8 inch. Handrails shall be placed to provide a minimum of 1½ inches knuckle clearance from the nearest adjacent surface. Handrails shall not interfere with the wheelchair or mobility aid maneuverability when entering or leaving the vehicle.

# 19. Air Travel

Below is a copy of **New Horizons for the Air Traveler with a Disability** published by the US Department of Transportation. The reader may obtain the document from the
Department of Transportation, Office of Consumer Affairs,
400 Seventh Street, SW,
Washington, DC. 20590
(202) 366-2220 or TT (202) 755-7687.

## Introduction

Access to the nation's air travel system for persons with disabilities has been an area of substantial dissatisfaction, with both passengers and the airline industry recognizing the need for major improvement. In 1986 Congress passed the Air Carrier Access Act, requiring the Department of Transportation (DOT) to develop new regulations which ensure that persons with disabilities will be treated without discrimination in a way consistent with the safe carriage of all passengers. These regulations were published in March 1990.

The DOT regulations, referred to here as the Air Carrier Access rules, represent a major stride forward in improving air travel for persons with disabilities. The rules clearly explain the responsibilities of the traveler, the carriers, the airport operators, and the contractors, who collectively make up the system which moves over one million passengers per day.

The new rules are designed to minimize the special problems that travelers with disabilities face as they negotiate their way through the nation's complex air travel system from origin to destination. This minimization is achieved:

By recognizing that the physical barriers encountered by passengers with disabilities can be vastly reduced by employing simple changes in layout and technology.

By adopting the principle that many difficulties confronting the passengers with hearing or vision impairments will be relieved if they are provided access to the same information as is available to all other passengers.

Through training of all air travel personnel who come in day-to-day contact with persons with disabilities, to understand their needs and how they can be accommodated quickly, safely, and with dignity.

This guide is designed to offer travelers with disabilities a brief but authoritative source of information about the new Air Carrier Access rules: the accommodations, facilities, and services that are now required to be available and accessible. It also describes features required by other regulations designed to make air travel more accessible.

The guide is structured in much the same sequence as a passenger would plan for a trip: the circumstances her or she must consider prior to traveling, what will be encountered at the airport, and what to expect in the transitions from airport to airplane, on the plane, and then airplane to airport.

**Planning the Trip**

The new rules sweep aside many restrictions that formerly discriminated against passengers with disabilities:

- A carrier cannot refuse transportation to a passenger solely on the basis of a disability.
- Air carriers may not limit the number of individuals with disabilities on a particular flight.
- All trip information that is made available to other passengers also must be made available to passengers with disabilities.
- Carriers must provide passage to an individual with a disability that may affect his or her appearance or involuntary behavior, even if this disability may offend, annoy, or be an inconvenience to crew members or other passengers.

There are a few exceptions:

- The carrier may refuse transportation if the individual with a disability would endanger the health or safety of other passengers, or transporting the person would be a violation of FAA safety rules.
- The carrier may refuse transportation if the plane has fewer than 30 seats and there are no lifts, boarding chairs, or other devices available which can be adapted to the limitation of such small planes, by which to place the passenger on board. Carrier personnel are not required to carry a mobility impaired person onto the aircraft by hand.
- There are special rules about persons with certain disabilities or communicable diseases. These rules are covered later in this appendix.
- The carrier may refuse transportation if it is unable to seat the passenger without violating the FAA Exit Row Seating rules.

There are new procedures for resolving disputes:

- All carriers are now required to have a Complaints Resolution Official (CRO) closely available to resolve disagreements which may arise between the carrier and passengers with disabilities.
- Travelers who disagree with a carrier's actions toward them can pursue the issue with the carrier's CRO on the spot.
- A carrier that refuses transportation to any person based on a disability must provide a written statement to that person within 10 calendar days, stating the basis for the refusal. The statement must include, where applicable, the basis for the carrier's opinion that transporting the person could be harmful to the safety of the flight.
- If the passenger is still not satisfied, he or she may pursue DOT enforcement action.

**Getting Advanced Information About the Aircraft**

Travelers with disabilities must be provided information upon request concerning facilities and services available to them. When feasible this information will pertain to the specific aircraft scheduled for a specific flight. Such information should include:

- Any limitations which may be known to the carrier concerning the ability of the aircraft to accommodate an individual with a disability;

- The location of seats (if any) with moveable aisle armrests and any seats which the carrier does not make available to an individual with a disability (e.g., exit rows);
- Any limitations on the availability of storage facilities in the cabin or in the cargo bay for mobility aids or other equipment commonly used by an individual with a disability;
- Whether the aircraft has an accessible lavatory.

Normally, advance information about the aircraft will be requested by phone. Any carrier that provides telephone service for the purpose of making reservations or offering general information must provide comparable services for hearing-impaired individuals, utilizing telecommunications devices for the deaf (TDDs) or text telephones (TTs). The TTs shall be available during the same hours that the general public has access to regular phone service. The response time to answer calls on the TT line shall also be equivalent to the response time available to the general public. Charges for the call, if any, shall be the same as charges made to the general public.

**When Advance Notice Can Be Required**

Carriers may require up to 48 hours advance notice and one hour advance check-in from a person with a disability who wishes to receive the following services:

- Transportation for an electric wheelchair on an aircraft with fewer than 60 seats;
- Provision by the carrier of hazardous materials packaging for the battery of a wheelchair or other assistive device;
- Accommodations for 10 or more passengers with disabilities who travel as a group;
- Provision of an on-board wheelchair on an aircraft that does not have an accessible lavatory (beginning no later than April 5, 1992) for persons who can use an inaccessible lavatory but need an on-board chair to do so.

Carriers are not required to provide the following services or equipment, but should they choose to provide them, may require 48 hours advance notice and a one hour advance check-in:

- Medical oxygen for use on board the aircraft;
- Carriage of an incubator;
- Hook-up for a respirator to the aircraft's electrical supply;
- Accommodations for a passenger who must travel on a stretcher.

Carriers may impose reasonable, non-discriminatory charges for these services. They must ensure the required service is provided if appropriate notice has been given and the service requested is available on that particular flight. If a passenger does not meet advance notice or check-in requirements, carriers must make a reasonable effort to accommodate the requested service, providing it does not delay the flight.

If a passenger with a disability provides the required notice but is required to fly on another carrier (for example, if the flight is canceled), the original carrier must, to the maximum extent feasible, provide assistance to the second carrier in furnishing the accommodation requested by the individual.

It must be recognized that even though the passenger has requested information in advance on the accessible features of the scheduled aircraft, carriers sometimes have to substitute a different aircraft at the last minute for safety, mechanical or other reasons. It also must be recognized that the substitute aircraft may not be as fully accessible – a condition that may prevail for a number of years. On-board wheelchairs must be available on certain aircraft by 1992, but it will take a number of years before movable aisle armrests are available on all aircraft with over 30 seats. Similarly, while accessible lavatories must be built into new wide-body aircraft, they will be put into existing aircraft only when such aircraft are undergoing a major interior refurbishment.

**When Attendants Can Be Required**

Carriers may require the following individuals to be accompanied by an attendant:

- A person traveling on a stretcher or in an incubator (for flights where such service is offered);
- A person who, because of a mental disability, is unable to comprehend or respond appropriately to safety instruction from carrier personnel;
- A person with a mobility impairment so severe that the individual is unable to assist in his or her own evacuation from the aircraft;
- A person who has both severe hearing and severe vision impairments which prevent him or her from receiving and acting on necessary instructions from carrier personnel when evacuating the aircraft during an emergency.

The applicability of one of these criteria may be cause for disagreement between the carrier and the passenger. In such cases, a carrier can require the passenger to travel with an attendant, contrary to the passenger's assurances that he or she can travel alone. In such a case, the carrier cannot charge for the transportation of the attendant. The carrier may designate, however, an individual of its own choosing to be the attendant.

The carrier can choose an attendant in a number of ways. The carrier could designate an off duty employee who happened to be traveling on the same flight to act as the attendant. The carrier or the passenger with a disability could seek a volunteer from among other passengers on the flight to act as the attendant. The carrier could provide a free ticket to an attendant of the passenger's choice for that flight segment.

The attendant so chosen would not be required to provide personal service to the passenger with a disability other than to provide assistance in the event of an emergency evacuation. This is in contrast to the case of the passenger that usually travels accompanied by a personal attendant, who would provide the passenger whatever service he or she requests.

In such cases, if there is not a seat available on the flight for an attendant, and as a result a person with a disability holding a confirmed reservation is denied travel on the flight, the passenger with a disability is eligible for denied boarding compensation.

For purposes of determining whether a seat is available for an attendant, the attendant shall be deemed to have checked in at the same time as the person with the disability.

**At the Airport**

Until recently, only those airport facilities designed, constructed, or renovated by or for a recipient of federal funds had to comply with federal accessibility standards. Even on federally-assisted airports, however, not all facilities and activities were required to be accessible. Examples are privately-owned ground transportation and concessions selling goods or service to the public.[14] As a result of the Air Carrier Access rules, and the Americans with Disabilities Act of 1990 (ADA), and implementing regulations, these privately-owned activities also must be made accessible.

In general, airports under construction or being refurbished must comply with ADA Accessibility Guidelines (ADAAG) and other regulations governing accessibility in accordance with a timetable established in the ADA. Thus, while there are still many changes to be made, the accessibility of most

---

[14]The accessibility features for over 500 airports are covered in a publication of the Airports Association Council International entitled **A Guide to the Accessibility of Terminals, Access Travel: Airports**, and may be obtained by writing the Consumer Information Center, Pueblo, CO 81009.

airports is improving. With few exceptions, these services should be available in all air carrier terminals within the next few years:

- Accessible parking near the terminal;
- Signs indicating accessible parking and the easiest access from those spaces to the terminal;
- Accessible medical aid facilities and travelers aid stations;
- Accessible restrooms;
- Accessible drinking fountains;
- Accessible ticketing systems at primary fare collection areas;
- Amplified telephones and text telephones (TTs) for use by person with hearing and speech impairments – there must be at least one TT in each terminal in a clearly marked accessible location;
- Accessible baggage check-in and retrieval areas;
- Accessible jetways and mobile lounges;
- Level entry boarding ramps, lifts or other means of assisting an individual with a disability on and off an aircraft;
- Information systems using visual words, letters or symbols with lighting and color coding and facilities providing information orally;
- Directional signs indicating the location of specific facilities and services.

## Moving Through the Airport

To further enhance the ease of travel for an individual with a disability, major airports will be required to make the following services accessible under new rules being put into effect in the next several years:

- Shuttle vehicles, owned or operated by airports, transporting people between parking lots and terminals buildings;
- People movers and moving walkways within and between terminals and gates.

By March 1993, all carrier facilities must include one accessible route from an airport entrance to ticket counters, boarding locations and baggage handling areas. Terminals must be designed so that the routes minimize any extra distance that wheelchair users must travel compared to other passengers to reach these facilities. Outbound and inbound baggage facilities must provide efficient baggage handling for individuals with a disability, and these facilities must be designated and operated so as to be accessible.

There must be appropriate signs to indicate the location of accessible services.

Carriers cannot restrict the movements of persons with disabilities in terminals or require them to remain in a holding area or other location while awaiting transportation and other assistance.

Curbside baggage check-in (available only for domestic flights) may also be helpful to passengers with a disability.

## Passenger Information

Carriers must ensure that individuals with disabilities, including those with vision and hearing impairments, have timely access to the same information provided to other passengers. Such information may include, but is not limited to:

- Ticketing details;
- Scheduled departure times and gates;
- Status of flight delays;
- Schedule changes;
- Flight check-in;
- Change of gate assignments;

- Checking and claiming of luggage.

This information must be made available upon request. An exception to this requirement prevails in instances when such information is to be supplied by a crew member, but providing it would interfere with the crew member's immediate safety duties.

A copy of the Air Carrier Access Act rules must be made available by carriers for inspection upon request at each airport.

As previously noted, any carrier that provides telephone service for the purpose of making reservations or offering general information shall also provide TT service. This service for people with speech and hearing impairments must be available during the same hours that the general public has access to regular phone service, with equivalent response times and charges.

**Security Screening**

An individual with a disability must undergo the same security screening as any member of the traveling public.

If an individual with a disability is able to pass through the security system without activating it, the person shall not be subject to special screening procedures. Security personnel are free to examine an assistive device that they believe is capable of concealing a weapon or other prohibited item. If an individual with a disability is not able to pass through the system without activating it, the person will be subject to further screening in the same manner as any other passenger activating the system.

Security screening personnel at some airports may employ a handheld device that will allow them to complete the screening without having to physically search the individual. If this method is still unable to clear the individual and a physical search becomes necessary, then at the passenger's request, the search will be done in private.

If the passenger requests a private screening in a timely manner, the carrier must provide it in time for the passenger to board the aircraft. Such private screenings will not be required, however, to a greater extent or for any different reason than for other passengers, but may take more time.

**Medical Certificates**

A medical certificate is a written statement from the passenger's physician saying that the passenger is capable of completing the flight safely without requiring extraordinary medical care.

A disability is not sufficient grounds for a carrier to request a medical certificate. Carriers shall not require passengers to present a medical certificate unless the person traveling:

- Is on a stretcher or in an incubator (where such service is offered);
- Needs medical oxygen during flight (where such service if offered);
- Has a medical condition which causes the carrier to have reasonable doubt that the individual can complete the flight safely, without requiring extraordinary medical assistance during the flight;
- Has a communicable disease or infection that has been determined by federal public health authorities to be generally transmittable during flight.

If the medical certificate is necessitated by a communicable disease (see next section), it must say that the disease or infection will not be communicable to other persons during the normal course of flight. The certificate shall state any conditions or precautions that would have to be observed to prevent transmission of the disease or infection to others.

Carriers cannot mandate separate treatment for an individual with a disability except for reasons of safety or to prevent the spread of communicable disease or infection.

## Communicable Diseases

As part of their responsibility to their passengers, air carriers try to prevent the spread of infection or a communicable disease on board an aircraft. If a person who seeks passage has an infection or disease that would be transmittable during the normal course of a flight, and that has been deemed so by the federal public health authority knowledgeable about the disease or infection, then the carrier providing transportation may:

- Refuse to provide transportation to the person;
- Require the person to provide a medical certificate;
- Impose on the person a condition or requirement not imposed on other passengers.

If the individual presents a medical certificate it must state any conditions or precautions that would have to be implemented to prevent the transmission of the disease during the flight. In that case the carrier shall provide transportation unless it is not feasible to act upon the conditions set forth in the certificate to prevent transmission of the disease.

## Getting On and Off the Plane

The safety briefing that carrier personnel provide is for the passengers' own safety and is intended for that purpose only. FAA regulations require that a safety briefing be given to all passengers before takeoff.

Carrier personnel may offer an individual briefing to a person whose disability precludes him or her from receiving the information presented in the general briefing, The individual briefing will be provided as inconspicuously and discreetly as possible. Most carriers choose to offer this briefing before other passengers board the flight if the passenger with a disability chooses to pre-board the flight. A carrier can present the special briefing at any time before takeoff that does not interfere with other safety duties.

Carriers may not test the individual about the material presented in the briefing, except to the same degree they test all passengers in the general briefing. A carrier cannot take any adverse action against the passenger on the basis that in the carrier's opinion the passenger did not understand the briefing.

Safety briefings presented to the passengers on video screens will have an open caption or an insert for a sign language interpreter, unless this would interfere with the video or would not be large enough to be seen. This requirement takes effect as old videos are replaced in the normal course of business.

## Handling of Mobility Aids and Assistive Devices

Assistive devices brought into the cabin by an individual with a disability shall not count toward a limit on carry-on items. To the extent consistent with various FAA safety regulations, passengers may bring on board and use ventilators and respirators, powered by non-spillable batteries.

Persons using canes and other assistive devices may stow these items on board the aircraft in close proximity to them, consistent with safety regulations. Carriers shall permit passengers to stow wheelchairs or component parts of a mobility device under seats, or in overhead compartments.

One folding wheelchair can be stowed in a cabin closet, or other approved priority storage area, if the aircraft has such areas and storage can be accomplished in accordance with FAA safety regulations. If the passenger pre-boards, stowage of the wheelchair takes priority over the carry-on items brought on by other passengers enplaning at the same airport, but not over items from previous stops.

Wheelchairs and other assistive devices must be given priority over cargo and baggage when stowed in the cargo compartment, and must be among the first items unloaded. Mobility aids shall be returned to the owner as close as possible to the door of the aircraft (consistent with DOT hazardous materials regulations) or at the baggage claim area in accordance with whatever request was made by the passenger before boarding.

If the priority storage accorded to mobility aids prevents another passenger's baggage from being carried, the carrier shall make its best efforts to ensure the other baggage arrives within four hours.

Due to the limited size of storage available on certain aircraft, some assistive devices will have to be disassembled in order to be transported (e.g., electric wheelchairs, other devices too large to fit in the cabin or in the cargo hold in one piece). When assistive devices are disassembled, carriers are obligated to return them to the passengers in the condition received by the carrier.

Carriers must transport battery-powered wheelchairs, except where cargo compartment size or aircraft air worthiness considerations do not permit doing so.

- Electric wheelchairs must be treated in accordance with both DOT regulations for handling hazardous materials, and DOT Air Carrier Access regulations, which differentiate between spillable and non-spillable batteries.

- *Spillable Batteries*- If the chair is powered by a spillable battery, the regulations stipulate that the battery must be removed unless the wheelchair can be loaded, stored, secured, and unloaded always in an upright position. When it is possible to load, store, secure, and unload with the wheelchair always in an upright position, and the battery is securely attached to the wheelchair, the carrier may not remove the battery from the chair.

- *Nonspillable Batteries* - It is never necessary under the DOT hazardous materials regulations to remove a nonspillable battery from a wheelchair before stowing it. There may be individual cases, however, in which a carrier is unable to determine whether a battery is spillable or nonspillable. DOT is issuing new rules covering the marking of such batteries.

The carrier may remove a particular unmarked battery from the mobility aid if there is reasonable doubt that it is nonspillable, and the conditions cited above for spillable batteries cannot be met. An across-the-board assumption that all batteries are spillable is not consistent with the Air Carrier Access rules.

In addition, a nonspillable battery may be removed where it appears to be damaged and leakage of battery fluid is possible.

*Establishing the Battery Type* - Compliance with DOT rules covering the marking of nonspillable batteries is sufficient to identify a battery as nonspillable for this purpose. In the absence of such markings, carrier personnel are responsible for determining, on a case-by-case basis, whether a battery is nonspillable, taking into account information provided by the user of the wheelchair.

- The battery of a wheelchair may not be drained.
- When DOT hazardous materials regulations require detaching the battery from the wheelchair, the carrier shall upon request provide packaging for the battery that will meet safety requirements.
- Carriers may not charge for packaging wheelchair batteries.
- Carriers may require passengers with electric wheelchairs to check-in one hour before flight time.
- If a passenger checks-in later than one hour before flight time, the carrier shall make a reasonable effort to carry his or her wheelchair unless it would delay the flight.
- Passengers may provide written instructions concerning the disassembly and assembly of their wheelchairs.

Carriers may not require a passenger with a disability to sign a waiver of liability for damage or loss of wheelchairs or other assistive devices. The carrier may make note of any pre-existing defect to the device.

On domestic trips, carrier's liability for loss, damage or delay in returning assistive devices cannot be greater than twice the liability limits established for passengers' luggage under DOT regulations. As of the publication of this booklet, the current limit for liability on assistive devices is $2,500 per passenger (i.e., two times the $1,250[15] limit for luggage).

This expanded liability does not extend to international trips, where the Warsaw Convention applies. For most international trips (including domestic portions of an international trip) the current liability is approximately $9.07 per pound for checked baggage and $400 per passenger for unchecked baggage.

**Boarding and Deplaning**

Properly trained service personnel who are knowledgeable on how to assist individuals with a disability in boarding and exiting must be available if needed. Equipment used for assisting passengers must be kept in good working condition.

Boarding and exiting most medium and large-size jet aircraft is almost always by way of level boarding ramps or mobile lounges which must be accessible. If ramps or mobile lounges are not used, a lifting device (other than a device used for freight) must be provided to assist persons with limited mobility safely on and off the aircraft. For large and medium size airplanes, hand carriage is not an appropriate method for enplaning or deplaning a passenger with a disability.

At present, however, there are few suitable devices to assist persons with limited mobility in boarding and exiting certain small aircraft. Lifting devices for smaller aircraft are now under development and will be put into place as soon as available.

Carriers do not have to hand-carry passengers on and off aircraft with fewer than 30 seats, if it is the only means of getting the person on and off the aircraft. Carrier employees may do so on a strictly voluntary basis.

In order to provide some personal assistance and extra time, the carrier may offer a passenger with a disability, or any passenger that may be in need of assistance, the opportunity to pre-board the aircraft. The passenger has the option to accept or decline the offer.

On connecting flights, the delivering carrier is responsible for providing assistance to the individual with a disability to reach his or her connecting flight and transportation between gates.

Carriers cannot leave a passenger unattended for more than 30 minutes in a ground wheelchair, boarding chair, or other device in which the passenger is not independently mobile.

**On the Plane**

Prior to the enactment of the Air Carrier Access Act of 1986, requirements that an aircraft be accessible were very limited. The new rules require that a new aircraft after April 1992 have the following accessibility features:

---

[15] As with any passenger baggage, this limit may be increased through Excess Valuation Insurance purchased through the individual airline. The passenger should also check his or her homeowner's or renter's insurance to determine whether it provides such coverage.

For aircraft with 30 or more passenger seats:

- At least one half of the armrests on aisle seats shall be movable to facilitate transferring passengers from on-board wheelchairs to the aisle seat;
- Carriers shall establish procedures to ensure that individuals with disabilities can readably obtain seating in rows with movable aisle armrests;
- An aisle seat is not required to have a movable armrest if not feasible or if the person with a disability would be precluded from sitting there by FAA safety rules (e.g., an exit row).

For aircraft with 100 or more seats:

- Priority space in the cabin shall be provided for stowage of at least one folding wheelchair. (This rule also applies to aircraft of smaller size, if there is a closet large enough to accommodate a folding wheelchair.)

For aircraft with more than one aisle:

- At least one accessible lavatory (with door locks, call buttons, grab bars, and level faucets) shall be available which will have sufficient room to allow a passenger using an on-board wheelchair to enter, maneuver, and use the facilities with the same degree of privacy as other passengers.

Also, after April 1992, aircraft with more than 60 seats must have an operable on-board wheelchair if:

- There is an accessible lavatory, or
- A passenger provides advance notice that he or she can use an inaccessible lavatory but needs an on-board chair to reach it, even if the aircraft predated the rule and has not been refurbished (see below).

An existing aircraft does not have to be made accessible until its interior is refurbished. At that time the relevant accessibility features shall be added.

Airplanes in the commercial fleet have their seats replaced under different schedules depending on the carrier. At the time when all seats are being replaced on an aircraft, half of the aisle seats must be equipped with movable aisle armrests.

Aircraft with fewer than 30 seats, in which seats are replaced, shall include 50 percent movable aisle armrests to extent they are not inconsistent with structural, weight, balance, operational or interior configuration limits.

Similarly, all aircraft undergoing replacement of cabin interior elements or lavatories must meet the accessibility requirements for the affected features, including cabin storage space for a folding wheelchair, and an on-board wheelchair if there is an accessible lavatory (unless prohibited by structural, weight, balance, or configuration limitations).

### Personnel Training

Carriers must now provide training for all personnel who deal the traveling public. This training shall be appropriate to the duties of each employee and will be designed to help the employee understand the special needs of travelers with disabilities, and how they can be accommodated quickly, safely, and with dignity. The training must familiarize the employees with:

- The Department of Transportation's rules on the provision of air service to an individual with a disability;
- The carrier's procedures for providing travel to persons with disabilities including the proper and safe operation of any equipment used to accommodate such persons;
- How to respond appropriately to persons with different disabilities, including persons with mobility, sensory, mental, and emotional disabilities.

## Seat Assignments

An individual with a disability cannot be required to sit in a particular seat, or be excluded from any seat except those prohibited by FAA safety rules, such as the FAA Exit Row Seating rule. For safety reasons, that rule limits seating in exit rows to those persons with the most potential to help in an orderly evacuation. The carrier cannot deny transport, but may deny specific seats to travelers who are less than age 15 or lack the capacity to act without an adult, or who lack sufficient mobility, strength, dexterity, vision, hearing, speech, reading or comprehension abilities to perform emergency evacuation functions. The carrier may also deny specific seats to a person with a condition or responsibilities, such as caring for small children, that might prevent the person from performing emergency evacuation functions, or cause harm to themselves in doing so.

A traveler with a disability may also be denied certain seats if:

- The passenger's involuntary behavior is such that it could compromise safety of the flight and the safety problem can be mitigated to an acceptable degree by assigning the passenger a specific seat rather than refusing service;
- The seat desired cannot accommodate guide dogs or service animals.

In each instance, carriers are obligated to offer alternative seat locations.

## Service Animals

Carrier must permit dog guides or other service animals with appropriate identification to accompany an individual with a disability on a flight. Identification may include cards or other written documentation, presence of a harness or markings on a harness, tags, or the credible verbal assurance of the passenger using the animal.

If carriers provide special information to passengers concerning the transportation of animals outside the continental United States, they must provide such information to all passengers with animals on such flights, not simply to passengers with disabilities who are traveling with service animals.

Carriers must permit a service animal to accompany a disabled traveler with a disability to any seat in which the person sits, unless the animal obstructs an aisle or other area that must remain clear in order to facilitate an emergency evacuation, in which case the passenger will be assigned another seat.

## In-Cabin Service

Air carrier personnel shall assist a passenger with a disability to:

- Move to and from seats as part of the boarding and exiting process;
- Open packages and identify food (but not in actual eating);
- Use an on-board wheelchair when available to enable the passenger to move to and from the lavatory;
- Move semi-ambulatory persons to and from the lavatory (as long as this does not require lifting or carrying by the airline employee);
- Load and retrieve carry-on items, including mobility aids and other assistive devices stowed on board the aircraft.

Carrier personnel are not required to provide assistance inside the lavatory or at the passenger's seat with elimination functions. The carrier personnel are also not required to perform medical services for an individual with a disability.

## Charges for Accommodations Prohibited

Carriers cannot impose charges for providing facilities, equipment, or services to an individual with a disability that are required by DOT's Air Carrier Access regulations. They may charge for optional services, however, such as oxygen and accommodations of stretchers.

## Compliance Procedures

Each carrier must have at least one Complaints Resolution Official (CRO) available at each airport during times of scheduled carrier operations. The CRO can be made available by telephone.

Any passenger having a complaint of alleged violations of the Air Carrier Access rules is entitled to communicate with a CRO, who has authority to resolve complaints on behalf of the carrier.

If a CRO receives a complaint before the action of the carrier personnel has resulted in a violation of the Air Carrier Access rules, the CRO must take or direct other carrier personnel to take action to ensure compliance with the rule. The CRO, however, does not have the authority to countermand a safety-based decision made by the pilot-in-command of an aircraft.

If the CRO agrees with the passenger that a violation of the rule occurred, he must provide the passenger a written statement summarizing the facts and what steps if any, the carrier proposes to take in response to the violation.

If the CRO determines that no violation has occurred, he or she must provide the passenger a written statement summarizing the facts and reasons for the decision or conclusion.

The written statement must inform the interested party of his or her right to pursue DOT enforcement action if the passenger is still not satisfied with the response. If possible, the written statement by the CRO must be given to the passenger at the airport; otherwise, it shall be sent to the passenger within 10 days of the incident.

Carriers shall establish a procedure for resolving written complaints alleging violations of any Air Carrier Access rule provision, If a passenger chooses to file a written complaint, the complaint must note whether the passenger contacted the CRO at the time of the alleged violation, including the CRO's name and the date of the contact, if available. It should include any written response received from the CRO. A carrier shall not be required to respond to a complaint postmarked more than 45 days after the date of an alleged violation.

A carrier must respond to a written complaint within 30 days of its receipt. The response must state the airline's position on the alleged violation, and may also state whether and why no violation occurred, or what the airline plans to do about the problem, The carrier must also inform the passenger of his or her right to pursue DOT enforcement action. Any person believing that a carrier has violated any provision of the rule may contact the following office for assistance:

Department of Transportation
Office of Consumer Affairs
400 Seventh Street SW
Washington, DC 20590
(202) 336-2220
TT (202) 755-7687

Our work is not yet done. At the time of publication of this booklet, there remained a number of accessibility issues unresolved. These include:

Accessible terminal transportation systems;
Boarding chair standards;
Lifts for persons unable to board small aircraft;
Accessible lavatories on narrow body aircraft;
Open captioning for in-flight movies and videos;
TT service on aircraft.

There are many others.

The Department of Transportation, along with groups representing people with disabilities and the air carrier industry, is dedicated to eliminating these barriers with all possible speed.

December 1991

# References

Bach, C.A., McDaniel, R.W. (1993). Quality of Life in Quadriplegic Adults: A Focus Group Study. **Rehabilitation Nursing**, 18, 364-367.

Blake, J.G. (1991). Therapeutic Recreation Assessment and Intervention with a Patient with Quadriplegia. **Therapeutic Recreation Journal**, 25, 71-75.

Blauvelt, C.T., Nelson, F.R.T. (1990). **A Manual of Orthopaedic Terminology.** St. Louis: C.V. Mosby Company.

Bond-Howard, B. (1993) **Introduction to Stroke**. Ravensdale, WA: Idyll Arbor, Inc.

Bovee, T. (1994, January 28). Many disabled who want to work can't afford to. **The Seattle Times** pp. A3.

Bullock, C.C., & Howe, C.Z. (1991). A Model Therapeutic Recreation Program for the Reintegration of Persons with Disabilities into the Community. **Therapeutic Recreation Journal**, 25, 7-17.

burlingame, j. & Blaschko, T.M. (1990). **Assessment Tools for Recreational Therapy**. Ravensdale, WA: Idyll Arbor, Inc.

Daniels, & Worthington (1972) **Muscle Testing Techniques of Manual Evaluation by Comparison** (Ed. 3). Philadelphia: WB Saunders Company.

DiGregorio, V.R. (Ed.) (1984). **Rehabilitation of the Burn Patient.** New York: Churchill Livingstone.

Dunn, J.K. (1981). Leisure Education: Meeting the Challenge of Independence of Residents in Psychiatric Transitional Facilities. **Therapeutic Recreation Journal**, 15, 17-23.

Engrave, L.H. (1992). Treatment of Pressure Ulcers. **Rehabilitation Spinal Cord Injury Update**, 2, Nov.

Equal Employment Opportunity Commission and the United States Department of Justice. (1991). **Americans with Disabilities Act Handbook.** Washington DC: Author.

Freed, M. (1984). Quality of Life: The Physician's Dilemma. **Archives of Physical Medicine and Rehabilitation**, 65, 109-111.

Gaule, K., Nietupski, J., & Certo, N. (1985). Teaching Supermarket Shopping Skills Using An Adaptive Shopping List. **Education and Training of the Mentally Retarded**, 20, 53-59.

Harborview Medical Center (1988). **Approved Nursing Diagnoses for Harborview Medical Center**. Unpublished manuscript/Nursing Document, Harborview Medical Center, Seattle, WA.

Haney, M., & Rabin, B. (1984). Modifying Attitudes Toward Disabled Persons While Socializing SCI Patients. **Archives of Physical Medicine and Rehabilitation**, 65, 431-435.

Hauber, F.E., et al. (1984). National Census of Residential Facilities: A 1982 Profile of Facilities and Residents. **American Journal of Mental Deficiency**, 8, 236-245.

Karam, C. (1989). **A Practical Guide to Cardiac Rehabilitation**. Rockville, MD: Aspen Publishers, Inc.

Kisner, C., & Colby, L. A. (1990). **Therapeutic Exercise Foundations and Techniques, Second Edition**. Philadelphia: F.A. Davis.

Krinksy, A. (1992). Therapeutic Recreation and the Homeless: A Clinical Case History. **Therapeutic Recreation Journal**, 26, 53-57.

McClain, L., Beringer, D., Kuhnert, H., Priest, J., Wilkes, E., Wilkinson, S., Wyrick, L. (1993) Restaurant Wheelchair Accessibility. **American Journal of Occupational Therapy**, 47, 619-623.

McClain, L., & Todd, C. (1990). Food Store Accessibility. **American Journal of Occupational Therapy**, 44, 487-491.

McInerney, C.A., & McInerney, M. (1992). A Mobility Skills Training Program for Adults with Developmental Disabilities. **American Journal of Occupational Therapy**, 46, 233-239.

Mulcahey, M.J. (1992). Returning to School After a Spinal Cord Injury: Perspective From Four Adolescents. **American Journal of Occupational Therapy**, 46, 305-312.

Patrick, G.D. (1986). The Effects of Wheelchair Competition on Self-Concept and Acceptance of Disability in Novice Athletes. **Therapeutic Recreation Journal**, 20, 61-71.

Payne, J.A. (1993). The Contribution of Group Learning to the Rehabilitation of Spinal Cord Injured Adults. **Rehabilitation Nursing**, 18, 375-379.

Peterson, C.A. & Gunn, S.L. (1984). **Therapeutic Recreation Program Design** (2nd Edition). Englewood Cliffs, NJ: Prentice-Hall, Inc.

Ragheb, M.G., & Beard J.G. (1992) Leisure Attitude Measure Manual. Ravensdale, WA: Idyll Arbor, Inc.

Salzberg, C.L., & Langford, C.A. (1981). Community Integration of Mentally Retarded Adults Through Leisure Activity. **Mental Retardation**, 19, 127-131.

Schutt, R.K. & Garrett, G.R. (1992). **Responding to the Homeless: Policy and Practice**. New York: Plenum Press.

Smith, S.H. (1985). A Five Year Follow-Up Review of the Harborview Medical Center Rehabilitation Service Community Integration Program (CIP). **Proceedings of the Intermountain Leisure Symposium, November 7, 1985.**

Stolov, W.C. (1992). New ASIA Standards for Classifying SCI. **Rehabilitation Spinal Cord Injury Update**, 2, Nov.

United States Architectural & Transportation Barriers Compliance Board. (1990). **American's with Disabilities Fact Sheet.** Washington DC: Author.

United States Architectural & Transportation Barriers Compliance Board. (1992). **Automated Guideway Transit (AGT) Systems Technical Assistance Manual.** Washington DC: Author.

United States Architectural & Transportation Barriers Compliance Board. (1992). **Buses, Vans & Systems Technical Assistance Manual.** Washington DC: Author.

United States Architectural & Transportation Barriers Compliance Board. (1992). **Commuter Rail Cars & Systems Technical Assistance Manual.** Washington DC: Author.

United States Architectural & Transportation Barriers Compliance Board. (1992). **High-Speed Rail Cars, Monorails & Systems Technical Assistance Manual.** Washington DC: Author.

United States Architectural & Transportation Barriers Compliance Board. (1992). **Intercity Rail Cars & Systems Technical Assistance Manual.** Washington DC: Author.

United States Architectural & Transportation Barriers Compliance Board. (1992). **Light Rail Vehicles & Systems Technical Assistance Manual.** Washington DC: Author.

United States Architectural & Transportation Barriers Compliance Board. (1992). **Over-The-Road Buses & Systems Technical Assistance Manual.** Washington DC: Author.

United States Architectural & Transportation Barriers Compliance Board. (1992). **Rapid Rail Vehicles & Systems Technical Assistance Manual.** Washington DC: Author.

United States Architectural & Transportation Barriers Compliance Board. (1992). **Trams, Similar Vehicles & Systems Technical Assistance Manual.** Washington DC: Author.

United States Department of Transportation (1991). **New Horizons for the Air Traveler with a Disability**. Washington DC: Author.

Wehman, P., & Schleien, S. (1981). **Leisure Programs for Handicapped Person: Adaptations, Techniques, and Curriculum**. Baltimore, University Press.

Welch, J., Nietupski, J., Hare-Nietupski, S. (1985) Teaching Public Transportation Problem Solving Skills to Young Adults with Moderate Handicaps. **Education and Training of the Mentally Retarded**, 20, 287-295.

Ylvisaker, M. (Ed.). (1985). **Head Injury Rehabilitation: Children and Adolescents**. Boston: College-Hill.